Textbook of
CONTACT LENSES

Textbook of
CONTACT LENSES

FIFTH EDITION

Rajesh Sinha
MD DNB FIACLE FRCS
Additional Professor
Cornea, Lens and Refractive Surgery Services
Dr Rajendra Prasad Centre for Ophthalmic Sciences
All India Institute of Medical Sciences
New Delhi, India

Vijay Kumar Dada
MS DOMS
Senior Consultant
Department of Ophthalmology
Sir Ganga Ram Hospital
New Delhi, India

Forewords

Paul Rose
Eef van der Worp
Neil Cox
José Manuel González-Méijome

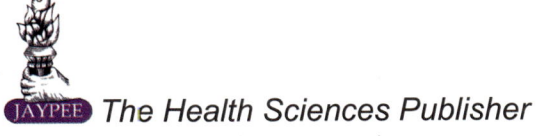

The Health Sciences Publisher
New Delhi | London | Philadelphia | Panama

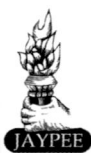 **Jaypee Brothers Medical Publishers (P) Ltd.**

Headquarters
Jaypee Brothers Medical Publishers (P) Ltd
4838/24, Ansari Road, Daryaganj
New Delhi 110 002, India
Phone: +91-11-43574357
Fax: +91-11-43574314
E-mail: jaypee@jaypeebrothers.com

Overseas Offices
J.P. Medical Ltd
83, Victoria Street, London
SW1H 0HW (UK)
Phone: +44 20 3170 8910
Fax: +44 (0)20 3008 6180
E-mail: info@jpmedpub.com

Jaypee Medical Inc.
325, Chestnut Street
Suite 412, Philadelphia,
PA 19106, USA
Phone: +1 267-519-9789
E-mail: support@jpmedus.com

Jaypee Brothers Medical Publishers (P) Ltd
Bhotahity, Kathmandu, Nepal
Phone: +977-9741283608
E-mail: kathmandu@jaypeebrothers.com

Jaypee-Highlights Medical Publishers Inc.
City of Knowledge, Building 235, 2nd Floor, Clayton
Panama City, Panama
Phone: +1 507-301-0496
Fax: +1 507-301-0499
E-mail: cservice@jphmedical.com

Jaypee Brothers Medical Publishers (P) Ltd
17/1-B, Babar Road, Block-B, Shaymali
Mohammadpur, Dhaka-1207
Bangladesh
Mobile: +08801912003485
E-mail: jaypeedhaka@gmail.com

Website: www.jaypeebrothers.com
Website: www.jaypeedigital.com

Inquiries for bulk sales may be solicited at: jaypee@jaypeebrothers.com

Textbook of Contact Lenses

First Edition: 1996
Fifth Edition: **2017**
ISBN: 978-93-86150-44-8
Printed at Sanat Printers

Dedicated to

The three special women in my life;
My mother Malti for her care and blessings
My wife Renu for her support
My daughter Suhani for her loving smile

– Rajesh Sinha

My Guruji
His Holiness
Saint Gurmeet Ram Rahim Singhji
Dera Sacha Sauda Ashram
Sirsa, Haryana

– Vijay Kumar Dada

Foreword

Thank you Professor Rajesh Sinha and Dr Vijay Kumar Dada for inviting me to write a foreword for *Textbook of Contact Lenses.*

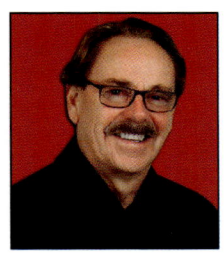

The last four decades have been an exciting time in the development of contact lenses considering that only 40 years ago our only option for fitting contact lenses to any eye including the irregular cornea, were polymethyl methacrylate (PMMA) corneal lenses, cut on manual lathes with secondary curves often applied by hand polishing, which often lead to inaccurate unrepeatable parameters.

Although surgical procedures for the irregular cornea have improved considerably over my career as a contact lens specialist, contact lenses still remain today, the first option for the correction of vision for the irregular cornea and should always be tried before surgery is considered.

In the early 70s, we accepted that about 1/3rd of keratoconus patients would eventually require a penetrating corneal graft no matter how well we managed and fitted them.

However, over the last 40 years, because of improvements in materials, designs and manufacturing techniques, this rate has dropped dramatically and today 15% or less of keratoconus patients in countries which have well-educated contact lens fitters, will end up ever requiring a graft as long as they are well managed.

With the advent of computerized lathes in the 1980s, which can cut nearly any imaginable shape into the back surface of a contact lens, this has allowed us to create designs which more accurately mimic the irregular profile of the keratoconus cornea. Add to this gas permeable materials with Dk's (oxygen permeability) now 100 and over, we can fit the irregular cornea more accurately today, and provide good tear exchange and adequate oxygen to meet the corneal demands, to avoid edema, which was often unavoidable with PMMA.

Also, these improved materials have allowed us to fit bigger lenses, e.g. scleral and semiscleral designs which require high oxygen permeable materials to provide sufficient oxygen to the cornea for normal daily wear.

Designs have also improved so that today even the inexperienced gas permeable (GP) fitter can often achieve a reasonable success rate fitting these challenging cases. The Rose K design is one such design which has taken the complexities out of fitting, reducing the number of variables, and subsequently the first fit success rate for the experienced fitter to over 80%.

Although these patients can often be challenging and require more time and effort than a regular contact lens fit, there is nothing more rewarding as an eye-care practitioner, than to be able to provide these patients with a level of acuity which allows them to lead a normal life.

Education and our knowledge of fitting the irregular cornea has also increased dramatically in recent years, and I am sure that this book will prove to be yet another useful tool in our understanding of how to manage and achieve the best possible fit for these challenging cases.

Paul Rose
BOpt BSc FNZSCLP
Consultant, Menicon

Foreword

The dynamics of our contact lens practice is changing dramatically and drastically. The most challenging thing is to comply with the individual needs of our patients. New technology can help us to do better: to define the ocular surface shape and to better analyze tear film quality for instance. However, all this would be worthless, if it was not for the knowledge of the eye care practitioner to interpret and apply that information. Without this knowledge, the eye care practitioner would not be able to make the right decisions.

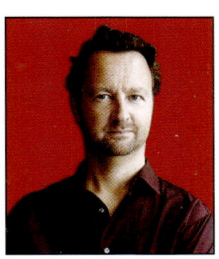

As an educator, as an editor of a number of international publications and as board member of a number of international contact lens conferences, it is clear that good and up-to-date knowledge is essential for a healthy contact lens practice. *Textbook of Contact Lenses* by Professor Rajesh Sinha and Dr Vijay Kumar Dada further adds to the ongoing quest for knowledge in our field. The book has a broad-spectrum range—to stay within the terminology of our field—of topics ranging from hypoxia and corneal physiology to keratoconus and scleral lenses; it not only looks at sports, colored lenses, basic-fitting approaches, lens material, but also at contact lens solutions; all with nice illustrations.

In this edition, the book updates itself regularly—to comply with the changes in our field—and it helps us in this way with the most fundamental task of an eye care practitioner: to provide the patient with the best possible optical solution for their visual requirement.

Eef van der Worp

BOptom PhD FAAO FIACLE FBCLA
Ex-Head, Department of Contact Lens
Hogeschool van Utrecht, The Netherlands
Adjunct Assistant Professor
Pacific University, College of Optometry
Oregon, USA
Adjunct Professor
University of Montreal
School of Optometry, Canada

Knowledge is power. Information is liberating. Education is the premise of progress, in every society, in every family.
– Kofi Annan

Foreword

It gives me immense pleasure to write a foreword to *Textbook of Contact Lenses* authored by Professor Rajesh Sinha and Dr Vijay Kumar Dada. This textbook will be very useful for both postgraduate students and experienced contact lens practitioners. The subject matter has been presented clearly and it is easy to understand.

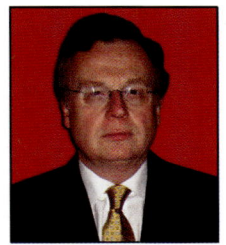

Over the last couple of decades, a lot of changes have occurred in the manufacturing and application of contact lenses. Materials have improved, fitting methodology has evolved, and the care systems have developed commensurately. We have witnessed the changes in soft lenses from the earlier generation hydrogel materials to current generation-refined silicone hydrogel lenses. Rigid gas permeable lenses have also evolved considerably, from the earlier generation low Dk to the current generation of high Dk lenses leading to increased success. The designs for keratoconus fitting have progressed with sophisticated manufacturing techniques producing corneal, semiscleral and scleral designs, utilizing high Dk materials. With all these changes, contact lenses have gained wider acceptance and the spectrum of usage has broadened. The book covers the basic understanding of contact lenses, available options, and deals with the recent advancements of the last decade.

This superb textbook by Professor Rajesh Sinha and Dr Vijay Kumar Dada covers all aspects of contact lenses with appropriate emphasis on fitting techniques. The material is well illustrated with excellent diagrams and colored illustrations. The book is a concise account, yet also comprehensive, and will prove to be a valuable reference guide for all practitioners. It represents an excellent resource for all those interested in current contact lens practice.

Neil Cox
FCOptom FAAO
Moorfields Eye Hospital
London, England, UK

Foreword

Contact lenses are amazing devices. In a thin layer of polymer can hold the properties to provide full correction of a variety of optical imperfections of the eye, well beyond the limits of other optical and surgical solution. More relevant is doing so with minimal interference with ocular physiology. Since their invention by the end of the 19th century, several steps have shaped glass, rigid polymer, hydrophilic polymer and hybrid materials towards the lenses, we fit today to our patients.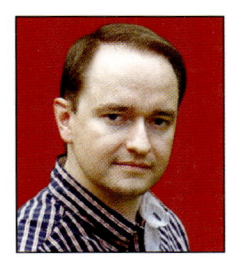

Particularly, there has been intense development over the last 15 years in the field of contact lenses. As a result of the advances in polymer science, miniaturization of electronics and computerized-controlled manufacturing, contact lenses are nowadays an essential part of the ophthalmic consultation and predictions are very exciting about their role in the future of several biomedical and technological applications.

An area that has been prolific in recent advances is the treatment of the irregular cornea that has benefitted from the rebirth of silicone hydrogel, hybrid lenses and corneoscleral and scleral supported lenses. This is indeed the area where contact lenses provide the highest benefit/risk ratio with dramatic benefits in terms of visual rehabilitation when surgical solutions are not viable, or further rehabilitation is required after surgical solutions have been performed.

Textbook of Contact Lenses is very timely to update the contact lens practitioners on these innovations. The 28 concise and well-illustrated chapters will become a source of daily consultation for medical and optometry students as well as contact lens practitioners.

Furthermore, not only the Indian but all the English reading audience will also benefit from this concise textbook. The book will be particularly helpful for those practitioners dealing with ectatic corneal diseases and traumatic abnormalities of the ocular surface.

I would like to congratulate Professor Rajesh Sinha and Dr Vijay Kumar Dada for bringing to us this piece of work.

José Manuel González-Méijome
OD PhD
Associate Professor (with Habilitation)
Clinical and Experimental Optometry Research Lab
Center of Physics (Optometry)
School of Sciences
University of Minho
Portugal

Preface to the Fifth Edition

Contact lens still remains a popular optical mode of correction for ametropia. There has been a constant change in the understanding of contact lens, its types and the care and maintenance over the years. Newer lenses with improved technology have come up which can have better tolerance as well as better visual performance. A lot of technological advances have taken place in the materials, designs and fitting methodology of contact lenses. The advent of silicone hydrogel material for soft lens has reduced the contact lens-induced hypoxia-related complications. The newer designs of contact lens especially for keratoconus has changed the overall scenario of contact lens industry. The multicurve Rose K lenses for all severity of keratoconus and the KeraSoft IC soft contact lenses for keratoconus have increased the spectrum of contact lens usage. The newer scleral and miniscleral lenses have made contact lens fitting possible even in large globus cones and grossly irregular cornea. Newer generation solutions for care and maintenance are available for the users. These solutions not only do better cleaning of contact lens but also provide greater compatibility with the ocular surface. Physiology of contact lens has been best understood and extensive work has been done to study the subacute inflammation during sleep. Physiological responses with regard to low Dk rigid and thick 2-hydroxyethyl methacrylate (HEMA) lenses have been clarified and their use cautioned more and more in the literature. Superiority of the new generation gas permeable lenses in daily and extended wear has been highlighted over other lenses. Use of toric lenses and their stabilization by various methods as well as the simplification in the fitting methodology have been described. New corneal measurements with the use of advanced topographic systems and its clinical application early in diagnosis of corneal pathologies and fabrication of contact lenses and distant teaching are amply clarified. After the study of contact lenses in Olympic athletes, necessity of fitting contact lenses in athletes for achieving better performance in sports and the use of specific design of lenses have been documented. Fitting of contact lens in infants and near adds with regard to age have been better understood and described. A new aspect of contact lens fitting after LASIK and radial keratotomy has been adequately discussed.

We have briefly introduced some newer subjects in *Textbook of Contact Lenses* which will serve to update the knowledge of contact lens practitioners and help them to do an excellent job in contact lens fitting.

Rajesh Sinha
Vijay Kumar Dada

Preface to the First Edition

This book on contact lens is primarily meant for postgraduates, general practitioners in ophthalmology, optometrists, ophthalmic assistants and for dispensing opticians who deal with contact lenses. This book also forms a brief but complete account for teachers engaged in postgraduate ophthalmic academics. The book is a handy manual for short-term contact lens workshop.

The book has chapters commencing with a historical background and relevant anatomical and physiological factors, indications and contraindications in Indian clients, patient's history examination and prognosis with fitting philosophies, follow-up and a detailed and up-to-date account of soft lenses. Every clinical chapter has been based on my personal clinical documentation and unpublished observations. The best treatment for each entity has been highlighted.

The book has an excellent display of colored photographs which forms a unique contact lens atlas next to the actual patient forming very useful material.

Four persons played a dominant role in shaping my ophthalmic and contact lens career: Professor Madan Mohan my teacher and mentor in ophthalmology has always been a source of inspiration; Professor LP Agarwal an excellent guide; Joseph W Soper my contact lens initiator; and Robert B Mandell who built the superstructure on the initial foundation.

I am indebted to the following eminent ophthalmologists; who encouraged me to continue the work, Professors PK Khosla, Y Dayal, Drs SK Angra, NN Sood, Professors Santokh Singh, Ishwar Chanda, T Selvam, Dr JM Pahwa, Professors MR Chadah, IS Roy and IS Jain.

I am most grateful to Drs RB Mandell and Harold Stein for permitting me to seek the guidance from their publications.

My Director Dr HD Tandon and Dean Dr P Chandra have always given appreciation and encouragement for all my academic pursuits.

My friends, Drs Srikant, Ramanjit Sihota and Raghu Ram, helped me in the final shaping for the manuscript. Illustrations by Mr Gian Singh and Miss Shakti Mittal provided a valuable support to my book.

Vijay Kumar Dada

Acknowledgments

We would like to put on record our grateful appreciations to all those who have helped us in writing *Textbook of Contact Lenses*.

We are thankful to Dr Vijay K Sharma, Dr Himanshu Shekhar and Dr Tarun Arora for helping in modifications and proofreading of the chapters. Our special appreciation goes to Professor Tanuj Dada for facilitating and helping to get the new edition published.

M/s Jaypee Brothers Medical Publishers (P) Ltd, New Delhi, India, deserves our special thanks for their efforts in publishing the 5th edition of the book.

The book is based on our experience of fitting contact lenses on various types of patients. This was not only meant for patient care but also for teaching of postgraduate students. We are extremely thankful to all our patients as fitting contact lenses on their eyes gave us huge experience. We are also thankful to the postgraduate students whose questions made us to think more that made us wiser. We are grateful to hundreds and thousands of students whom we have been privileged to teach during this period. Their questions and critical comments have contributed significantly to the content, style, and configuration of the book. We also thank our colleagues, especially Professor Jeewan Singh Titiyal, who is a stalwart in this field and with whom we had the privilege to share our experiences and knowledge of contact lens.

We are thankful to our family members who have been very supportive through thick and thin and who encouraged us to write the textbook on contact lenses. Finally, we would like to thank the almighty for making us capable of writing a book that will help the postgraduate students as well as contact lens practitioners.

Contents

CHAPTER 1

Evolution of Contact Lenses

INTRODUCTION

The contact lens that appears like a small wafer is designed to rest on the cornea or sclera usually for correction of refractive errors. The concept of contact lenses was borne as early as in 1500 although it took a few centuries for true contact lenses to be commercially available. The credit for conceiving the idea of contact lenses goes to Leonardo da Vinci (Fig. 1.1). In 1508, he sketched out several ideas for neutralizing the cornea through contact with fluid. He understood that corneal power could be altered by submerging the eye in a glass bowl filled with water (Fig. 1.2). Essentially, he described the principles of a contact lens without describing something we would actually recognize as a contact lens. More than a century later, Rene Descartes (1636) described a glass tube filled with liquid and attached to the eye. This was hardly a contact lens; but again, the principle of corneal neutralization was clear. Thomas Young 1801 is credited with the concept of changing the eye's dioptric power, utilizing the principle of fluid neutralization. He fitted a microscope lens at one end of a glass tube ¼ inch long, filled the tube with water, and then applied this to the eye. His device may be said to be the antecedent of hydrodiascope as well as contact lenses.

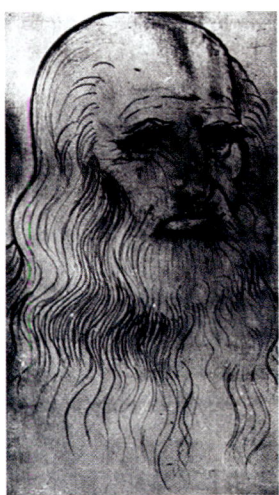

Fig. 1.1 Leonardo da Vinci

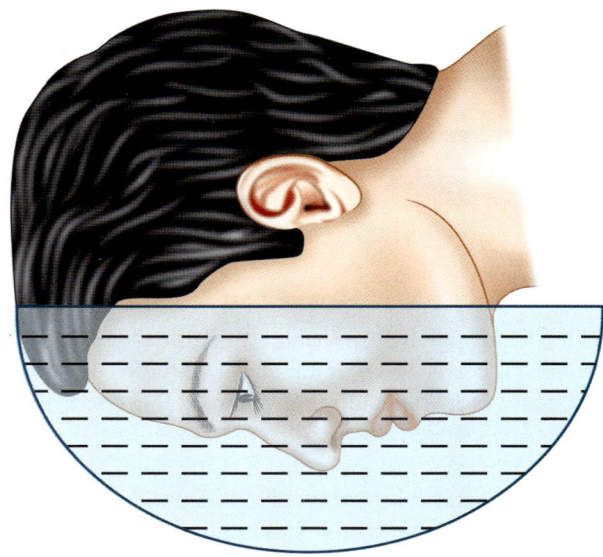

Fig. 1.2 Submerging the eye in a glass bowl filled with water to alter corneal power

EVOLUTION

The first written description of a device approximating a contact lens is believed to date to 1823. Sir John Herschel, an English astronomer, proposed "some transparent animal jelly contained in a spherical capsule of glass applied to the surface of the eye" to correct irregular astigmatism. He also suggested that a mold of the cornea might be taken and impressed on some transparent medium. He thought that it is possible that "a temporary distinct vision" might be obtained through one of these methods, but it is not known whether Herschel ever tried to put his ideas into practice. In the late 1880s, at least three men are thought to have independently invented the first contact lens. Adolf Eugen Fick, a Swiss ophthalmologist, and Eugene Kalt, a French ophthalmologist, devised glass lenses with the goal of correcting corneal abnormalities. Eugen Fick called his contact lens Kontakt Brille. It was a small cap of thin glass made up of a spherical segment with concentric and consequently parallel faces. The space between the lens and the eye was filled with a liquid of the same refractive index as that of the cornea. He made a series of plaster mouldings, first on rabbit's eyes and then on human cadaver eyes; cups of blown glass were then shaped on these mouldings. He discovered that a well chosen shape can adhere to the eyeball. He also investigated a number of solutions to be used between the eye and the lens. He fitted the patients with corneal and scleral lenses, the scleral flange providing better support and distribution of the lens weight than his original corneal lens alone.

E. Kalt, in 1888, treated two patients with keratoconus, with corneal lenses. Unlike Fick's corneal lenses, Kalt's pressed against the cornea instead of arching over the center of the cornea.

Around the same time, August Muller, a German medical student who wanted to correct his own high myopia, also produced a glass lens. These first contact lenses were crude by modern standards, made of blown glass bubbles or ground and polished glass, and were primarily scleral designs that covered much of the eye. They were heavy and unwieldy and let no oxygen through to the cornea. Patients could tolerate the lenses only briefly and usually suffered from signs and symptoms of corneal hypoxia rather quickly. Nevertheless, the improvement in visual acuity that a piece of glass on the eye could provide was encouraging.

Between 1890 and 1935, there were no developments of any great consequence. Two German companies, Karl Zeiss Optical Works and Mueller Co., as well as small labs in the US and elsewhere, continued to make glass contact lenses but demand was very limited. In 1889, Muller Gladbach of Wishaden corrected his own refractive error of 14D with a type of corneal glass contact lens. However, he could hardly wear the lenses for more than 30 minutes. He recognized that the cause of the intolerance was not the lens on a cornea but the crushing of the conjunctival vessels by the rough edge of the lens. He attempted to solve the difficulty, but finally gave up. Muller was the first to use the term corneal lenses but his lenses would be termed scleral today. In 1887, the German ophthalmologist Eugen Fick constructed and fitted the first successful contact lens. He described fabricating afocal scleral contact shells, which rested on the less sensitive rim of tissue around the cornea, and experimentally fitting them initially on rabbits, then on himself, and lastly on a small group of volunteers. These lenses were made from heavy blown glass and were 18–21 mm in diameter. Fick filled the empty space between cornea and glass with a dextrose solution. Fick's lens was large, unwieldy, and could only be worn for a couple of hours at a time.

The contact lenses so far described had poor optical surfaces and often gave bad visual acuity. Their primary objective was therapeutic. They were individually blown in glass. Sulzer, also of the same period, made scleral lenses by grinding from solid glass in much the same way as glass spectacle lenses were grounded. These scleral lenses, blown either to a shape after the method of Muller or grounded to a two-curve spherical design by Carl Zeiss of Jena, were then used up to beginning of the 20th century.

The twentieth century saw the full refinement of the contact lenses that we enjoy today. Many modern day manufacturing techniques and man-made products (such as plastics and silicone) go towards making contacts that the body can easily tolerate and which are much more comfortable to wear for extended periods.

In 1929, Heine described a method of fitting contact lenses by means of a trial set consisting of a large number of contact lenses, made for him by Zeiss. Glass contact lenses used so far were usually of the scleral type, the weight and irregular surfaces of the corneal type precluding their proper adherence to the cornea, thus restricting their use. In 1929, Joseph Dallos, a Hungarian physician, developed methods of taking molds from living human eyes so that glass lenses could be made to conform more closely to individual sclera. Glass-blown scleral lenses remained the only form of contact lens until the 1930s when polymethyl methacrylate (PMMA or Perspex) was developed, allowing plastic scleral lenses to be manufactured for the first time. In 1936, William Feinbloom, a New York optometrist, introduced the use of plastic for contacts. He made a lens having a glass corneal portion and a plastic scleral portion. Its lightness, workability and comfort with ocular tissue were advantageous factors.

Rohm and Hass Company (USA) in 1936 introduced transparent methyl methacrylate. The same year, John Mullen and Theodore Obrig developed techniques for making scleral lenses of the new substance by the much simpler process of turning it on a lathe. These lenses could be shaped and reshaped at low temperatures, scraped, routed drilled or buffed, quickly finished to a high polish and made thinner than was possible with fragile glass. Obrig is also known for introducing the use of fluorescein in ultraviolet light for checking the fitting of contact lenses over the cornea.

Scleral lenses used so far usually led to temporary corneal edema and to clouding just a few hours after lens insertion. In 1943, Bier introduced a minimum clearance fluidless, performed contact lens called the transcurve lens as it included a transitional curve between the scleral and corneal curves. He perforated these lenses to allow ingress and egress of natural tears, thus greatly ameliorating the corneal clouding. In 1946, Nissel in England used a similar wide-angle lens, which differed in having a flat transition between the corneal and scleral porions.

The first corneal plastic contact lens was introduced in 1947 by Kelvin Tuohy. It was approximately 11 mm in diameter and 0.4 mm thick, the back curve being flatter than the corneal curvature by 1.50 diopters. In 1950, an Oregon optometrist, Dr George Butterfield, designed a corneal lens. The inner surface of this lens followed the eye's shape instead of sitting flat, increasing comfort and eye tolerability. This also reduced problems with image and peripheral vision distortion in certain prescription types.

In 1951, Sohnges of Germany, Dickinson of England and Neill of USA simultaneously introduced the micro-corneal contact lenses about 9.5 mm in diameter 0.2 mm thick and fitted 3–4 D flatter than the corneal curvature. The diminished size, thickness, and greater curvature permitted better tear circulation to the cornea. Hence, they were much better tolerated. In 1955 Norman Bier introduced a new principle of fitting the contact lens spoken of as "contouring the cornea", paralleling the cornea or "corneal alignment". It implies that the contact lens has multiple inside radii, the lens thus being in contact with the cornea quite uniformly except at the very periphery of the lens. Corneal contact lenses now being constructed were small and thin, and they were either parallel to the cornea or vault its apex in which case they are called apical clearance lenses. They were now fitted as small as 7–8 mm in diameter.

During 1960's in Prague, Czechoslovakia, Otto Wichterle and Drahoslav Lim experimented with contact lenses made of a soft, water-absorbing plastic they had developed. This was the major step leading to the soft and disposable lenses that we have today. The water absorption helped with eye dryness problems that could lead to irritations, eye tiredness and focusing problems. The polymers from which soft lenses are manufactured improved over the next 25 years, primarily in terms of increasing the oxygen permeability by varying the ingredients. In 1972, British optometrist Rishi Agarwal was the first to suggest disposable soft contact lenses.

In 1979 Rigid gas permeable (RGP) contact lenses made of co-polymers PMMA and silicone became available for commercial distribution. Many silicone-acrylate lenses became available at this time. Gas permeability allows the eye to maintain its natural moisture and to refresh its surface tear layer without hindrance. The 1980s saw the development of tinted daily wear soft lenses which became available for commercial distribution. This was one of the first soft colored contact lenses in the market. In 1982 bifocal daily wear soft contact lenses became available for commercial distribution.

In 1998, an important development in soft lenses was the launch of the first silicone hydrogels into the market by CIBA VISION in Mexico. These new materials combined the benefits of silicone, which has extremely high oxygen permeability, with the comfort and clinical performance of the conventional hydrogels which had been used for the previous 30 years. These lenses were initially advocated primarily for extended (overnight) wear although more recently, daily (no overnight) wear silicone hydrogels have been launched.

An important development in the history of gas permeable contact lenses started when in 1989, Paul Rose of New Zealand began developing the Rose K keratoconus lenses. After testing 700 lenses and 12 different designs, he produced a set of 26 lenses from which all patients could be fitted. A further two years were spent to perfect the lens design before it was launched in the New Zealand market. In 1995, Rose K lens gained approval from the Federal Drug Administration (FDA) of America. Since then, advances in technology have resulted in the introduction of the Rose K2 lens, the Rose K2 Irregular Cornea (IC) lens, the Rose K2 Post Graft (PG) lens, and the Rose K2 NC lens for nipple cones designed for patients with specific conditions. These conditions include pellucid marginal degeneration, keratoglobus, LASIK-induced ectasia and patients who have undergone penetrating keratoplasty.

APPENDIX

Nomenclature

Contact lens specification can be better understood by the practitioners if a uniform nomenclature is used. The author has used the following in this text.

- *Contact lens blank:* A circular button of plastic 12.55 mm diameter, 7.50 mm thick (Fig. 1.3).
- *Semi-finished blank:* A blank where base curve has been generated and polished.
- *Semi-finished contact lens or uncut lens:* A contact lens with proper front and back curves which are polished, but still need edging. Steps B and C are done on the lathe (Fig. 1.4) and polisher (Fig. 1.5).
- *Finished contact lens:* A properly edged semi-finished contact lens (Fig. 1.6).

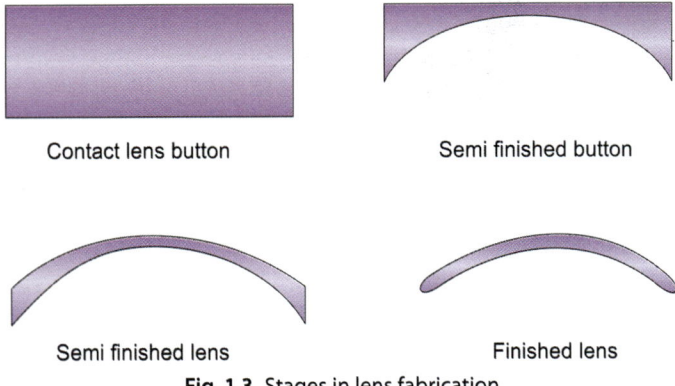

Contact lens button   Semi finished button

Semi finished lens   Finished lens

Fig. 1.3 Stages in lens fabrication

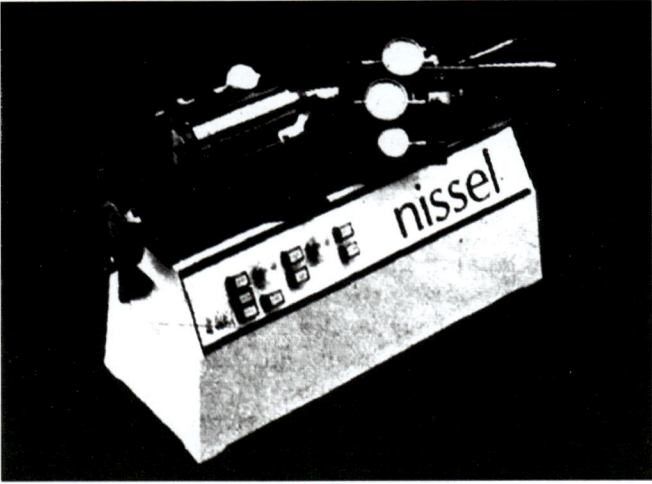

Fig. 1.4 Contact lens lathe

- Diameters
  - *Overall diameter (OD):* The dimension across the physical boundary of the lens, expressed in mm (Fig. 1.6).
  - *Optic zone (OZ):* The dimension of central optic zone of the lens meant to focus the rays on the retina.
- *Curves*
  - Base curve (BC) or central posterior curve (CPC) on the back surface to fit the front surface of cornea.
  - Peripheral posterior curves (PPC) are concentric to the BC, and usually two in number, i.e. intermediate posterior curve (IPC) and peripheral posterior curve (PPC). They are meant to serve as reservoirs of tears and to form a ski for lens movements.
  - Front curve (FC) or central anterior curve (CAC) is the central zone on the front surface corresponding to the optical zone, and its curvature determines the lens power.

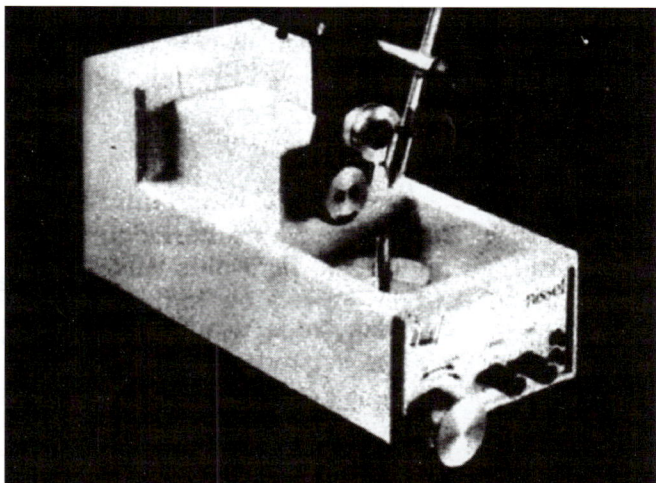

Fig. 1.5 Polishing machine

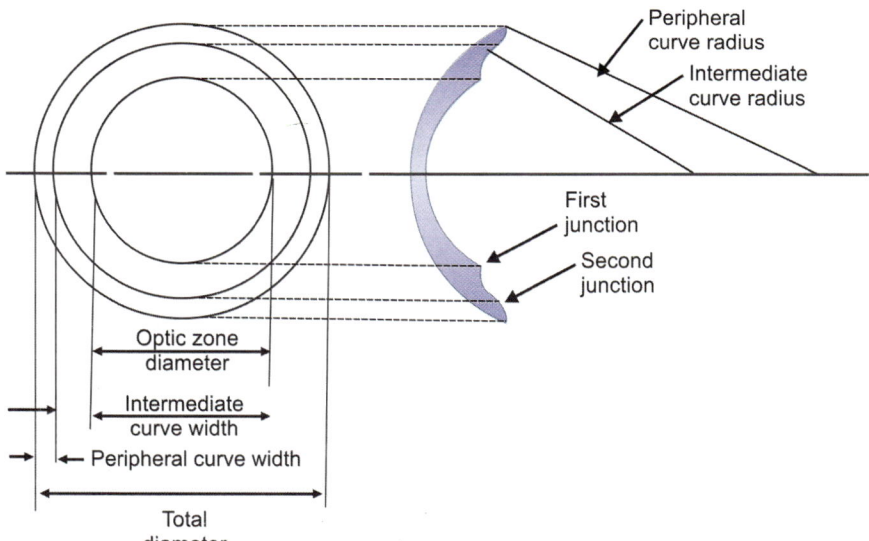

Fig. 1.6 Parts of contact lens

- Peripheral anterior curves (PAC) which are two in number are curves on the front surface. The intermediate anterior curve (IAC) is only fabricated in high minus and high plus lenses. The peripheral anterior curve (PAC) is slope going to the edge of the lens.

  NB: The radii of all curves are expressed in mm or diopters.

- Edge is the union of front and back curves at the periphery (Figs 1.7A and B)
- Power is always described as the back vertex power.

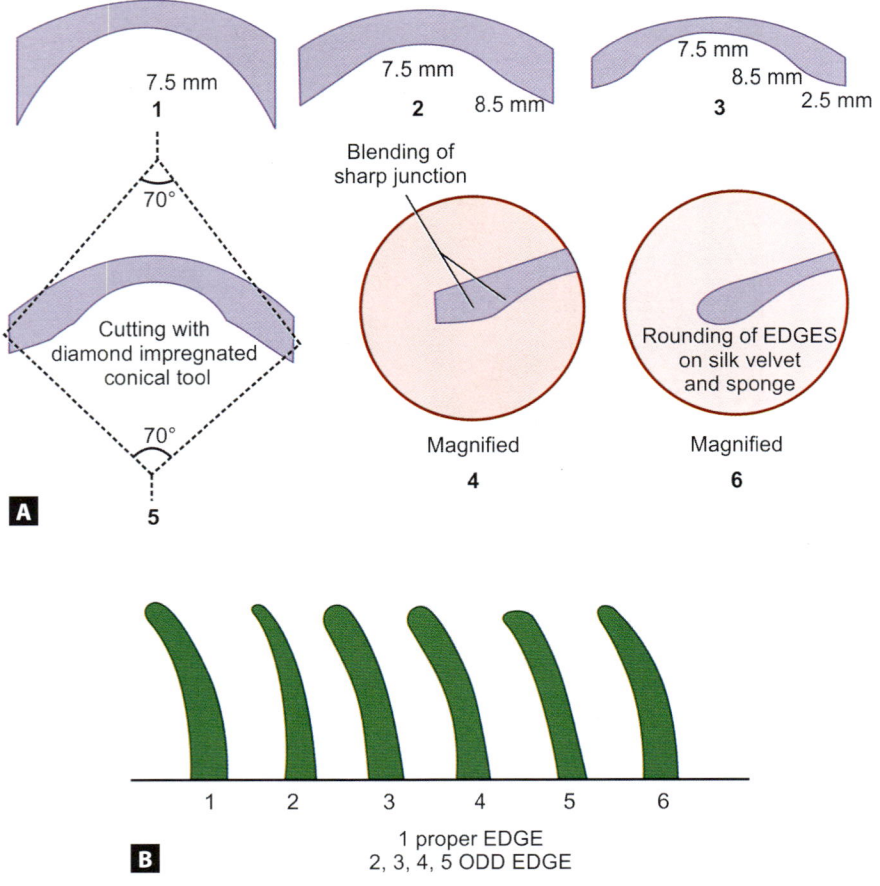

Figs 1.7A and B Contact lens edge

- *Blend:* This is curve to knock off the sharp junction between two curves and has a value between the two surrounding curves.
- Thickness is usually measured in mm at the center of the lens.
- Tint is the color of the lens with each color having light, medium and dark shades.
- *Corneal zones:* The cornea can be divided keratometrically into three zones:
  1. Apical zone, centrally located 3–9 mm in diameter (usually), and the most steep and most uniform in curvature.
  2. Limbal zone, in the peripheral part of cornea where the mires of keratometer appear doubled.
  3. Transitional zone joining apical and limbal zones.

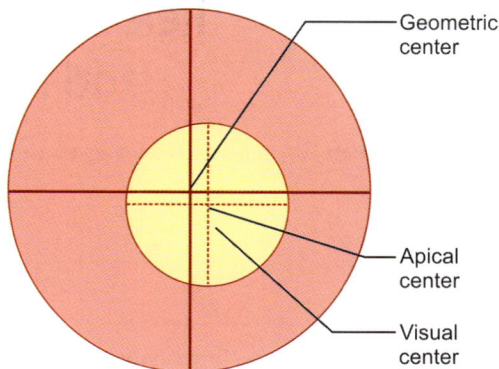

Fig. 1.8 Geometric, apical and visual centers of cornea

- *Corneal centers (Fig. 1.8):* Cornea has three centers:
    1. Geometric center, the intersection of widest and shortest diameter of the cornea.
    2. Apical center, the intersection of the widest and the shortest diameter of the apical zone.
    3. Visual center, the point on the cornea which transmits the visual axis.
- "K" refers to the flatter of the two meridian in keratometry.

CHAPTER 2

Relevant Anatomy and Physiology

INTRODUCTION

The eyeball has three layers enclosing the inner contents. The outermost layer is the corneo-scleral layer that has a protective function. The cornea is a transparent avascular connective tissue that acts as the primary infectious and structural barrier of the eye. Together with the overlying tear film, it also provides a proper anterior refractive surface for the eye. The primary concern of the cornea lies in its optical function imparting 40–45 diopters to the eye, almost ¾ of its total power.

The cornea has an aspheric shape with a diameter of 10.5 mm. It is 0.54 mm thick in the center and 1.0 mm at the periphery with a radius of curvature of (7.94 mm) 43.50D. In an average adult, the horizontal diameter of the cornea is 11.5–12.0 mm and about 1.0 mm larger than the vertical diameter. It has five layers (Fig. 2.1) which are epithelium (5–90 µm), Bowman's layer (8–14 µm), stroma, Descemet's membrane (6–10 µm) and endothelium (4.5 µm).

The shape of the cornea is prolate meaning flatter in the periphery and steeper centrally which creates an aspheric optical system. Corneal shape and curvature are governed by the intrinsic biomechanical structure and extrinsic environment. Anterior corneal stromal rigidity appears to be particularly important in maintaining the corneal curvature. Organizational differences in the collagen bundles of the anterior stroma may contribute to a tighter cohesive strength in this area and may also explain why the anterior curvature resists change to stromal hydration much more than the posterior stroma, which tends to develop folds more easily. Stromal hydration also appears to affect the corneal response to strain and shear forces.

EPITHELIUM

The epithelial surface of the cornea creates the first barrier to the outside environment and is an integral part of the tear film–cornea interface that is critical to the refractive power of the eye. This outermost corneal layer consists of non-keratinized, stratified epithelium, which is mounted on a fine basement membrane and anchored by filaments extending into the underlying collagen. Columnar basal cells are next to the basement membrane, and two or three rows of small interlocked wing cells are mounted on the basal cells. Two or three layers of surface squamous cells cap the wing cells. Thus, the epithelium is divided morphologically into three layers: superficial or squamous cell layer, middle or wing cell layer, and deep or basal cell layer. The superficial cells contain a long nucleus and the cytoplasm has mitochondria, glycogen granules, Golgi apparatus,

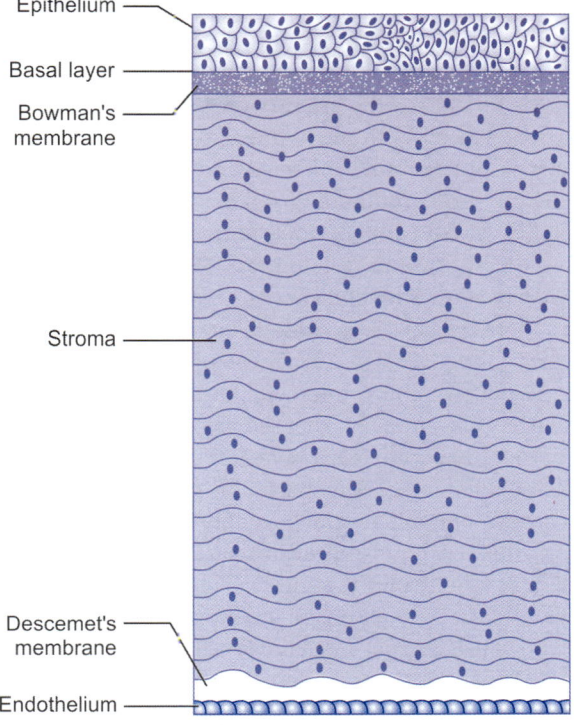

Epithelium

Basal layer

Bowman's
membrane

Stroma

Descemet's
membrane

Endothelium

Fig. 2.1 Layers of cornea

endoplasmic reticulum and abundant tonofibrils. On electron microscopy they show microvilli towards the outer surface, which serve to retain the precorneal tear film. The middle 2–3 layers of wing or umbrella cells are named so because they send projections to the sides. Their contents are the same as those of superficial cells. Basal cells are long attached to the basement membrane below by hemidesmosomes, and to each other by desmosomes. Mitosis is seen in the basal layer. The daughter cells becoming wing cells which then migrate to become superficial cells. This period of epithelial turnover is about 7 days. The basement membrane is secreted by the epithelium. It is constituted of tightly packed filaments. It is separated from basal cells by a translucent zone and has regularity towards the basal cells but fades indistinctly into Bowman's zone. During scraping of the epithelium this membrane is left behind, but in edema and inflammation it tends to separate from the Bowman's membrane. This is periodic acid Schiff (PAS) positive and is regenerated if injured. It is destroyed by proteolytic enzymes like trypsin and chymotrypsin. The epithelium derives most of its glucose and protein from the anterior chamber.

The air-tear film interface, together with the underlying cornea, provides two-thirds of the total refractive power of the eye. The corneal epithelium and overlying tear film have a symbiotic relationship both anatomically and physiologically. The mucinous layer of the tear film, which is in direct contact with the corneal epithelium is produced by the conjunctival goblet cells and interacts closely with the corneal epithelial cell glycocalyx to allow hydrophilic spreading of the tear film with each eyelid blink. Loss of the glycocalyx from injury or disease results in loss of tear-film stability and subsequent breakdown of the ocular optical system. The tear film is the primary protector of the corneal surface from microbial invasion, as well as from chemical, toxic, and foreign-body damage. The tear film also supplies immunological and growth factors that are critical for epithelial health, proliferation, and repair. Corneal epithelial cells have an average lifespan of 7–10 days and routinely undergo orderly involution, apoptosis (programed cell death), and desquamation. This process results in complete turnover of the corneal epithelial layer every week as deeper cells replace the desquamating superficial cells in an orderly, apically directed fashion. The most superficial corneal epithelial cells form a mean of 2–3 layers of flat polygonal cells. These cells have extensive apical microvilli and microplicae, which in turn are covered by a fine, closely apposed, charged glycocalyx layer. These surface cells maintain tight junctional complexes between their neighbors, which prohibit tears from entering the intercellular spaces. This can be demonstrated clinically by observing a healthy epithelial surface's ability to repel dyes such as fluorescein and rose bengal. This barrier also prevents toxins and microbes from entering deeper corneal layers. Beneath the superficial cell layer and just anterior to the deepest basal layer of the epithelium are the suprabasal or wing cells. This layer is 2–3 cells deep and consists of cells that are less flat than the overlying superficial cells but possess similar tight lateral intercellular junctions.

Very small corneal epithelial wounds are covered in about three hours by adjacent basal cells, which send out pseudopodia to blanket the area. With larger corneal epithelial wounds, cells from all layers of the surrounding epithelium advance and flatten to cover the wound. Initially, the newly regenerated epithelium is very susceptible to damage, but a tight adhesion is established in only a few days if the basement membrane is largely intact. At first the epithelium is only a couple of layers thick and will regain normal thickness within several weeks. The superficial layer has a tight junction complex among laterally adjacent cells, and this produces a barrier that resists fluid flow through the epithelial surface.

The impairment of oxygenation by a tightly fitted contact lens causes depletion of glycogen, increase in lactic acid and accumulation of fluid. This leads to intercellular edema, formation of cyst, the cellular attachment to the basement membrane loosens and cells may rupture to be cast off in sheets to form erosion. This results in stromal edema which epithelial cells normally prevent. Epithelial edema is called Sattler's veil. When the size of intercellular edema becomes more than half the wave length of light, scatter occurs. Chronic edema may be associated with fibrosis and vascularization which may further add to the scatter.

BOWMAN'S LAYER

Bowman's layer (or Bowman's membrane) lies just anterior to the stroma and is not a true membrane but rather the acellular condensation of the most anterior portion of the stroma. This smooth layer is approximately 15 μm thick and helps the cornea maintain its shape. When disrupted, it will not regenerate and can form a scar.

Stroma

The corneal stroma provides the bulk of the structural framework of the cornea and comprises roughly 80–85% of its thickness. The collagen fibers are arranged in parallel bundles called fibrils, and these fibrils are packed in parallel arranged layers or lamellae. The stroma of the human eye contains 200–250 distinct lamellae, each layer arranged at right angles relative to fibers in adjacent lamellae. The peripheral stroma is thicker than the central stroma, and the collagen fibrils may change direction to run circumferentially as they approach the limbus. This highly organized network reduces forward light scatter and contributes to the transparency and mechanical strength of the cornea. An additional feature of the stroma is that the ultrastructure within the organization of the lamella appears to vary based on the depth within the stroma. Deeper layers are more strictly organized than superficial layers, and this difference accounts for the greater ease of surgical dissection in a particular plane as one approaches the posterior depths of the corneal stroma. This variation in stromal organization also accounts for the differences in response to corneal edema, as mentioned previously. Descemet folds are the result of asymmetric swelling of the posterior stroma imposed by the structurally more rigid anterior cornea and structural restriction imposed by the limbus. Stromal swelling is therefore directed posteriorly and results in relative flattening of the posterior surface, which can push Descemet's membrane into multiple folds that become visible as striae.

Ground substance in corneal stroma consists of mucoproteins and glycoproteins. A disturbance of the ratio of mucoprotein and glycoprotein is reported in keratoconus. Keratocytes are long irregular cells with the nucleus occupying its central portion. They have a Golgi apparatus, ribosomes, endoplasmic reticulum, and mitochondria. They show great activity after stromal injury and form irregularly arranged collagen fibers resulting in opacity. Cells and vessels migrate from the limbus and settle down.

Descemet's Membrane

The posterior boundary of the stroma is lined by a homogeneous membrane called Descemet's membrane. It is 6–10 μm thick and can be separated easily form the stroma and the endothelium. This is thick in the periphery, it is PAS positive. Though it curls, it is not elastic. It is formed by collagen fibrils and amorphous material. Fibers have nodes on them and are arranged in the geometric shape of equilateral triangles. It is resistant to chemical and inflammatory insults. Unlike Bowman's membrane it is replaced by the endothelium on destruction.

ENDOTHELIUM

The intact human endothelium is a monolayer, which appears as a honeycomb-like mosaic when viewed from the posterior side. There are 5,00,000 endothelial cells. Each is 4–5 μm thick and 18–20 μm wide and they are arranged in a single layer. Microvilli project into the anterior chamber. Intercellular spaces are tortuous, and cells are joined by adhesive thickenings. There is a large oval nucleus and the cytoplasm shows mitochondria, Golgi apparatus, endoplasmic reticulum, and ribosomes. Normally, it serves as a barrier to aqueous. The endothelial layer of the cornea maintains corneal clarity by maintaining adequate stromal hydration and ensuring that it remains in a relatively deturgescence state.

Blood Supply of the Cornea

Although the normal human cornea is avascular, it relies on components of the blood to remain healthy. These components are supplied by tiny vessels at the outermost edge of the cornea as well as components supplied by end branches of the facial and ophthalmic arteries via the aqueous humor and tear film.

Nerve Supply

Corneal nerves enter through the middle or superficial third of the sclera. They run towards the center and then branch to rich plexus under Bowman's layer from where they go up into the intercellular spaces. The endothelium and Descemet's layers are devoid of nerves. After corneal grafting, sensation is not fully recovered for 6–12 months. Reduced sensitivity after contact lens wear may not be due to adaptation alone, but to atrophic changes in nerve endings caused by trauma, pressure and chronic corneal edema.

CORNEAL METABOLISM

The cornea gets most of its oxygen from the atmosphere through the precorneal tear film. It is also supplied by palpebral and limbal vessels, and by the aqueous. The partial pressure of oxygen in the tear film is 155 mm of mercury in open eye and on lid closure it falls to 50 mm of mercury. The pressure of oxygen essential for corneal metabolism and proper epithelial functioning is 12–20 mm of mercury. Both aerobic and anaerobic processes are present in the cornea. Glucose, the main nutrient comes mainly from the aqueous. Glucose is utilized by (a) the Embden-Meyerhof pathway (Fig. 2.2) to pyruvic acid and then into lactic acid or through the Krebs cycle into carbon dioxide and water or (b) pentose phosphate or hexose monophosphate shunt into carbon dioxide and water. Compared to the epithelium and the endothelium, stroma has very little of glycolytic activity. Interference of oxygen supply to the cornea leads to depletion of glycogen, accumulation of lactic acid and corneal haziness. Lactic acid concentration rises in the aqueous and in the tears in contact lens wearers because it diffuses out both anteriorly into the tears and posteriorly into the aqueous. Corneal thickness is increased and the curvature is changed.

A piece of cornea put in water or hypotonic solution swells up. Normally corneal dehydration is maintained by (a) continued evaporation of tears (b) hypertonicity of teats (c) metabolic endothelial and epithelial pump. The latter two mechanisms are more important. The endothelial dysfunction is evident in glaucoma and in endothelial dystrophy where all corneal layers get water-logged ultimately.

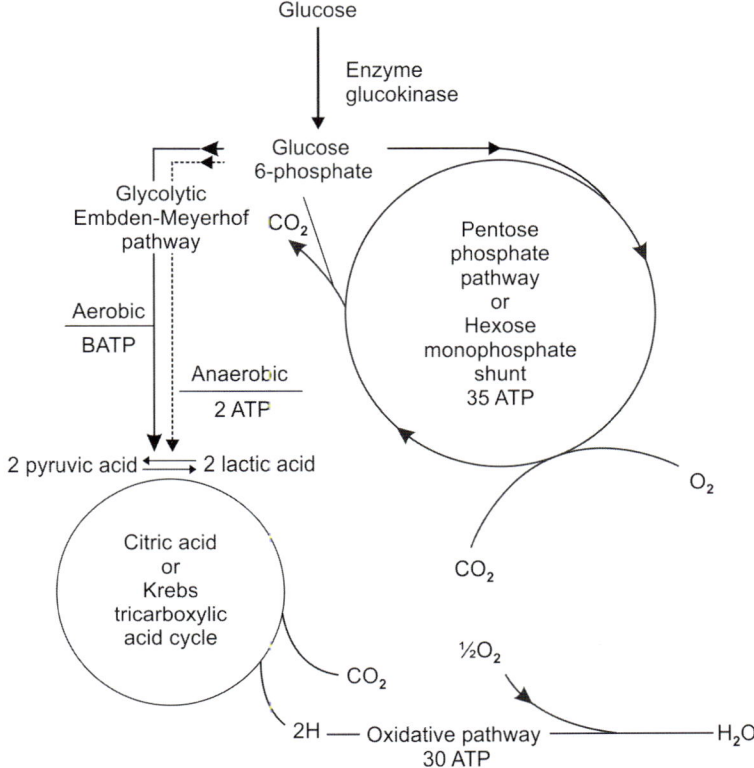

Fig. 2.2 Embden-Meyerhof pathway

Corneal transparency is due to uniformity in the arrangement of collagen which does not allow light to scatter. Hydration disturbs the collagen matrix spacing and the refractive index becomes less uniform. Regarding permeability, the epithelium and endothelium are resistant barriers to water but not to lipids and the stroma allows free exchange of water.

Lid

The most anterior structures affecting contact lens fit are the eyelids. The eyelids have three main functions. These are:
1. Protection of the globe
2. Distribution of the tear film
3. Production of tears

The eyelids contain many of the structures for producing the tear film. Among these are the meibomian glands which produce the outer lipid layer of the tear film with their openings at the lid margin. The lacrimal glands are located in the superior and temporal aspect of the underside of the lid and produce the aqueous component. As the lid blinks it spreads the tear film over the surface of the eye toward the lacrimal ducts positioned on the upper and lower lid margins. While some of the tears are lost to evaporation the majority drain out of the eye through the openings, called puncta, into the nasolacrimal duct.

During the pre-fit evaluation it is important to examine the lids and lid margins. They should be free of debris and inflammation. The under-surface of the lid should be smooth and uniform in color and texture. Patients that exhibit signs of chronic allergies or blepharoconjunctivitis are unlikely to be successful contact lens wearers. Follow-up exams should monitor the lids as well. One common complication observed with contact lenses is giant papillary conjunctivitis (GPC). GPC is a hypersensitivity reaction most commonly diagnosed in soft contact lens wearers. The underside of the lid becomes red and irritated developing a cobblestone-like texture.

Conjunctiva

The conjunctiva is divided into two main sections: the palpebral, lining the undersurface of the lids, and the bulbar covering the sclera. It is a translucent mucous membrane that is not easily observable unless irritation of the eye is present. The conjunctiva provides a smooth interface between the lid and eye during blinking. It has two layers: an epithelial and stromal layer. The epithelium crosses at the limbus and is continuous with the corneal epithelium. Goblet cells, which produce the mucoid bottom layer of the tear film, are also located in conjunctiva.

Contact lens wearers may experience conjunctival injection if a lens does not fit properly. Excessive mechanical irritation can cause the loosely attached tissue to become edematous and inflamed.

The conjunctiva is also susceptible to inflammation of a viral, bacterial or allergic nature. These conditions always contraindicate contact lens wear and must be carefully screened for at every visit.

Tears

Tears are secretions of the lacrimal glands. They serve optical, protective, nutritional, and wetting functions. They collect waste products of the epithelium and stroma, i.e. carbon dioxide, water, and dead cells. The major part of the oxygen supply of the cornea is supplied from the atmospheric oxygen dissolved in the tears. Healthy tear film is essential for a successful contact lens wear.

Tears include (a) the serous component which comes from the lacrimal gland (b) the lipoid component from the meibomian glands and (c) the mucoid component from the goblet cells (Fig. 2.3). The tears contain 98–99% water. They are isotonic in the closed eye and hypertonic in the open eye. The refractive index is 1.33%. Potassium concentration is several time higher and chloride only little more than blood serum. Protein content in the tear is 0.2–0.6%.

Lysozyme present in the tear constitutes 4% of proteins and it breaks the cell wall of bacteria by breaking the linkage between N-acetylglucosamine and

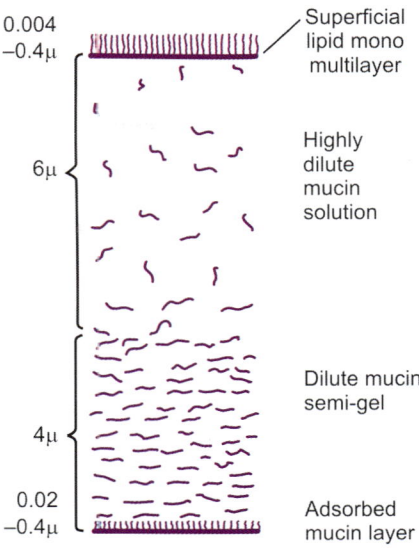

Fig. 2.3 Layers of tear film

M-acetylmuramic acid. It acts best at a pH of 7.4. Other nonlysosomal antibacterial components are also present in the tears.

The tear is produced as a rate of 1.2 microliters per minute. Women secrete more tears and this may be a reason why women tolerate contact lens better.

Tear production is governed by various factors. It is only at 6 months of age that the serous component begins to attain normal levels in the eyes and before that its production is minimal and it is lacking within first four weeks. So before 6 months of age it is possible but not advisable to get contact lenses. Older people produce less tears than young.

Physical and mental fatigue decrease tears and so it is inadvisable to persist with contact lenses, late in the evening. Quantitatively tears are best measured by the dilution of dye. The Schirmer test is a crude test. A 20 × 5 mm filter paper strips is put in lower fornix by the short end. Wetting of 10 mm or more after 5 minutes is considered as normal. This determines the reflex secretion as well. If this test is done with local anesthesia, basic tear flow is determined. Drugs like antihistamines and beta-blockers reduce tear secretions and should be cautiously used in contact lens wearers.

The lacrimal gland is supplied by sensory sympathetic and parasympathetic nerves which branch from sphenopalatine ganglion and 7th cranial nerve. Afferent fibers go along the 5th nerve and efferent fibers leave via sympathetic and parasympathetic. The sympathetic controls the normal and the parasympathetic controls the reflex or excessive lacrimation. The stimuli may come from the periphery or brain, (emotional tears; hypothalamus).

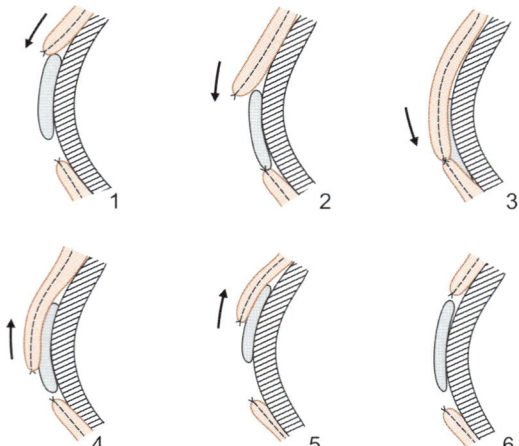

Fig. 2.4 Excursion of contact lens during blink

Each blinks lasts for 0.3 second and most people blink 12 times a minute. Contact lenses can significantly affect blinking because of physical irritation. Excursion of the contact lens during blinks is shown in Figure 2.4. Tears exchange with each blink; 1–2% in soft lenses and 10–20% in rigid lenses.

The tear film has a positive role in contact lens wear. Tears fill up the corneal irregularities in irregular astigmatism as in corneal opacities. Tears help in lens positioning by their capillarity and viscosity. It also helps in the evaluation of cornea lens relationship. In dry eye, tears make the cornea more hydrophobic which conserves the tears and in soft contact lens wear, tears help in keeping up its integrity. Tears help in the circulation of nutrients and the elimination of waste products removal lowering the evaporation rate, disturbing tonicity and traumatizing the epithelial cells.

CORNEAL OXYGEN UPTAKE AND LENS PERMEABILITY

Whether a contact lens can supply adequate amount of oxygen to the cornea can be known by:

- Comparing the oxygen uptake of the cornea before and after the contact lens wear with the use of polarographic electrode. Here the curve obtained after the use of contact lens can be compared with standard curves of several oxygen concentrations. The oxygen consumption after the lens removal is expressed as "Equivalent Oxygen Percentage" (EOP). This can be compared with the normal oxygen percentage which is 21%. The pressure exerted by this is 21% of atmospheric pressure, i.e. 760/21 = 159 mm Hg. A 7.5–21% (average 10%) of oxygen must be supplied to the cornea for its proper metabolic function. Normal consumption of oxygen is 4–5 mL per square cm of cornea per hour.
- By comparing the percentage of corneal swelling with the use of a standard lens for a known period.

- Permeability of the lens material can be known by the intervention of a lens between two chambers. The chamber with oxygen transmits it and the electrode on the other side senses transmission. Permeability is known by multiplying transmission with lens thickness. This is a better term as it is independent of thickness. 'DK' is the expression for oxygen permeability and DK/L or DK/T is used for oxygen transmissibility. 'D' represents coefficient for oxygen diffusion in the lens material and 'L' or 'T' stands for lens thickness 'K' stands for solubility coefficient of oxygen of the material.

Physiology of the Closed Eye

There is a shift in the nature and the composition tear film in eye after an overnight lid closure. *The closed eye shows:*
- IgA rich tears
- Increase in albumin levels
- Activation of plasminogen
- Conversion of complement C_3 to C_{3c}
- Increase in the number polymorphs
- Increase in vitronectin

This is an indicator of subclinical inflammation. Hence wearing of contact lens during sleep is not advisable.

CHAPTER 3

Contact Lenses: Indications

Prescribing and fitting contact lenses have become an integral part of today's comprehensive ophthalmology practice. Majority of the people are using contact lenses for cosmetic purposes. Other reasons for wearing contact lenses include occupational preferences, sports and therapeutic uses. Their growing importance makes it appropriate to inquire into the origins and development of these valuable ophthalmic resources.

In the author's survey of 4000 cases, two-thirds were females and one-third cases were males. Sixty percent of the lenses were cosmetic and 40% optical where visual acuity was better with contact lenses than with the glasses. The ratio of the cosmetic to optical contact lens fittings in males was 1:2 and in females 2:1.

For the group as a whole the order of magnitude was as follows, in terms of indications (Table 3.1).

With extensive use of contact lenses, fitters must have a clear concept of contact lens superiority for various indications. Unthinkingly fitting contact lenses for each and every optical problem can only cause trouble. This chapter clarifies the advantage of contact lenses in various indications. Before fitting, the patient must be properly classified.

OPTICAL

- *Myopia:* As compared to glasses, contact lenses are better because of larger image, better transmission, little marginal aberration, larger field, brighter perception, avoidance of rim interference, etc. (Fig. 3.1). In myopia contact

Table 3.1 Indications of contact lens	
	Percentage
Myopia	72.0
Aphakia	13.8
Keratoconus	5.0
Corneal opacities	4.0
Anisometropia	1.6
High regular astigmatism	1.4
Hyperopia	1.2
Mixed astigmatism	0.8
Albinism	0.2

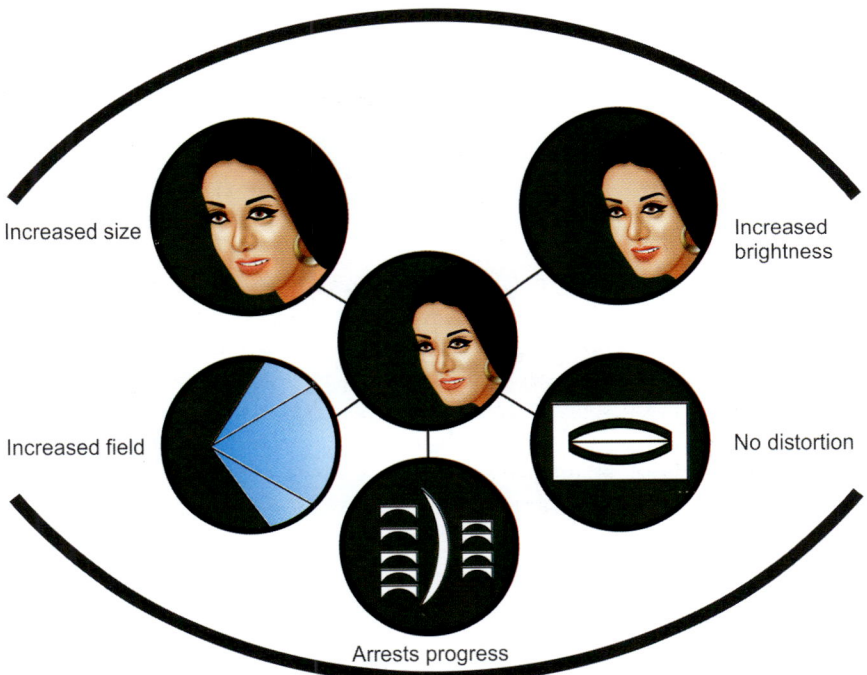

Fig. 3.1 Advantages of contact lenses over glasses in myopia

lenses are a little superior to glasses as contact lenses may affect the axial length. Before giving contact lenses the error of over-correction usual in myopia may be excluded. The author has found a decrease in myopia in 77% cases after 3 years of lens wear.

- *Hyperopia:* Optically better corrected with contact lenses due to larger field, less marginal aberrations, better transmission, brighter image, little rim interference and exerts less accommodation and less convergence compared to spectacles (Fig. 3.2). There is more convergence in spectacles due to base out prisms which the eye faces during convergence.
- *Astigmatism:* A corneal lens fills up the irregularities of the astigmatic surface; the irregular surface of the cornea is thus replaced by regular surface of contact lens. Even with a regular cornea the author found that 6.4% cases of astigmatism improve only with contact lenses.
- *Presbyopia:* A hyperope exerts less accommodation with contact lenses: minor presbyopic correction in hyperopia can therefore be delayed for a few years with contact lenses. The reverse is true for myopia; with contact lenses presbyopia will be precipitated in pre-presbyopic age.
- *Keratoconus and irregular astigmatism:* The mode of action while using the contact lenses is the same as in regular astigmatism. The contact lens has no effect on the basic course of the disease.
- *Aphakia:* Contact lenses are better due to smaller magnification (7% compared to 25% in spectacles), wider field, lesser marginal aberration, absence of Jack

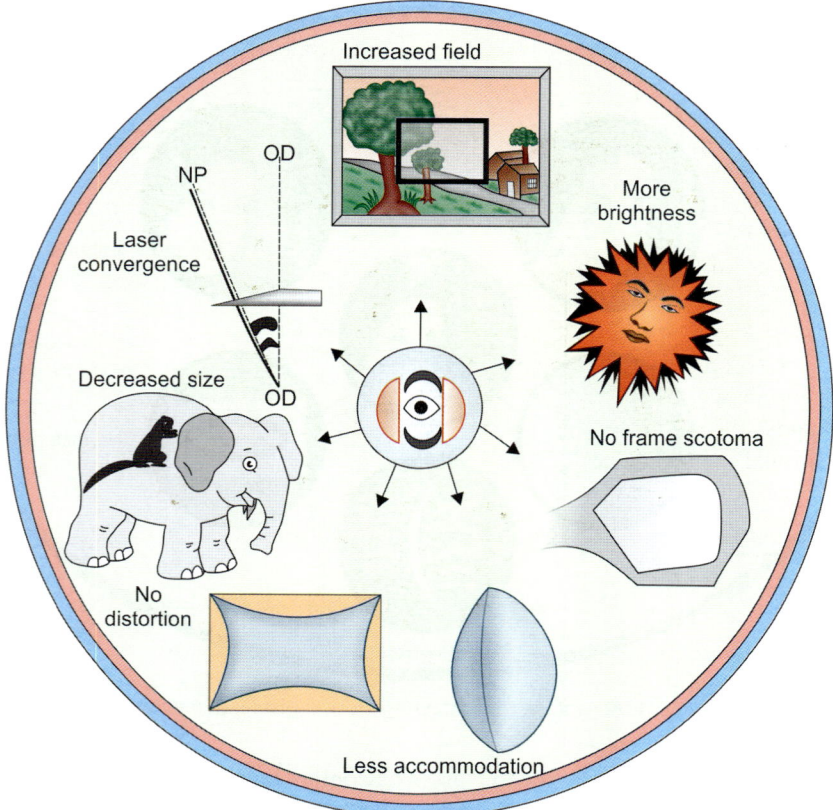

Fig. 3.2 Advantages of contact lenses over glasses in hyperopia

in box phenomenon, more transmission, brighter field, lesser convergence, and better chances of binocularity compared to correction by spectacles.

- *Anisometropia and aniseikonia:* These anomalies of refractive origin are best corrected by contact lenses which bring the image size of defective eye nearer to an emmetropic eye. This helps to establish binocularity. Vertical prism imbalance of anisometropic glasses during up and down gaze is avoided. Contact lens also provides a large field, and a brighter and clearer image due to absence of aberration.

- *Albinism:* Contact lenses are better as they correct the associated myopia and astigmatism, and are also better for the same reasons as in high myopia and astigmatism. Transmission may be retarded through a darker contact lens. Lenses with opaque scleral part and lenses with multiple holes in optical area are a better aid.

- *Aniridia:* Contact lens better corrects the associated ametropia. Transmission may be reduced through darker tint or painted iris lenses. There is immediate improvement in photophobia.

- *Nystagmus:* Contact lenses improve performance through better correction of the associated refractive anomaly and also decrease the amplitude of nystagmus.

THERAPEUTIC

Soft lenses and flush fitting shells have been found useful in the following diseases:
- Corneal burns
- Indolent ulcers
- Bullous keratopathy
- Stevens-Johnson syndrome
- Neuroparalytic keratitis
- Exposure keratitis
- Corneal edema
- Corneal graft
- Pemphigus
- Keratoconjunctivitis Sicca
- Descemetocele
- Trichiasis
- Symblepharon (a scleral shell is given after cutting adhesions)
- Leaking wounds
- Small traumatic corneal wounds
- Recurrent erosions
- Dry eyes.

In recent years, soft lenses are gaining ground over rigid lenses, the later however remain superior in providing better visual activity.

Sauflon, Permalens and Bausch and Lomb soft lenses have also been used for therapeutic purposes. The author has reported excellent results with soft lenses in (a) Desiccating diseases like pemphigus, keratoconjunctivitis sicca and Stevens-Johnsons syndrome. Preservative free artificial tears are used with the soft lenses for a week or two (b) Neuroparalytic cornea after 5th nerve lesions, keratoplasty, corneal herpes and acid or alkali burns in which soft lenses afford excellent protection, (c) Bullous keratopathy in which 5% hypertonic saline is used with the soft lenses, (d) Medication like pilocarpine and iododeoxyuridine therapy has been found to be more efficacious when the medicines were incorporated in or instilled over the soft lenses, (e) In symblepharon after operation to avoid adhesions and to protect cornea. The author has also reported good results in epithelial dystrophies with recurrent erosions, indolent ulcers, bullous keratopathy, dry eyes in early stages, herpetic exposure and neuroparalytic keratitis and post-operatively in lid surgery, leaking wounds and post-operative indolent filamentary keratitis. Soft lenses are routinely fitted in operation theater in all cases of photorefractive keratectomy (PRK), phototherapeutic keratectomy (PTK) and collagen cross linking (CXL) of an ectatic cornea.

COSMETIC

- Unsightly corneas or eyeballs can be hidden by the painted or tinted contact lens. A deformed eye with useful vision is corrected by a painted lens with clear pupil, which bears the optical correction.
  Prosthetic: Here contact lenses may be:
  - *Scleral* when it may be used as
    - Prosthetic haptic with clear optic or vice versa
    - Occlusion of pupil as in complicated cataract with retinal dysfunctions or clear pupil as in aniridia.
    - Partial prosthetic in partial aniridia and peripheral corneal opacities.
    - Ptosis props
    - Orbital prosthesis
  - *Corneal*: Extra limbal corneal lenses for anirdia
- *Actors:* Natural color of the iris can be covered by using iris painted soft contact lenses which may be blue, light gray or green.

OCCUPATIONAL

- *Temperature variation:* Fogging of spectacles is avoided while shifting from cold or hot and humid temperature as contact lenses are at same temperature as the body.
- News casters and television actors are enabled to avoid reflection that occurs with spectacles.
- *Sports:* Contact lenses have an advantage because of better performance due to wider field, better optics and lesser hazards of serious injury compared to spectacles.

DIAGNOSTIC

Contact lenses are used in the following instruments where they are used to neutralize cornea to pick-up its potentials, or as marker.

- *Gonioscopy*: This is to see angle, and to operate on angle in infantile glaucoma (Fig. 3.3).
- *Fundoscopy*: Has a high minus central lens, which neutralizes the cornea so that fundus can be viewed directly. It is much more comfortable if soft lens is placed underneath.
- *Electrodiagnostic procedure*: Electrode incorporation is used in the lens to pick potentials at the corneal plane. Gold, silver or platinum wires can be used. Scleral lens with electrode or electrode sandwiched between two soft lenses are used in electroretinography and its finer components like early receptor and oscillation potentials.

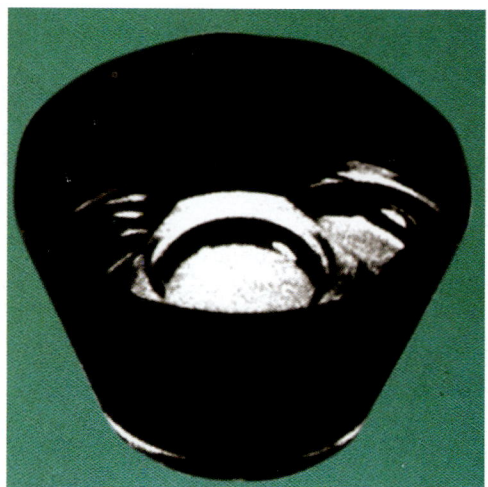

Fig. 3.3 Gonioscope

RESEARCH

Contact lens may be used in research for:
- Stimulating accommodation with minus lenses.
- Relaxing accommodation with positive lenses.
- Noting the eye movements by seeing movements of reflected light from a mirror attached to the front surface of scleral lens.
- Temperature measurements
  - By implanting thermostat through a haptic lens. This is a small ceramic device which creates different electrical potentials with changes in temperature.
  - It is also done by noting changes in color of heat sensitive crystals laminated within the contact lens.
- Measurement of lid pressure through planting a transducer on the front surface of haptic lens.
- Getting a stabilized retinal image through a scleral lens, used to neutralize small involuntary movements of the eye.
- Study of surface tension after alternation of lens parameters.
- Experimental studies on animals for occlusion, hemianopic effects to stimulate or relax accommodation and protection of the eye under anesthesia.

CHAPTER 4

Contact Lens: Contraindications

Before fitting a contact lens, the following conditions must be looked into. Contact lenses should be withheld till the pathology is completely treated. The contraindications may be classified into following broad groups.

- **Palpebral**
  - Stye
  - Chalazion of upper lid
  - Trichiasis
  - Entropion
  - Ectropion
  - Squamous blepharitis
  - Ulcerative blepharitis
- **Conjunctival**
  - Chronic hyperemia
  - Acute bacterial and viral conjunctivitis
  - Allergic conjunctivitis
  - Vernal conjunctivitis
  - Symblepharon
  - Pterygium
- **Corneal**
  - Epithelial dystrophies
  - Pannus formation
  - Corneal ulcer
  - Keratitis
- **Paralysis of fifth nerve**
- **Dry eye**
- **Exophthalmos**
- **Medications**
- **Other ocular conditions**
  - Scleritis
  - Episcleritis
  - Acute or chronic iritis
  - Cyclitis
  - Choroiditis
  - Uncontrolled diabetes
  - Glaucoma with bleb
- **Occupation**

- **Nonmedical causes**
  Nonmedical factors which may affect the successful use of contact lenses are:
  – Motivation
  – Sex
  – Complexion
  – Type and extent of refractive error
  – Degree, sign and site of astigmatism
  – Corneal toricity
  – Visual acuity without glasses

PALPEBRAL

- *Stye:* It is an acute staphylococcal infection of the gland of Zeis. Contact lens fitting may result in infection of minor abrasions (violent ulceration may ensure) resulting in corneal ulceration.
- *Chalazion of the upper lid:* It is responsible for induction of false astigmatism. Contact lens fitting will further add to irritation.
- *Entropion and trichiasis:* In this case, contact lens fitting adds to the irritation. The upper lid is incapable of performing its physiological function of properly picking up the lens. Removal of lens also becomes difficult as posterior lid margins are rounded.
- *Ectropion:* The contact lens does not get support of the involved lid causing further irritation. Removal of lens is difficult.
- *Squamous blepharitis:* The lens remains coated with thick oily secretion of the meibomian gland and the vision remains blurred.
- Ulcerative blepharitis is an infective inflammation of the lid. With contact lens, there are more chances of corneal infection through minor abrasions.

CONJUNCTIVAL

- *Chronic hyperemia* due to minor irritation is further aggravated by the use of contact lens.
- *Acute infective conjunctivitis:* With the contact lens, the condition may spread to the cornea, causing ulceration. Even as it is the condition may persist longer due to the contact lens irritation.
- *Allergic or vernal conjunctivitis:* Contact lens causes intolerable irritation to a patient with conjunctival allergy, and the duration of allergic conjunctives is prolonged due to contact lens wear with more chances of corneal abrasion. A patient may be or can become allergic to contact lens or its solutions.
- Symblepharon is a contraindication, when it is extensive and progressive. It interferes with lid actions during blinking or lens removal.
- *Pterygium:* Contact lens may irritate the pterygium head, and even a regressed one might become vascularized. It is better to treat it before fitting contacts lens, and the pterygium may be shown to the patient otherwise he will feel that the contact lens is responsible for its causation.

PARALYSIS OF FIFTH NERVE

This results in lack of sensation in the cornea. Any trauma due to contact lens or a foreign body may result in a severe ulceration, without the patient feeling it.

DRY EYE

Even though some contact lens materials are better for the dry eye patients, working with dry eye patients can be time consuming and not always successful. Mild to moderately dry eye patients may succeed; however, patients with severe dry eye probably will not. Of course, some dry eye patients are willing to wear their lenses on a part-time basis or just for social occasions. The fitter should always provide samples of a rewetting drop at the dispensing visit.

CORNEAL

- *Epithelial dystrophies:* With abnormal epithelial cell, contact lens may cause abrasion and even ulceration.
- *Pannus formation:* Is a subepithelial infiltration with vascularization of the cornea. Irrespective of the causal factor, contact lens tends to activate the condition by massaging blood into the defunct vessels.
- *Corneal ulcer and keratitis:* Any active inflammation of cornea will flare-up due to mechanical trauma and continued irritation caused by hard contact lenses.
- Keratitis sicca is a desiccating condition of the conjunctiva and cornea. Use of the contact lenses over such corneas can cause abrasion, infection and ulceration. Violent and indolent infections leading to blindness have been repeatedly documented in these dry eyes.

EXOPHTHALMOS

In this case, the upper lid does not reach the limbus and the lens does not get picked up.

MEDICATIONS

Some medications, systemic and topical, are directly and/or indirectly responsible for contact lens intolerance. Symptoms range from ocular dryness to discomfort and decreased vision. Some may even cause photophobia (light sensitivity). Some medications can cause a reduction in blink rate, such as antihistamines, anticholinergics, muscle relaxants, antidepressants and tranquilizers. The fitter should always ask for medication information when taking the complete history. The problems associated with these medications have to be explained to the patients.

OTHER OCULAR CONDITIONS

- Inflammatory conditions like episcleritis, scleritis, acute or chronic iritis, cyclitis, and choroiditis are likely to be aggravated by continued irritation caused by the contact lens. The patient does not tolerate contact lens in an irritated eye.
- *Uncontrolled diabetes:* These are poor subjects for contact lenses. They are more prone to bacterial fungal infection of the eye which is difficult to control. These patients show delayed healing.
- *Glaucoma with bleb:* The authors have seen eyes being lost due to the opening of the bleb by the injury caused by the edge of the corneal contacts lens. Soft lens can be fitted over the bleb.

OCCUPATION

Certain occupations can be contraindication to contact lenses. Mechanics work around a lot of grease, oil and fumes. Their fingers are never quite clean and are very rough. Soft lenses are definitely not a good choice. Construction workers battle the elements and flying debris. Gas permeable (GP) contact lenses and flying debris in the workplace do not work well together. However, wearing lenses after working hours for sports and social wear should not be a problem.

OTHER FACTORS

After practicing contact lens fitting for over a decade, the authors would share their experience with other practitioners particularly in respect of failure. It is obvious that motivation is the most important factor, and when it is lacking failure is most likely to occur. *Other generalizations which may be made are that failures are more common in:*
- Males than females
- Fair persons than dark
- Female aphakes than male
- Hyperopes than myopes
- Spherical corneas than astigmatic
- Astigmatism more than 4.00 D
- Extra corneal astigmatism
- Patients with better vision with glasses
- Low myopia
- Patients with larger pupils.

CHAPTER 5

Materials for Contact Lenses

Several materials have been used in fabrication of contact lenses. The first material used was glass, however, owing to its brittle nature, it was soon dropped. With the progress of polymer science and technology a large number of polymeric materials have been made available for preparation of these lenses, which brought a rapid revolution in the contact lens industry. Stress was laid on the development of materials with higher stability, flexibility, oxygen permeability and biological tolerance.

Polymeric materials denote compounds whose molecules are made up by repetition of some simpler units known as monomers. The characteristic properties of polymers like high viscosity, long range elasticity and high strength depend upon their large size and molecular weight. Thus polyethylene is a waxy solid of molecular weight in the range 1000–5000 but becomes a brittle solid if the molecular weight is greater than 10,000. In general the molecular weights of the polymers are high and lie in the range 10^4–10^7. However, the useful range of molecular weight is not the same for all polymers but is dependent on the composition of other polymer chain and its ultimate use.

Material used in the manufacture of contact lenses should ideally have the following characteristics:

- Should be biologically inert.
- Should be nonselective in the absorption of metabolites and toxins and not take part in enzymatic activity.
- Should not exhibit strong molecular adhesive forces.
- Should not show excessive electrophoretic osmotic properties.
- Should have little friction effect between the surface of the material and the eye tissues.
- Should have high gas permeability.
- Should be compatible with the surface eye tissue electrical charges without a change of properties.
- Should not change its properties within normal biological range of pH.
- Should not excite an inflammatory or immune response even if buried in the tissues over a long period of time.

Fitting and wearing behavior of the lens can be assessed from the following:

- Specific gravity
- Micropenetration (hardness)
- Elasticity

- Plasticity
- Tensile strength
- Water absorption
- Surface wettability
- Stress and strain
- Gas permeability
- Gas permeability of lens relative to thickness
- Thermal conductivity
- Coefficients of size related to 7° (Linear expansion)
- Coefficients of size relative to water (Linear expansion)
- Refractive index
- Optical quality
- Light transmission %
- Material purity
- Polymer stability

The process of conversion of monomers to high molecular weight material is called polymerization. Based on the method of polymerization various polymers can be classified into two groups (a) addition polymers (b) condensation polymers. In addition polymers monomers add on to one another and have the molecular formula of structural unit identical with that of monomer from which they are derived, e.g. (1)

$$CH_2 = CH_2 \underline{\hspace{3cm}} (CH_2 - CH_2 -)_{11}$$
(ethylene)   (Polyethylene)

In condensation polymers monomers condense with each other with the elimination of simple molecules usually water and the molecular formula of the structural unit is not identical with the monomer, e.g. (2)

$$H_2N(CH_2)_6NH_2 + HOOC(CH_2)_4COOH \underline{\hspace{3cm}} (HN(CH_2)_6$$
(Hexamethylenediamine) adipic acid $\underline{\hspace{1cm}}$ $(HNOC(CH_2)_4CO)_{11} \underline{\hspace{0.5cm}} + nH_2O$
Nylon66

If all the repeat units in a polymer are of the same chemical composition the resulting polymer is known as homopolymer. If two or more types of repeated units are present in the polymer then the term copolymer is used.

Copolymers can be either of (i) alternative type or (ii) block type. In alternating copolymers, two more different repeat units occur alternately along the chain, e.g. copolymers of styrene and maleic anhydride and styrene/acrylonitrile, etc. In block copolymers distinct blocks of monomers alternate with each other in the polymer backbone. Polymer properties can be tailored as per requirement by copolymerization of monomers of different characteristics, for example, polymethylacrylate is soft and rubbery whereas polymethylmethacrylate is relatively strong and hard. By copolymerization, materials can be prepared with hardness intermediate between the two.

A polymer can be of linear, branched or of cross-linked type. Linear polymers are straight-chained ones and are also known as one-dimensional polymers. Branched polymers have long or short branches on the back-bone of the polymer. The branches may be of 5 or 6 carbon atoms as in high pressure polyethylene or they can be very long.

The cross-linked or network polymers are extended polycyclic structures of bridged, fused, or spirolinked rings. They are prepared by polymerizing monomers having functionality greater than two. They can also be prepared by cross linking two linear polymers. These three dimensional polymers may be ordered or disordered, may be gels or microgels and have limited solubility.

Polymers to be used as contact lenses should be of high purity. Commercially available monomers used in plastic industry have inhibitors to prevent autopolymerization prior to the manufacturing process. These inhibitors are intolerable in biomaterials (contact lenses) and there is a necessity for their removal. Hence, the raw materials used for these polymers are of high purity and are tested for impurities by using such techniques as infrared and ultraviolet spectroscopy, thin layer, liquid gas or gel permeation chromatography, viscosity, specific gravity, nuclear magnetic resonance spectroscopy, refractive index analysis, electrical constant, etc.

Once the raw material is purified, it is polymerized either chemically or using radiation. Radiation-induced polymerization is desirable because it avoids the use of chemical initiators which are usually toxic. The initiation of polymerization takes place at the radical centers. In chemical polymerization the free radicals are generated with the help of catalysts such as benzyl peroxide.

In radiation-induced polymerization, radical centers are generated with the help of high energy radiation such as UV radiation. Polymerization should be carried out up to completion, to avoid large quantities of monomer being left in the end-product. However, small quantities of monomer are always left which are not incorporated in the polymer. The unreacted monomer and other undesirable molecules which might be present must be removed by extraction. Such materials, if left in the plastic can leak out in the eye and cause undesirable toxic effects.

Material can be polymerized into a variety of shapes such as rods, sheets or buttons which are later on cut into desired types of lenses. The shaped plastics may have areas of stress within them which could cause warpage of contact lenses during manufacture. To prevent this, material is annealed above its glass transition temperature (Tg) usually 55–85°C for 24–72 hours and then cooled very slowly to eliminate any stress.

The polymers used for contact lenses are classified broadly into three categories (a) hard (b) hydrophobic flexible (c) soft. This classification is based on the way the finished lens fits in the eye. Some of the materials which are used now having a potentiality for further development would be dealt with here.

Polymethylmethacrylate (PMMA): This is one of the most commonly used materials for hard contact lenses. It can be prepared by polymerizing methyl methacrylate in presence of a cross linking agent such as ethylene glycol dimethacrylate (EDMA).

It has got good optical properties and is nontoxic. PMMA has excellent moulding and machining qualities but is practically impermeable to oxygen. Therefore, the lenses fabricated from this material can be used only for limited time. Due to this reason it is no longer used in contact lens practice.

The oxygen permeability and other properties of a PMMA can be improved by copolymerizing methyl methacrylate with other monomers. Methyl methacrylate-styrene and methyl methacrylate alpha methylstyrene, copolymers have been used for the manufacture of the contact lenses. Compared to PMMA these materials have higher light transmission, higher refractive index and a lower density.

The physical properties of PMMA and its copolymers are given in Table 5.1.

POLY (4-METHYL-1 PENTENE)

This is a thermoplastic material and has the repeat unit structure as shown below:

This polymer has high transparency to light, low density, high melting-point and useful mechanical properties such as retention to form and stability even near the melting point. Some of the physical properties and summarized in Table 5.1. One the greatest advantage of this polymer is its oxygen permeability which is 650 times more than PMMA. This may be because of the less dense structure of the polymer due to the presence of bulky side group.

STYRENE-ACRYLONITRILE COPOLYMER

Poly (Styrene) is a highly transparent (90% transmission) material and has got excellent moulding and good machining properties, but due to its brittleness, it is not recommended for the manufacture of contact lenses.

But the copolymers of styrene (70%) and acrylonitrile (30%) have higher strength, rigidity and chemical resistance than Poly (styrene). This polymer has good transmission (88%) and a refractive index of 1.56–57. It has got moulding as well as machining properties and has a use as contact lenses.

ACRYLONITRILE-BUTADIENE-STYRENE-COPOLYMERS

Acrylonitrile-butadiene-styrene-copolymers (ABS) plastics are derived from acrylonitrile, butadiene and styrene. It is obtained by copolymerizing these monomers and usually grafting technique is followed for such preparation. Grafting of acrylonitrile and styrene is usually done into polymerized butadiene. By changing the various parameters during copolymerization, the properties of the resulting copolymer can be varied over a wide range. Transport grade polymer are available. This material has good balance of tensile strength, impact resistance, surface hardness and heat resistance and has a refractive index of 1.538. Physical properties are hardly affected by moisture.

Table 5.1 Modern rigid gas permeable (RGP) materials

Material name	Manufacturer	Dk	Colors	UV filter	Wetting angle	Specific gravity	Chemical make-up	Index of refraction
Alberta S–66		66	Blue	Yes	8.6	1.16	PSF	1.475
Boston® 7	B and L	49	Blue	Yes	54	1.22	Fluorosilicone acrylate	1.428
Boston EO®	B and L	58	Blue, ice blue, electric blue green, gray, brown	Yes	49	1.23	Fluorosilicone acrylate	1.429
Boston® Equalens®	B and L	47	Blue, electric blue, clear	Yes	30	1.19	Fluorosilicone acrylate	1.439
Boston® Equalens® II	B and L	85	Blue	Yes	30	1.24	Fluorosilicone acrylate	1.423
Boston ES®	B and L	18	Blue, ice blue, green, gray, brown	Yes	52	1.22	Fluorosilicone acrylate	1.443
Boston® II	B and L	14	Blue, green, clear	No	20	1.13	Silicone acrylate	1.471
Boston® IV	B and L	26	Blue, clear	No	17	1.1	Silicone acrylate	1.468
Boston RXD®	B and L	45	Blue, ice blue	Yes	39	1.27	Fluorosilicone acrylate	1.435
Boston® XO	B and L	100	Blue, ice blue, green	Yes	49	1.27	Fluorosilicone acrylate	1.415
Boston® XO2	B and L	141	Blue, ice blue, green	Yes	50	1.19	Fluorosilicone acrylate	1.424
Flosi	Lagado Corporation	26	Blue, clear, gray, green	Yes	23.5	1.12	Fluorosilicone acrylate	1.455
Fluorex 300	GT Laboratories	26.5	Blue, green, gray	No	12.6	1.11	Fluorosilicone acrylate	1.465
Fluorex 500	GT Laboratories	49.8	Blue, green, gray	No	13.3	1.1	Fluorosilicone acrylate	1.460
Fluorex 700	GT Laboratories	70	Blue, green, gray	No	15.3	1.1	Fluorosilicone acrylate	1.457
FluoroPerm® 30	Paragon Vision Sciences	30	Blue, majestic blue, green, gray, clear	Yes	12.8	1.14	Fluorosilicone acrylate	1.466
FluoroPerm® 60	Paragon Vision Sciences	60	Blue, green, gray, brown, clear	Yes	14.7	1.15	Fluorosilicone acrylate	1.453

Contd...

Contd...

Material name	Manufacturer	Dk	Colors	UV filter	Wetting angle	Specific gravity	Chemical make-up	Index of refraction
FluoroPerm® 92	Paragon Vision Sciences	92	Blue, green, gray, clear	Yes	16	1.1	Fluorosilicone acrylate	1.453
FluoroPerm® 151	Paragon Vision Sciences	151	Blue	Yes	42	1.1	Fluorosilicone acrylate	1.453
FluoroPerm® HDS	Paragon Vision Sciences	58	Blue, green	Yes	14.7	1.16	Fluorosilicone acrylate	1.449
Hybrid FS	Contamac US, Inc.	31	Blue, glacier blue, green, gray, clear	No	0	1.183	Fluorosilicone acrylate	1.447
Hydro2®	Innovision, Inc.	50	Blue, ocean blue, green	No	<5	1.146	Fluorosilicone acrylate	1.463
Menicon Z	Menicon America, Inc.	163	Blue	Yes	24	1.2	Fluorosilicone acrylates	1.440
Novawet		55	Blue	No	14	1.05	HSS	1.470
ONSI-56	Lagado Corporation	56	Blue, green, gray, onsure (Blue-violet)	Yes	7.2	1.206	Fluorosilicone acrylate	1.452
OP-2	Stellar Contact Lens, Inc.	16	Blue, green, brown, clear	No	18	1.12	Fluorosilicone acrylate	1.470
OP-3	Stellar Contact Lens, Inc.	30	Blue, green, brown, clear		15.5	1.12	Fluorosilicone acrylate	1.470
OP-6	Stellar Contact Lens, Inc.	60	Blue, green		23	1.11	Fluorosilicone acrylate	1.470
Optimum Classic	Contamac US, Inc.	26	Blue, glacier blue, green, gray	Yes	12	1.189	Roflufocon	1.453
Optimum Comfort	Contamac US	65	Blue, glacier blue, green, gray	Yes	6	1.178	Roflufocon	1.441
Optimum Extra	Contamac US	100	Blue, glacier blue, green, gray	Yes	3	1.166	Roflufocon	1.433
Optimum Extreme	Contamac US	125	Blue, green	Yes	6	1.155	Roflufocon	1.433
Paragon HDS®	Paragon Vision Sciences	58	Blue, crystal blue, green, forrest green	Yes	14.7	1.16	Fluorosilicone acrylate	1.449
Paragon HDS® HI	Paragon Vision Sciences	22	Blue, green	Yes	44	1.12	Fluorosilicone acrylate	1.54

Contd...

Contd...

Material name	Manufacturer	Dk	Colors	UV filter	Wetting angle	Specific gravity	Chemical make-up	Index of refraction
Paragon HDS® 100	Paragon Vision Sciences	100	Blue, green	No	42	1.1	Fluorosilicone acrylate	1.442
Paragon Thin	Paragon Vision Sciences	29	Blue, clear, green	Yes	12.8	1.14	Fluorosilicone acrylate	1.466
ParaPerm® EW	Paragon Vision Sciences	56	Blue, green, clear	No	26	1.07	Silicone acrylate	1.467
ParaPerm® O2	Paragon Vision Sciences	15.6	Blue, green, clear	No	23.1	1.12	Silicone acrylate	1.473
PMMA		0	Blue, green, gray, brown, clear			1.19	Mm	1.490
SGP 1	The Lifestyle Company, Inc.	18.5	Blue, green	No	30	1.12	Silicone acrylate	1.471
SGP 2	The Lifestyle Company	43.5	Blue, green, brown	No	31	1.07	Silicone acrylate	1.471
SGP 3	The Lifestyle Company	43.5	Blue, green	No	20	1.13	Fluorosilicone acrylate	1.471
Tyro 97—Large Diameter	Lagado Corporation	97	Blue, green, gray, green	Yes	23	1.087	Fluorosilicone acrylate	1.44

POLYCARBONATE

The polymer is prepared by reacting phosgene with aliphatic and aromatic dihydroxy compounds by a scheme of reaction.

It is very clear and has high impact-resistance, toughness and high refractive index. It is more prone to scratching than PMMA. It is specially used for the manufacture of high power contact lenses.

POLYSULFONES

These are prepared by the reaction between sodium salt of 2.2 bis (4-hydroxy phenyl) propane and 4.4'-dichlorodiphenyl sulfone.

It is transparent and has high heat resistance and can be moulded or extruded to various shapes. The material has relatively low water absorption and is resistant to most chemicals and has a potentiality as contact lens material.

CELLULOSE ACETATE BUTYRATE

This is a class of thermoplastics prepared by various treatments of purified contact or special grades of wood cellulose. Cellulose, which has got three free hydroxyl groups in the repeat unit can be converted to cellulose acetate butyrate (CAB) with acetic anhydride and butyric anhydride. CAB used for the manufacture of contact lenses contains 26–39% butyryl and 12–15% acetyl group. It is hard, stiff, strong, tough and has excellent moulding and machining properties.

HYDROPHOBIC FLEXIBLE MATERIALS

These materials can be stretched to at least twice the original length and after release of stretching force, return back nearly to their original length. These are generally called elastomers or rubbers. The properties of the elastomers can be changed by copolymerization with other monomers.

Silicon rubber is a potential candidate for contact lens material. Due to the flexibility of Si-O-Si bonds, the material is highly permeable to oxygen. Light transmission of silicon rubber is about 91% and refractive index 1.439. But unfortunately, it is a strong hydrophobic material and without a hydrophilic coating, contact lenses made of this material are not only optically poor but also very uncomfortable to the wearer.

Styrene-butadiene block copolymer is yet another material for use in contact lenses. Due to the combination between a rubber (butadiene) and a thermoplastic (styrene), it has unique properties. The material is soft and highly elastic. It has got a refractive index of 1.62–1.55 and absorbs very little water.

Ionomers can also be used in preparation of hydrophobic flexible lenses. These are a class of polymers characterized by the presence of both covalent and ionic bonds. The polymer chains usually polyethylene are cross linked by ionic bonds. Carboxy groups provide the anionic portion of the cross links and metal ions the cationic. It has good transparency, improved solvent resistance and a refractive index of 1.51. The material is quite flexible, soft and has low density. The material has good chance for hydrophobic flexible contact lens material. But it degrades when exposed to UV light due to ionic cross-linking. But grades are available which are stable to UV light for at least one year.

SILICONE AND FLUOROSILICONE ACRYLATE

The first modern gas permeable (GP) lenses to gain wide acceptance were made of an oxygen permeable material called silicone acrylate (SA). These lenses were introduced in the late 1970s under the brand name Polycon and had a Dk value of 12. Since then, new gas permeable lens materials have been developed that provide greater oxygen transmissibility, enabling even overnight wear of GP contacts. Initially, increased oxygen permeability was achieved by adding more silicone to the lens materials. However, this ultimately caused GP lenses to become more fragile and caused them to dry out and accumulate lens deposits more easily. Eventually, fluorine was added to GP lens polymers to solve these problems. Today's fluorosilicone/acrylate GP lenses are optimized for oxygen permeability, lens stability and surface wetting characteristics. In order to improve the surface hydrophilicity of fluorosilicone acrylate rigid gas permeable (RGP) contact lens, low temperature nitrogen plasma was used to modify the *lens* surface. Because of their hardness and because they do not fluctuate significantly in their water content, gas permeable contacts generally have superior optical characteristics and provide sharper vision than soft lenses.

SOFT MATERIALS

The hydrogel polymers have been used as base for soft contact lenses. The term "hydrogel" refers to a coherent three dimensional polymeric network that can imbibe large quantities of water without its dissolution. In these materials the large water uptake occurs because of the presence of certain hydrophilic groups such as hydroxyl group in the monomers used.

The soft contact lenses in contrast to hard contact lenses are not dimensionally stable and swell in water to form a pliable soft lens. The presently available soft contact lenses are mostly based on poly (2-hydroxyethyl methacrylate) (PHEMA). It is essentially a three dimensional network and swollen in an aqueous media. Hydron, Soflens, Geltakt and Spofalens are all different names of contact lenses made of PHEMA. The polymers have unique properties depending on the preparative condition. For example, PHEMA can be made into a homogeneous hydrogel which is brittle in dry state but soft and pliable when wet in water.

An essential difference between hard PMMA lenses and soft hydrophilic lenses must be emphasized here. The hard lenses are dimensionally stable, but soft lenses are used in a state of equilibrium swelling that is easily disrobed by changes in its environment. Medication variations in tear flow, changes in atmospheric conditions, etc. would affect the swelling, determining size, shape, and fitting of the lens as well as optical properties. However, the effect of hydration on hard lenses in negligible.

Soft lenses based on PHEMA are resistant to biodegradation or attach by any enzyme present in the normal or abnormal tear and withstand sterilization which can be either chemical or thermal. In addition of this these are resistant to spontaneous oxidation (auto-oxidation).

In general hydrogels for contact lenses are made by copolymerization of certain hydrophilic monomers with a cross-linking agent and also by copolymerization and cross-linking of a hydrophilic monomer with a hydrophobic monomer to obtain a desired combination of equilibrium swelling.

The polymeric network consists of hydrophilic polymer chains, joined by the bridges of cross-linking compound. The number of repeating units on the main polymeric chains. These cross-links are responsible for the coherent structure of the system. A covalently cross-linked hydrophilic polymer cannot dissolve, but it will swell by absorbing water. The tendency to swell, caused by the osmotic pressure of the polymer segments, is opposed by elastic retractive forces arising as the chains between the cross-links elongate. Ultimately equilibrium between the forces is reached. This is referred to as equilibrium swelling of the gel under given conditions. This equilibrium swelling should occur equally in all three dimensions. This is important in maintaining the optical quality of a particular lens.

The amount of water that hydrogel can absorb depends on the number of hydrophilic groups and on its kind. It also depends upon the amount of cross-links in the network (i.e. cross link density). In general, the larger the amount of water that a hydrogel can absorb higher is its permeability to water and water soluble molecules, the lower is the strength of the gel, and more sensitive the gel becomes to its environment.

The degree of swelling of a gel can be changed by varying the chemical composition of the polymer, cross-link density, pH, temperature pressure (hydrostatic pressure and osmotic pressure and on chemical composition of the solution soaking the gel). The degree of swelling can be tailored by copolymerizing a hydrophilic monomer with a hydrophobic monomer.

The presently available soft contact lenses are made either from silicone hydrogel or HEMA or copolymers of HEMA and vinyl pyrrolidone. Glyceryl (2, 3-dihydroxypropyl methacrylate) is another transparent hydrogel which can be cross-linked with tetraethylene glycol dimethacrylate (TEGDMA) to form a thermosetting plastic. Propylene glycol monoacrylate is a cross-linked hydrogen with TEGDMA as the cross-linking agent. Copolymers of propylene glycol monoacrylate are also used to prepare the soft contact lenses. Graft copolymers of vinyl pyrrolidone onto silicone rubber are other candidates for hydrogel contact lenses. The material is made by irradiating an already cured room temperature vulcanizing silicon rubber in the presence of oxygen. The irradiated rubber is then allowed to swell in vinylpyrrolidone and heated. Poly (vinylpyrrolidone) grafted

Table 5.2 Soft contact lens material

Material	Trademark	USAN council and other names	Company
Poly (2-HEMA)	Hydron	–	Hydron Europe Inc. National Patent Dev. Crop. (USA)
	Geltakt	Spofa lens Ergon	Spofa, Ergon Co. (Czechoslovakia)
	Soflens	Polymacon	Bausch and Lomb (USA)
	Welcon	–	Titmus-Eurocon (Germany)
	Medigel 38	–	Medicornea (France)
	Profil H	–	Essilor (France)
	Hydrolens	–	Hydroptives, Inc. (USA)
Poly (2-HEMACo-EMA)	Semi soft 38	–	Nippon Contact Lens Research Institute (Japan)
Poly (HEMA Co-EA)	Semi soft 31	–	–
Poly (2-HEMA co-Vinyl Pyrrolidone)	Hydrocurve	Helfilcon A	Soft Lens Inc. (USA)
Poly (Vinyl Pyrrolidone-g-2-HEMA)	Softcon	Vifilcon A	Warner Lambert American Optics (USA)
Poly (MMA-Co vinyl Pyrrolidone)	Sauflon	Molluter	Belgravia Optical Co (UK)
Silicon-g-Vinyl-Pyrrolidone	–	–	Essilor (France)
Poly (2-HEMA-Co Methacrylic acid-co-Vinyl pyrrolidone)	Perma lens	Decarle	Cooper Vision Labs (UK)
Poly (Methyl methacrylate Co-acrylic) and	Bioplex	–	Hydrophilics International (USA, Israel)
Poly (Glycerylmethacrylate Co-methylmethacrylate)	–	Comfilcon A CS-151	Corneal Sciences Inc (USA)
Poly (Glycidylmethacrylate Co-vinylpyrrolidone) and/or Poly-(Giycidylmethacylate-Co-2 Hydroxyethlymethacrylate)	Aquafleed Theraflex	–	Union Optics (USA)
Blend of poly vinylpyrrolidone and Poly (2-hydroxyethylmethacrylate)	–	Ewell	Kontur Kontact (USA)
Poly (2-hydroxyethylmethacrylate)	Menicon soft	N and N lens	Tokyo Contact Lens I (Japan)
Co-vinyl-acetate-Co-N (1,1 dimethyl)	Hiflica 515		New Optical Co (Canada)
Silicone rubber	Silicon	–	Dow Corning Mueller-Welt USA
Silicone–vinylpyrrolidone	–	–	Essilor (France)
Cellulose acetate butyrate	–	RX-56	Rynoc Scientific (USA)

Table 5.3 Monomers and United States Adopted Name (USAN) for common hydrogel contact lens materials

Commercial name	Manufacturer	USAN	Water content	Monomers	FDA group
Frequency 38	CooperVision	Polymacon	38.0	HEMA	I
Optima FW	B and L	Polymacon	38.0	HEMA	I
Preference	CooperVision	Tetrafilcon	42.5	HEMA, MMA, NVP	I
Biomedics 55	Ocular Sciences	Ocufilcon D	55.0	HEMA, MA	IV
Focus (1–2 weeks)	CIBA Vision	Vifilcon	55.0	HEMA, PVP, MA	IV
1-Day Acuvue	Vistakon	Etafilcon	58.0	HEMA, MA	IV
Acuvue 2	Vistakon	Etafilcon	58.0	HEMA, MA	IV
Proclear Compatibles	CooperVision	Omafilcon	62.0	HEMA, PC	II
Soflens 66	B and L	Alphafilcon	66.0	HEMA, NVP	II
Focus Dailies	CIBA Vision	Nelfilcon	69.0	Modified PVA	II
Soflens One Day	B and L	Hilafilcon	70.0	HEMA, NVP	II
Precision UV	CIBA Vision	Vasurfilcon	74.0	MMA, NVP	II

Abbreviations: HEMA, 2-hydroxyethylmethacrylate; MA, methacrylic acid; MMA, methyl methacrylate; NVP, *N*-vinyl pyrrolidone; PC, phosphorylcholine; PVA, polyvinyl alcohol; PVP, polyvinyl pyrrolidone; USAN, United States Adopted Name.

Table 5.4 Silicone-hydrogel lens materials

Proprietary name	PureVision	Focus night and day	Acuvue advance
United States adopted name	Balafilcon A	Lotrafilcon A	Galyfilcon A
Manufacturer	Bausch and Lomb	CIBA Vision	Vistakon
Centre thickness (@–3.00 D) mm	0.09	0.08	0.07
Water Content	36%	24%	47%
Oxygen permeability (x 10–11)	99	140	60
Oxygen transmissibility (x 10–9)	110	175	86
Modulus (psi)*	148	238	65
Surface treatment	Plasma oxidation, producing glassy islands	25 nm plasma coating with high refractive index	No surface treatment. Internal wetting agent (PVP)
FDA Group	III	I	I
Principal monomers	NVP, TPVC, NCVE, PBVC	DMA, TRIS, siloxane macromer	Unpublished

Abbreviations: DMA, *N,N*-dimethylacrylamide; HEMA, 2-hydroxyethylmethacrylate; MA, methacrylic acid; NVP, N-vinyl pyrrolidone; TPVC, tris-(trimethylsiloxysilyl) propylvinyl carbamate; NCVE, *N*-carboxyvinyl ester; PBVC, poly[dimethylsiloxyl] di [silylbutanol] bis[vinyl carbamate]; PVP, polyvinyl pyrrolidone.

* Modulus data provided by Johnson and Johnson.

depends on the preirradiation dose, dose rate as well as on the temperature of grafting.

Other types of hydrogel of potential use for contact lenses are the polyelectrolyte complex hydrogels. In polyelectrolyte complexes, polymers are held together in a three-dimensional network by ionic charge between two oppositely charged polymers. Complexes of poly-vinylbenzyltrimethyl ammonium chloride (VBTAC) with poly (styrene sulfonate) NASS have been studies as a possible contact lens materials. When these two compounds are placed in a solution, they ionize and then the two polymers with many ionized units along them, come together like a zip so that the opposite charges are opposing. The water content can be varied between 30% and 75% depending on the concentration of VBTAC and NASS. The refractive index varies with water content and is 1.52 at 30% water content and 1.38 at 75% water content.

Table 5.2 summarizes few of the contact lens materials along with their trade names.

We investigated a series of copolymers for soft contact lenses. Co-polymer was synthesized using a combination of a hydrophilic monomer (HEMA) and hydrophobic monomer (MA, EA, MMA). By varying the composition of the two types of monomers in the initial monomer feed, we could regulate the water uptake of the resulting polymer (Table 5.2). We investigated the biological tolerance of these polymers by implanting them subcutaneously and in the anterior chamber of rabbit eye. They did not show any inflammatory reactions. These results thus indicate that the polymer samples are biocompatible.

The lenses prepared from these polymers retained their shape and clarity on keeping them in water or saline. These results thus indicate the potentiality of HEMA-alkyl acrylate copolymers for soft contact lens preparation (Table 5.3).

SILICONE HYDROGEL MATERIAL

Silicone hydrogel lenses are the latest development in soft contact lens materials. Silicone hydrogel contact lenses first appeared commercially in 1998 and since then have shown tremendous growth. Silicone hydrogel contact lenses represent a breakthrough over traditional hydrogel soft contact lenses, because silicone lets so much oxygen (essential for a healthy cornea) pass through the lens. These lenses offer exceptional oxygen transmission and durability. In silicone-hydrogel materials, silicone rubber is combined with conventional hydrogel monomers. The silicone component of these lens materials provides extremely high oxygen permeability, while the hydrogel component facilitates flexibility, wettability and fluid transport, which aids lens movement. Three silicone hydrogel lens materials are currently commercially available, with their major features being summarized in Table 5.4.

Newer materials are evolving in order to improve corneal oxygenation during contact lens wear and provide better comfort and wear ability to the contact lens user.

CHAPTER 6

Contact Lens Patients: Initial Visit

Preliminary assessment is essential for guiding the fitter and the patient regarding reaction to contact lens. This will go long way in determining success or failure of a fit. Many factors determine whether a patient is a good candidate for the use of contact lenses. First, a detailed history and ocular examination are necessary prior to fitting a contact lens.

HISTORY

The history collects information about the patient's general medical health, ocular health, personal hygiene, environmental hygiene, family history of eye disease, and previous use of contact lenses. Motivation is one of the most important factors for the success of fitting. Patients with moderate to high refractive errors may be better candidates for contact lens wear than those with low degrees of refractive error. A good way to make this judgement is to evaluate the number of hours per day that the patient wears glasses. Patients who are minimally dependent on glasses in general have a low degree of success with contact lens fitting. Poorly motivated patients frequently may not care for their contact lenses adequately and may not adapt to the lenses, particularly rigid gas permeable lenses. Patients are motivated to wear contact lens if they see better than glass and if their cosmetic appearance improves with contact lenses as in high myopia especially in marriageable age in girls.

History must elicit the reasons for getting contact lens which may be optical (for better vision), therapeutic (for treatment of disease), cosmetic (to hide blemish), occupational (to help in task performance), diagnostic (to facilitate diagnosis) and research (to induce myopia or hyperopia in experimental studies). It should be further clarified that diagnostic, therapeutic and research indications are usually the decisions of the fitter.

History must elicit surgery performed for eye diseases and any injury otherwise sustained. It is essential to avoid contact lens fitting for at least 3 months after surgery or injury, however, a soft lens may be given right on the operation table to promote healing as after epithelium debridement in recurrent erosions, photorefractive keratectomy (PRK), phototherapeutic keratectomy (PTK) and corneal cross linking or for optical purpose or to act as a splint.

Contact Lens History

The following contact lens information should be obtained:
- Types of contact lens previously worn
- Success and complications with previous lenses
- Reasons for the use of contact lens (cosmetic, spectacle intolerance, aphakia, keratoconus, improvement of visual acuity)
- Patient occupation (to determine if the patient is exposed to chemical products or works in a dirty or dusty environment)
- Previous refractive correction
- Type of sports and recreational activities.

OCULAR HEALTH

One must ask about the following issues:
- Any previous ocular injury
- Lid infection
- Meibomitis
- Conjunctivitis
- Cataract
- Glaucoma (including family history)
- Dry eye
- Any surgery to the eye or ocular adnexa
- Previous contact lens use
- Drug allergy
- Medication intolerance

GENERAL HEALTH

Allergies

The patient should be questioned about allergies to medications, foods, and other substances. The allergic patient is more susceptible to adverse reactions to contact lenses and their maintenance products.

Diabetes

In moderate or severe cases of diabetes, there is occasionally corneal hypesthesia, leading to a greater propensity for corneal erosion and infection. Diabetic patients are not candidates for extended-wear contact lens use.

Pregnancy and Menopause

Pregnant women with water retention may become intolerant to well tolerated and well fitted contact lens. In general, contact lens fitting should be avoided during pregnancy. Some patients in menopause may present significant changes in the quality and quantity of the lacrimal tear film that may cause contact lens intolerance.

Chronic Respiratory Disease

Patients with chronic respiratory disease such as asthma, sinusitis, and other similar conditions may have difficulty in fitting a contact lens. During respiratory crisis they may have conjunctival hyperemia, tearing, light sensitivity, and generalized discomfort that is aggravated by the use of contact lenses.

Psychological Conditions

It is essential that the contact lens wearer be sufficiently responsible to follow medical instructions, including information about the duration of wear, contact lens maintenance, understanding of the signs and symptoms of contact lens–related problems, the risks of contact lens wear, and an understanding of when prompt assistance must be obtained.

Medication Use

The contact lens wearer must be informed also of the medications, either topical or systemic (such as nasal decongestants, diuretics, benzodiazepines, immunosuppressants, etc.), that may alter the tear film and that may contraindicate or make contact lens use difficult for the patient.

EXAMINATION

Ophthalmic Examination

Vision

The visual function includes a record of visual acuity and refraction. Assessment of binocularity is of the utmost importance in unilateral aphakia, high refractive errors and in pre-presbyopia; in the latter two accommodation may also be tested. Field examination should be done especially in cases of high myopia, aphakia and glaucoma.

Corneal Curvature

The procedure most commonly employed conventionally has been the manual or automated keratometry, which measures the central corneal curvature. The videokeratography assesses the central as well as the peripheral cornea. The slit scanning topography system, scheimpflug imaging system like Pentacam and anterior segment optical coherence tomography (OCT) that have emerged in recent times are very useful tools to aid in performing contact lens fitting.

Biomicroscopy

The biomicroscope is used to evaluate the lid, conjunctiva, tear film, cornea, iris, pupil, and anterior chamber. The expert should try to look for any defect in the integrity of epithelium, stroma and endothelium. Dry spots shown up by the break-up of the tear film when lids are retracted must be excluded. A bleb at the limbus should be evaluated for its external communication; it may be a contraindication for corneal contact lenses. Iritis must be controlled and tension lowered within normal limits before fitting any contact lens.

Tear Film Evaluation

Quality and quantity are both important. The usual tests which are done include Schirmer's test in which wetting of a filter paper strip placed in lower fornix is measured. Normally, it should not be less than 10 mm after 5 minutes.

Tear breakup time (BUT) is another useful tool to assess the tear film. BUT should not be less than 10 seconds. It is actually the time taken for the appearance of first dark spot over the cornea after instillation of a drop of fluorescein in the cul-dé-sac. *A complete list of tests of evaluation of tears includes:*

- Schirmer test I, II and III
- BUT
- pH
- Lysozyme content
- Ceruloplasmin content
- Kurihashi thread test
- Dye dilution test
- Rose Bengal staining
- Conjunctival biopsy
- Lacrimal gland biopsy

Measurement of Palpebral Aperture Height

The opening of the normal palpebral fissure ranges from 7 mm to 13 mm (average is approximately 10 mm). The size of the palpebral fissure may contribute to or detact substantially from stabilization of the lens, especially rigid gas permeable contact lenses. Measurement of the palpebral aperture height is done at the slit lamp, with the patient looking at the examiner's ear.

Lid Tone

Lids that are extremely tense or tight may alter the movement of the contact lens. There is no precise clinical method to measure lid tension. One can estimate lid tension by grasping the lid between the index finger and thumb and pulling it away from the globe. It can then be classified as loose or tight. Studies have found a relation among lid tension, palpebral aperture height, and contact lens fitting characteristics (Fig. 6.1).

Blinking

The examiner should evaluate the frequency and thoroughness of the blink. An incomplete blink may change the movement of the lens on the eye and the distribution of the tear film, with consequent desiccation of the cornea and/or conjunctiva and lens intolerance. Normal frequency of blinking is 12–15 times per minute, which is increased with head movement and is diminished during states of attention, such as reading, watching television, driving, and computer use.

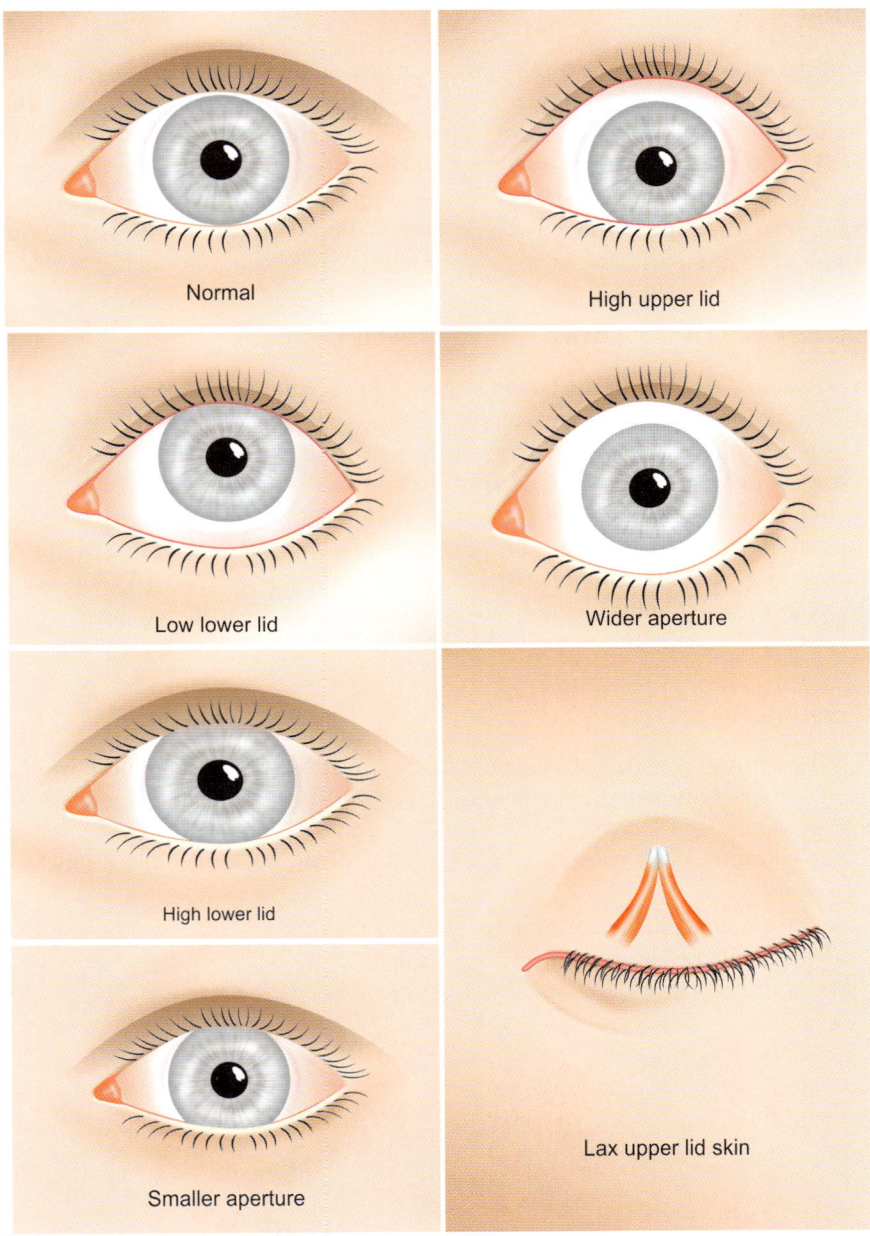

Fig. 6.1 Lid related factors affecting contact lens fitting

Corneal Diameter

The average horizontal diameter is approximately 11.7 mm (varying generally between 11 mm and 12.5 mm). The vertical diameter is approximately 1 mm less. This is an important measurement in the determination of lens diameter.

Corneal Sensation

Corneal sensation may be diminished in systemic diseases such as—diabetes, intrinsic eye disease (e.g. herpes simplex keratitis), and also in pregnancy, the menstrual cycle, the use of topical or systemic medications, or as a result of corneal surgery. Contact lens wear may also induce decreased corneal sensation. Contact lens wearers with decreased corneal sensation may be more prone to corneal erosion and/or infection. Corneal sensation can be grossly evaluated using a wisp of cotton or, more precisely, with the esthesiometer of Cochet-Bonnet.

EXTERNAL EXAMINATION

It is essential to confirm the leading points of the patient's history and to know what may not be known to the patient.

The face may be examined for acne, rosacea, and lids for infective or irritative disorders like squamous or ulcerative blepharitis, trachoma, wart, herpes, stye, meibomianitis, chalazion, nevus and scar (Fig. 6.2). Conjunctiva should be examined for nevus especially at limbus, pterygium, pinguecula bitot's spots, concretions, scarring, and neovascularization in the cornea (Fig. 6.3). A careful preferably photographic record of all these examinations is essential.

A record of all these observations helps in check-up and in medicolegal aspects.

Consultation

It is desirable, also as an opportunity for clarification which the patient would want to seek about the contact lenses. It also helps the fitter to know more about the patient.

- Ability to wear—A successful contact lens fit should satisfy the following criteria:
  – It should work for a minimum period of 8 hours.
  – It should be comfortable; except for slight awareness

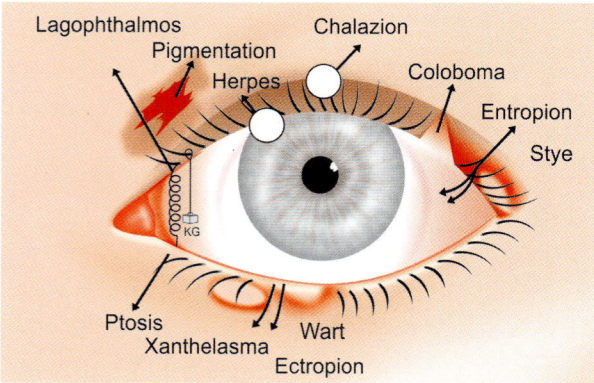

Fig. 6.2 Face and lid lesions to be noted during external examination before contact lens fitting

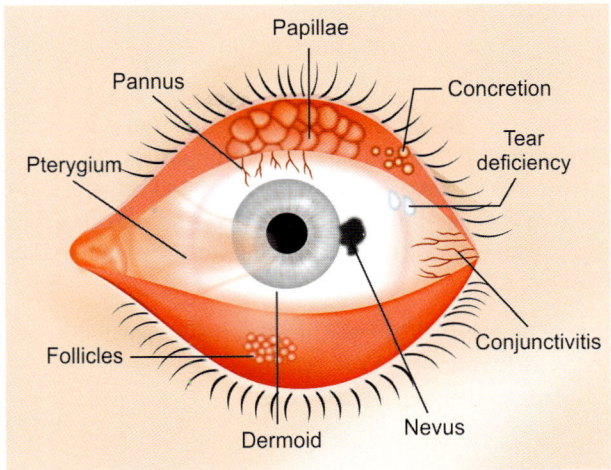

Fig. 6.3 Conjunctival lesions to be noted during external examination before contact lens fitting

  – It should give good vision, preferably better than glasses but vision may sometimes deteriorate in astigmatism; especially with spherical soft lenses.
  – It should give a normal appearance, i.e. there should not be any redness, squint, excessive blinking or abnormality of head posture; and
  – There should be no significant change in ocular tissues like staining edema and curvature.
- *Appearance:* Corneal and soft lenses can rarely be seen. Scleral lens may be apparent.
- *Period of adjustment:* Adjustment takes any time from 2 days to 2 months, depending upon restoration of tonicity of tears and cessation of excessive volley of nerve impulses from the lid margins.
- *Safety:* Patient is usually worried about safety but serious injury has never been reported even when the contact lens was found broken in the eye.
- *Occupation:* In certain areas like acting in TV, theater and movie, contact lens greatly helps also as a cosmetic aid. Odd light reflections from spectacles are avoided.
- *Driving:* Law permits driving with contact lenses but a bad lens, like bad glasses may distract attention and may cause accident.

Air crew are not permitted to wear contact lenses except in experienced monocular aphakes. However, air hostesses can use them provided the unaided vision is 6/18 or better. Contact lens is contraindicated in mining, sand blasting, drilling and in any atmosphere with irritating fumes. In sports it is helpful in gymnastics, boating, archery, tennis, fencing, golf, squash and badminton. A tightly fitted hard lens, a scleral lens or a soft lens is preferred in sports as they do not get easily displaced. A duplicate pair should be available with the individuals involved in body sport where contact lenses are likely to get dislodged, displaced or lost.

Myopia control: The authors have documented a decrease in myopia in 77% of the patients under 22 years of age after a fitted period of 3 years. However, the subject is still controversial amongst fitters.

Life of contact lens: The life of contact lens depends upon the wearing regimen. The disposable lenses are for their specific time period. The yearly soft lenses and the gas permeable lenses are for one year. Soft lenses start showing deposits in few months, deposits get denatured in 15 days and need intensive laboratory cleaning. It is best to use monthly disposable lenses to achieve most hygienic contact lens wear.

Losses: It is quite common for gas permeable lenses especially among children, during the first year. In author's clinic, 30% of ordered lenses were duplicates for replacement of damaged or lost lenses.

PROGNOSIS

Preliminary assessment can give an idea about future success or failure. *The following points deserve attention:*

- *Motivation:* Motivation means the urge or desire to get contact lenses, the purpose being to see well or to look well. Females fare better; amongst males, funicular apaches fare better. Lenses may be discontinued when the purpose like an interview or marriage is served.
- *Personality:* People who are confident, dominating and more careful about their health, do not fare as well as expected. Reverse is true for timid personalities.
- *Former contact lens wearer:* These patients are a little fussy. Failure of the previous lens must be ascertained before the fit is started; otherwise failure may be repeated.
- *Monocular wearer:* This is usually a failure due to comparison of the fitted eye with the normal eye. Relative success has been found in monocular aphakes.
- *Manual dexterity:* Some old people may fall in handling contact lenses due to lack of manual dexterity.
- *Hygiene:* Patient with unhygienic habits is likely to invite trouble, and so he should be advised against wearing contact lens.
- *Refractive errors:* Low refractive errors are usually unsuccessful because vision without correction is fairly satisfactory. High myopes do not tolerate well due to physical discomfort of the odd lens design. Hyperopes do well if they are dependent on spectacles. Those who have high astigmatism also do well. Gain in vision is the prime motivating factor.
- *Binocularity:* There may be change from phoria to tropia with contact lenses. They may be much more obvious if the patient was using vertical prisms in spectacles.
- *Accommodation:* There is more demand on accommodation in myopes and in pre-presbyopic age. This may cause asthenopia (eye strain). After contact lenses a high myope may find reading problem for 2–3 weeks due to demand on accommodation which he has never used.

- *Anatomical considerations:* The following anatomical features have been found unfavorable
  - Tight upper lid
  - Low lower lid
  - Large palpebral fissure
  - Large pupil
  - Low upper lid tone
  - Spherical cornea
  - Fair complexion.

CONTACT LENSES: FUNDAMENTAL PRINCIPLES

These include basic lens type, fitting philosophies fitting methodology; and also certain physical phenomena which affect lens positioning.
- *Lens type:* This relates to construction of lenses. A large variety of lenses are being used. They may be classified according to:
  - *Material:* Hard, soft, gas permeable and silicone
  - *Construction:* Monocurve, bicurve, tricurve, multicurve aspheric and offset.
  - *Size:* Corneal and scleral.
  - *Purpose:* Bifocal, tinted, fenestrated, nonrotational cosmetic, therapeutic,
  - Sports, underwater wettable lenticular and others.
- *Fitting philosophy:* This includes various methods to achieve particular dimensional and baring corneal lens relationship.
- *Fitting methods:* Relates to contact lens specification.

General Requisites

- It should be comfortable, without immediate or long-term adverse effects, without imparting any abnormal look to the eye and ensuring minimal 8 hours wearing time.
- Optical requisites
  - Visual acuity should be at least the same as with spectacles.
  - Pupil should be adequately be covered with the contact lens (at least ¾). Hence abnormalities in pupil size and shape can result in patient dissatisfaction (Fig. 6.4).
  - Weight of lenses should be evenly distributed over entire cornea. Lens should not put its weight on a particular point otherwise epithelial damage will occur. Author has seen development of corneal opacities in flatly fitted lenses due to pressure on particular corneal area.

Forces Affecting Lens Fit

Lens positioning is a balance between two opposing forces which are trying to adhere or eject the lens from the eye. This may be:
- *Fluid attraction:* This is capillarity and is inversely proportional to the thickness or tear film. More tears under a flat lens cause less capillarity and more movement.

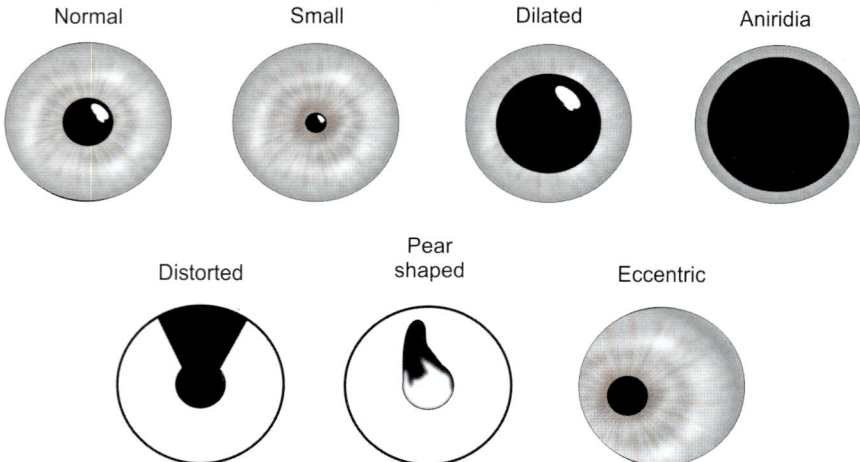

Fig. 6.4 Abnormality in pupil size and shape

- *Gravity:* Center of gravity should be towards the anterior chamber if stability of lens is desired. A thin lens, a minus lens, a bigger lens and steeper lens are therefore, found to be more stable.

Tear Pump

Ultimate corneal oxygenation in polymethyl methacrylate (PMMA) lenses is a function of the tear pump, which is dependent on blink rate, percentage of tear exchange, and volume of tears under the lens. Normally, tear pump can supply 1–3% oxygen to the cornea. A decrease in blink rate from one per second to one every four seconds decreases the corneal oxygen uptake by 40%. A little volume of tears under the lens is essential because alignment fit does not furnish adequate exchange of tears; 20% exchange with each blink will provide adequate oxygenation. Exchange with soft lenses is one tenth compared to hard. Besides oxygen supply pump serves another important function of drainage of debris and metabolic wastes.

Initial Response of Lens Wear

Adaptation to lenses usually takes a fortnight. This is associated with demonstrable decrease in lid margin sensitivity. Corneal response during adaptation is diagnostic of ultimate fitting prognosis. This can be judged by extent of corneal swelling as measured by pachymetry, keratometry or slit lamp. Slit lamp fails to pick swelling if it is less than 4–6%. Keratometer does not register swelling if it is between the two mires and also due to the fact that contour of the swelling is aspheric. Hence, the pachymetry is the best way. Mandel has documented three types of responses in adaptation. A swelling of 2–4% on the first day is due to hypotonic tears and this returns back to normal on the same day; 5–8% swelling indicates additional anoxia, and corneal swelling does not return to the base line. Even after the adaptation is over, swelling will not touch the base line. Swelling above 8% indicates a severe corneal oxygen deprivement and is an intolerable lens situation.

Lens Parameters and Cornea

- A lens with a diameter of 7.8 mm and base curve of 42.50 will nicely contour a spherical cornea of 43.00 diopters.
- Reduction in diameter from 10 mm to 8 mm reduces the lens size by 36% and exposes the cornea more by 20%. This results in better oxygenation. A small sized lens being interpalpebral will lack corneal moulding effect of upper lid pressure.
- Edge of a lens should be optimum, i.e. 0.12 mm unfinished. A thicker or thinner edge is intolerable physically and physiologically.

CHAPTER 7

Keratometry and Corneal Topography

The ophthalmometer (Keratometer) was first designed during the first half of the 19th century by Helmholtz (who also designed the ophthalmoscope) to measure the difference in refractive power between the two principle meridians of curvature of the cornea. This is completed by comparing the radius of curvature of the corneal meridians. The dioptric value difference between the two corneal meridians is interpreted as the amount of corneal astigmatism. As early as in 1840, it was determined that the factors that created the total refraction of the eye were the curvature of the cornea, the position of the crystalline lens, and the distance of the retina from these two refracting surfaces. The keratometer was improved in Paris, in 1884 by Drs Javal and Schiotz, making it practical to use during the refractive eye examination.

PRINCIPLE OF KERATOMETRY

Cornea acts as a convex mirror; a virtual erect image of the mires is formed 4 mm behind the cornea. The size of the mires is 64 mm (Bausch and Lomb [B and L] keratometer) and image size is 3.00 mm. The distance between the cornea and the mires is 75 mm. Mires have variable separation in the same instrument depending upon the radius of curvature of cornea. Mires of different instruments have variable separation for the same corneal curvature.

The keratometer is designed to measure the image size which is converted into radius of curvature by the optics of the instrument. Image size can be measured with calipers but the motion of the eye presents a problem which is obviated by doubling the image and further helped by magnification. The image is magnified 1.304 times by the objective and magnified finally to 6.197 times by the eyepiece.

There are certain assumptions:
- U or object distance is taken to be very large.
- Refractive index 1.3375.
- Posterior surface of cornea is parallel to the anterior.

Keratometer produces double images which can be approximated:
- By varying the size of the object as in keratometers of Haag-Streit (Fig. 7.1) and Universal
- By varying separation between the two fixed sized images as in Bausch and Lomb (Fig. 7.2) and CI Ophthalmometer.

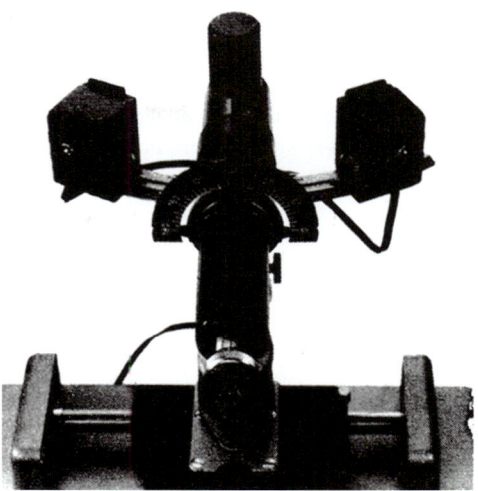

Fig. 7.1 Haag-Streit keratometer

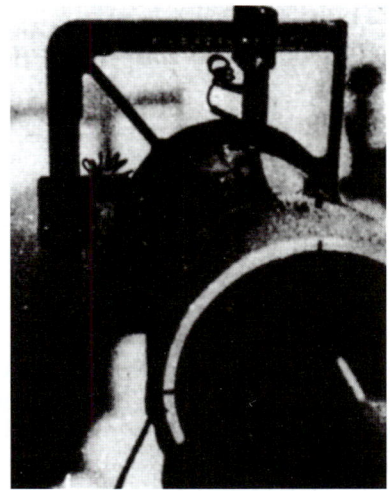

Fig. 7.2 Bausch and Lomb ophthalmometer

Doubling Systems

- *Universal and Javal-Schiotz type:* Here, doubling is achieved by Wollaston prism which consists of two doubly refracting prisms of quartz. Mires are green and red for finer distinctions.
- *CI ophthalmometry:* Image separation of fixed size object is controlled by biprism which is moved further and nearer to the cornea.
- *Bausch and Lomb keratometer:* In addition to the use of prisms for separation (a) Two small holes are used for forming images by Scheiner principle, and (b) Two larger holes are part of the doubling system.

- Essentially, the doubling system of the keratometer involves interruption by the prisms of a part of the bundle of rays from the images. Separation between the doubled images can be increased or decreased by moving the prisms further or nearer to the image plane in Bausch and Lomb keratometers.
- In Haag-Streit keratometer, separation is controlled by increasing or decreasing the size of the object.

Calibration of the Keratometer

Before using a keratometer it is better to assess its accuracy, best judged by measuring a steel ball of known radius of curvature. Balls are usually of the following dioptric value; 37.00 D (9.13 mm), 36.62 D (8.73), 40.25 D (8.38), 42.50 D (7.94), 44.75 D (7.54) and 47.25 D (7.14).

A graph is plotted between the actual keratometer readings and expected keratometer readings. If all the points do not lie on the diagonal, the keratometer is defective and the entire graph must be consulted for the actual value.

Correction

- By knowing the error using steel balls correction factor can be added or subtracted from readings of the defective keratometer. However, the keratometer may not be uniform in its error at higher and lower ranges.
- The dial of the keratometer (B and L) may be readjusted after loosening the screw, but the error may be different in vertical and horizontal positions.
- A steel ball is placed before the keratometer and its value is set on the scale or dial. The mires are then focused by clockwise and anticlockwise movements of the eyepiece through trial and error. When mires are in focus, calibration is complete.

Following disadvantages may be however be noted:
- This method takes away individual's own adjustment for relaxation of accommodation because the eyepiece is now fixed at one place.
- Minor insignificant error creep in due to the variation in magnification caused by movement of the eyepiece.
- The calibration can either be done for horizontal or vertical if both meridians show error, one will be left uncorrected.

Increasing the Accuracy

- Focus the hair cross of Bausch and Lomb and black line of Haag-Striet by taking out the eyepiece anticlockwise and bring it in clockwise position till the lines are first focused.
- Always occlude the eye which is not being examined: Otherwise this becomes the fixing eye and your readings may be picking up an eccentric point on the cornea.
- Bausch and Lomb keratometer was made extremely accurate by employing vernier type of alignment by Shick. Sides of the upper and center of the lower

'minus' mires were covered with black electric tape. The center of the one plus and 3 free sides of the other 'plus' mire were similarly covered with black tape. The end point of mires is then noted by accuracy of vernier acuity.

Bausch and Lomb Keratometer

This keratometer measures curvature from 36.00 D to 52.00 D. By placing –1.0 or +1.25 lens in front of the objective, the range can be extended from 30.00 to 61.00 diopters. Extended range reading after the use of +1.25 and –1.00 may be taken as follows:

- Use Mandel's table where you can feed the value on the scale and get the actual value.
- *Direct method:* If you use +1.25 add +9.00 to the reading of the scale. Similarly, 6.00 D is deducted from the scale when –1.00 D sph is placed before the objective.
- A graph is plotted between the scale reading along ordinate and the actual value of the steel ball along abscissa by placing + 1.25 and –1.00 D in front of the objective.

Use of the Keratometer

- *Adjustment of the instrument:*
  - Light is put on, and a white paper is held before the objective. The eyepiece is moved all the way out and then moved in till the hair and black line is just focused. The instrument is then individually objected.
  - Calibration is done with steel balls.
  - Accuracy is enhanced in every steep or very flat corneas which are usually pathological by using +1.25 or –1, over the objective.
- *Adjustment of the patient:*
  - Patient is requested to put his chin on the chin rest and head against the head rest. The chin is raised or lowered to bring the canthus in line with the black line of B and L outer keratometer or the white notch of the Haag-Streit keratometer.
  - Left eye is covered with eye occluder.
  - The instrument is raised or lowered till the patient pupil and the projecting knob and notch of the instrument are at same level.
- *Taking the reading of the cornea:*
  - Having covered the left eye, the patient is asked to look into the instrument with the right eye. The instrument is moved forward and backward till the mires are accurately focused. The dial is then moved till mires are approximated. In Bausch and Lomb one plus mire should overlap the other plus mire and it should appear as one plus mire. In Haag-Streit, red and green mire should just touch and the black line in the center should be straight (Figs 7.3 to 7.5). This requires three adjustments:
    1. Movement of instrument as a whole to keep the mires focused.
    2. Adjustment of mire size or mire separation by knob.

3. Adjustment of axis by tilting the instrument along anteroposterior axis to accurately overlap mires.

When these three procedures are completed, the value of the horizontal meridian is read from the dial of Bausch and Lomb or the scale of Haag-Streit. The mires are then approximated along the vertical meridian. In Bausch and Lomb the minus mires are made to overlap while the end point of Haag-Streit is the same as detailed earlier.

– The same procedure is repeated for the left eye by covering the right eye. The observer may notice the following phenomena on the cornea.

♦ Mires in Bausch and Lomb are a perfect sphere. This indicates a spherical cornea.

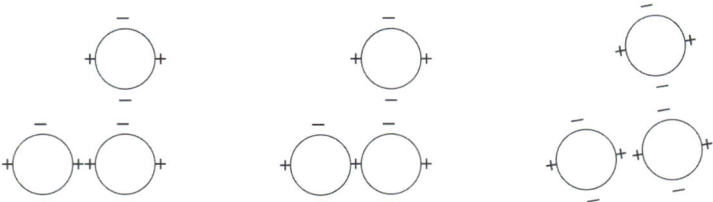

Fig. 7.3 Mires shapes and alignment for various keratometers

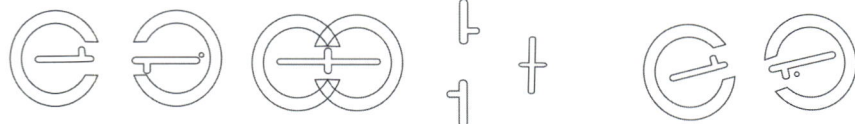

Fig. 7.4 Mires shapes and alignment for various keratometer

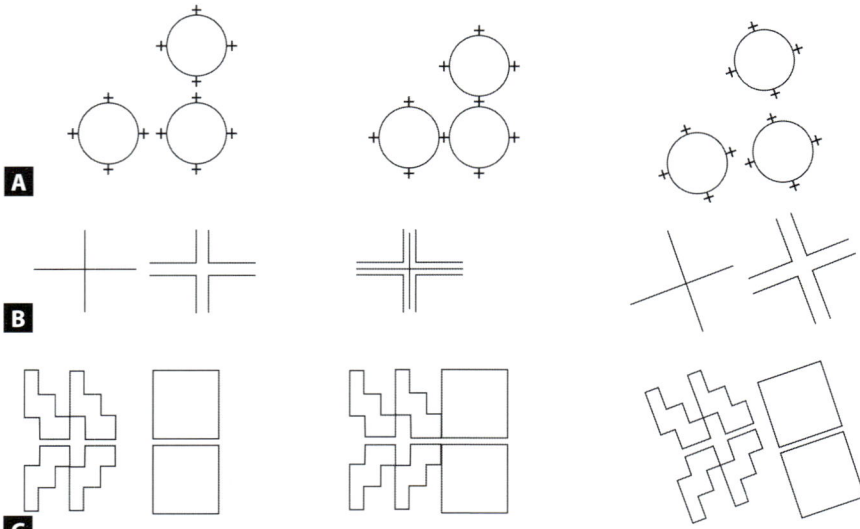

Figs 7.5A to C Mires shapes and alignment for various keratometers

- Mires may be horizontally oval. This indicates 'with the rule' toricity.
- Mires may look like a vertical oval. This indicates against the rule toricity.
- Mires may be irregular or doubled. This indicates an anterior surface irregularity of the cornea.
- Mires may pulsate. This is indicative of keratoconus.

Value of the Keratometer

For contact lens practitioners, the keratometer is valuable in a variety of situation.
- *High astigmatism:* In higher astigmatism the value of the keratometric cylinder is usually the same as that of refraction cylinder. This is a guide in prescription in opaque media where retinoscopy is not possible.
- Irregular corneas due to corneal opacity, keratoconus, dystrophies can be diagnosed at an early stage by keratometer.
- In aphakics it is of great help to know the axis and value of the corneal cylinder.
- *Opaque media:* Keratometry is a valuable guide to prescription both for sphere and cylinder.
- In children and persons of low intelligence keratometry can guide the prescription of glasses.
- Keratometer determines the progression of curvature changes of conical corneas.
- It helps to find the nature and extent of the refractive error. Taking normal reading to be 43.50 higher and lower reading indicate myopia and hyperopia. In anisometropia, if keratometric readings are similar, the error is axial and not refractive.

Relation of Corneal Toricity and Spectacle Cylinder (Based on Detailed Analysis of 300 Cases) (Table 7.1)

An idea of entire topography of cornea can be had by any of the following methods:
- Topogometry
- Rasterstereography
- Photokeratoscopy
- Placido disc
- Color coded photokeratogram

Table 7.1 Variable relationship between keratometric and spectacle cylinder

Sr. No.	Keratometric cylinder	Spectacle cylinder	Percentage
1.	With the rule	With the rule	41.67%
2.	With the rule	Nil	32.67%
3.	With the rule	Against the rule	14.33%
4.	Against the rule	Against the rule	8.00%
5.	With the rule	Oblique	1.50%
6.	Oblique	Oblique	1.83%

- Color coded computerized topography
- Slit scanning topography and Scheimpflug imaging

CORNEAL TOPOGRAPHY AND CONTACT LENS FITTING

Computerized corneal topography is a unique corneal modelling system which can read the entire corneal surface. It prints out the analysis of sixteen concentric circles composed of 3000 points spread over the entire corneal surface as color coded map, as curves on a graph, and as numerical value display chart at varies distances on axis in the cornea.

This system though expensive, is absolutely essential for understanding the response of cornea to contact lens and surgery. Even before this it tells about the exact (1) shape of cornea at various places, (2) it helps to diagnose corneal disease, (3) it helps to plan surgery, (4) helps to decide the exact placement of incisions in kerato-refractive surgery, (5) helps to analyse the result of surgery, (6) guides the surgeon to improve his skills by seeing the postoperative results, (7) helps to compare the data with others, (8) helps to fit contact lenses.

Keratometer has its Limitations

- Keratometer only tells average of two points 3 mm apart
- It fails to read and shape of corneal beyond 1.5 mm of the corneal center
- It miserably fails to guide the surgeon about incision placement. It will not read the effect of the tight suture or suture removal in the periphery.

Computerized Corneal Modelling System in Contact Lens Fitting

By using the software program available with the instrument the design of the contact lens can be finalized by getting the desired fluorescein pattern on the monitor. It will also be possible to see the change in fluorescein pattern on the monitor due to changes in the lens diameter and lens base curves. It is possible to get a desired fit as alignment, mild and moderate apical clearances.

We may transmit the topographic data and the laboratory at distance will transmit the various pattern and the ideal can be choses. Topographic data can only give static fit information and not the desired dynamic fit as true for trial lens fit.

Color coded photokeratograms: The use of the computer in the zone of photokeratometry has been used by S Klyce to give isometric color prints. Their greatest value is to describe visually the contours of the abnormal cornea such as keratoconus, after keratoplasty and refractive surgery. The fitting of a contact lens can be assisted by knowing where steep and flat zones are evident and their extent. Furthermore, the change in the color contour print can help evaluate clinical progress.

A definite correlation is seen with the base curve of contact lens and the 3 mm and 5 mm curvature as seen in slit scanning topography. This helps in reducing the number of trial lenses used and thereby reduces the total chair time.

PENTACAM

Principle

Theodor Scheimpflug, a cartographer of the Austrian navy, first introduced the Scheimpflug principle. It describes an optical imaging condition, which allows documentation of an obliquely tilted object with the maximally possible depth of focus and minimal image distortion under given conditions. *The Scheimpflug principle states that higher depth of focus can be achieved if subject plane, lens plane and image plane are moved in such a way that they cut each other at a point of intersection which is known as Scheimpflug intersection* (Fig. 7.6). Normally, the lens and image (film or sensor) planes of a camera are parallel and the plane of focus (PoF) is parallel to the lens and image planes. If a planar subject is also parallel to the image plane, it can coincide with the PoF, and the entire subject can be rendered sharply. If the subject plane is not parallel to the image plane, it will be in focus only along a line where it intersects the PoF. When an oblique tangent is extended from the image plane, and another is extended from the lens plane, they meet at a line through which the PoF also passes, referred as Scheimpflug line. With this condition, a planar subject that is not parallel to the image plane can be completely in focus.

The Pentacam obtains images of the anterior segment by a rotating Scheimpflug camera measurement (Fig. 7.7). The various models of Pentacam is classified in Table 7.2.

The camera is a digital CCD camera with synchronous pixel sampling. The light source consists of UV-free blue light emitting diode (LED's) with a wavelength of 475 nm. The system integrates two cameras. One is located in the center for the purposes of detection of the size and orientation of the pupil and to control fixation. The second is mounted on rotating wheel to capture images from the anterior segment. It is a complete picture from anterior surface of the

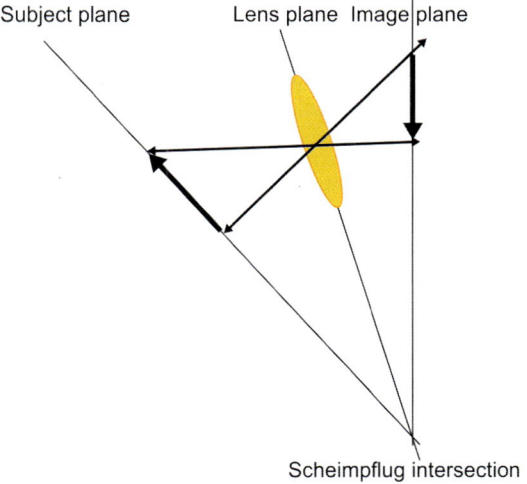

Fig. 7.6 Scheimpflug principle

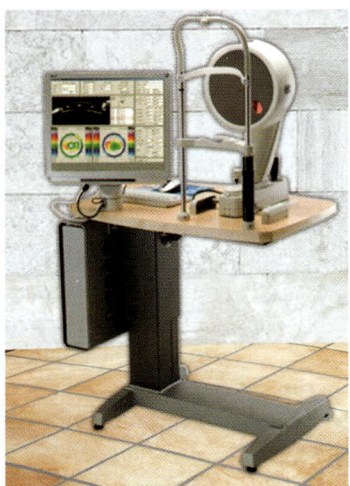

Fig. 7.7 Pentacam

Table 7.2 Various models of Pentacam		
Pentacam (Basic)	*Pentacam (Classic)*	*Pentacam (HR)*
Qualitative analysis of cornea	All features of basic plus Various software package	All features of classic plus
Glaucoma screening— Pachymetry based corrected IOP, anterior chamber angle, depth and volume determination	**Software package— Refractive** Calculation of corneal thickness progression for early keratoconus detection	Sharp Scheimpflug images for precise representation of implants, corneal rings, opacities for lens and cornea.
Topography based keratoconus detection and classification	**Software package—Cataract** Comprehensive cataract analysis (3D densitometry) and PNS (Pentacam nucleus staging)	Precise imaging for determining positions of pIOLs and IOLs in reference to centering and tilting. Optional 3D pIOL simulation software including aging prediction
Additional software upgrade module can be used to upgrade basic into classic model	Zernike analysis and corneal wavefront, e.g. for the selection of aspheric IOLs and determination of higher order aberrations	Belin/Ambrosio Enhanced ectasia Holladay report and Holladay EKR (equivalent keratometer readings) for optimized IOL calculation in postrefractive patient eyes. Contact lens fitting

cornea to the posterior surface of the lens. This rotating process supplies pictures in three dimensions and also allows the center of the cornea to be measured precisely. The slit images are photographed on an angle from 0° to 180° to avoid shadows from nose. Every picture is a complete image through the cornea at a specific angle, combination of such slit images creates a real 360° image of the anterior segment. The software utilizes a ray tracing algorithm to construct and calculate the anterior segment. It acquires a total of 50 images in approximately two seconds, extracting 2,760 true elevation points from these images which in turn generates 138,000 true elevation points for both the corneal front and back surfaces, from limbus to limbus, including the center of the cornea, a major advantage over keratometers and Placido-based corneal topographers. The measurement process lasts less than two seconds and minute eye movements are captured and corrected simultaneously.

CLINICAL INTERPRETATION AND USES

Curvature Map/Corneal Power Map

Before interpreting curvature map, it should be kept in mind that there is wide spectrum of normality of human cornea. Curvature map gives information about pattern, symmetry and skewing of axis of anterior surface of cornea. *Various pattern seen include:*

Pattern 1: Round, where the steepest part of the cornea is round but decentered.

Pattern 2: Oval, where the steepest part of the cornea is oval and may be centered or decentered.

Pattern 3: Superior steep (SS), where the steepest part of the cornea is localized in the upper part of the cornea.

Pattern 4: Inferior steep (IS) where the steepest part of the cornea is localized inferior to the apex of the cornea.

Pattern 5: Irregular, where the corneal surface takes no particular shape.

Pattern 6—Symmetric bow-tie (SB): This pattern may be indicative of normal astigmatism or very rarely a symmetrical type of keratoconus (Fig. 7.8).

Pattern 7—SB/SRAX: Also called "lazy 8" pattern. That is a symmetric bow-tie with angulation (skewing). Angulation is considered clinically significant when it exceeds 21°.

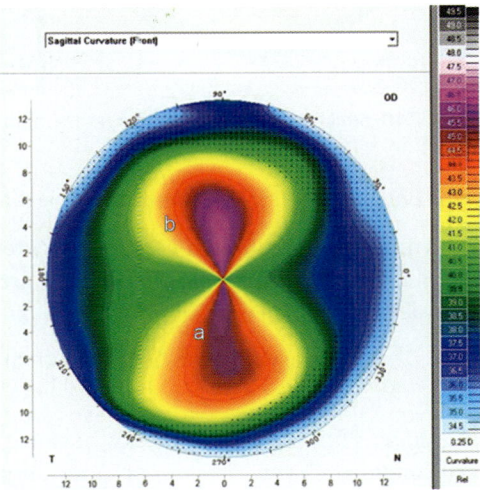

Fig. 7.8 Symmetric bow-tie (SB) pattern on curvature map

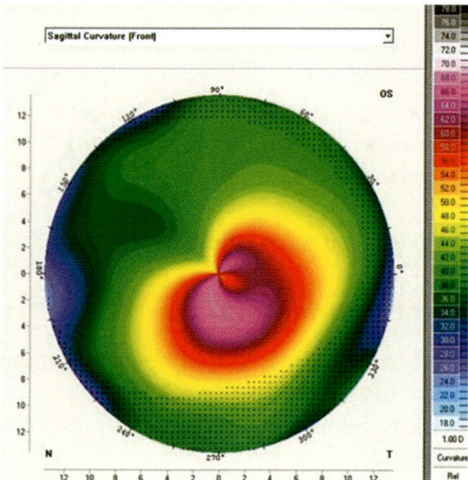

Fig. 7.9 Asymmetric bow-tie with skewed radial axis (AB/SRAX)

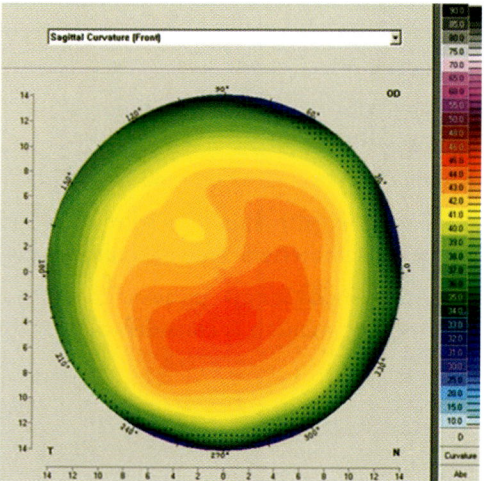

Fig. 7.10 Smiling face pattern on curvature map

Pattern 8—Asymmetric Bow-tie (AB)/IS: Asymmetric bow-tie that is inferiorly steep.

Pattern 9—AB/SS: Asymmetric bow-tie that is superiorly steep. This pattern is the reverse of pattern 8. If the difference is more than 2.5D, precaution should be taken when taking the decision.

Pattern 10—AB/SRAX: That is an asymmetric bow-tie with angulation between the two segments (Fig. 7.9).

Pattern 11—Smiling face: This is certainly risky because it often leads to postoperative ectasia, and might be an indicator of keratoconus (Fig. 7.10).

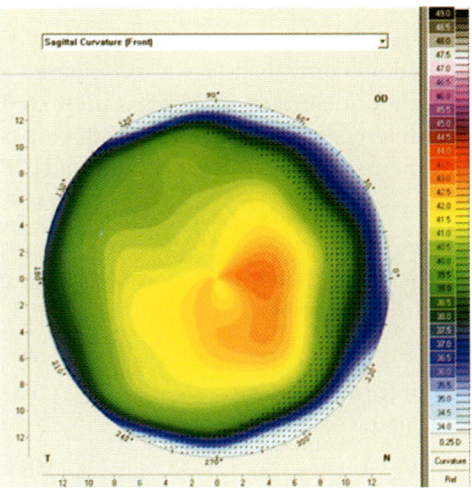

Fig. 7.11 Junctional pattern on curvature map

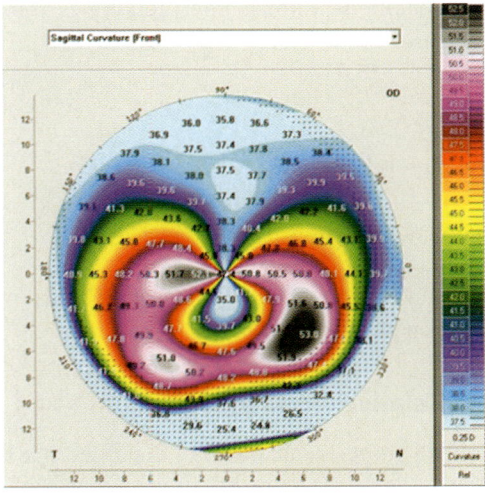

Fig. 7.12 Claw or "kissing birds" pattern on curvature map

Pattern 12—Junctional: It is a circular shape, where the two segments are connected laterally. It is a subject of suspicion (Fig. 7.11).

Pattern 13—Vortex pattern: It is also known as the "Nazi Logo". This is an indicator of corneal instability, and it may precede keratoconus.

Pattern 14—Claw pattern: It is also known as "kissing birds" and is seen in pellucid marginal degeneration (PMD) (Fig. 7.12).

Generally the two eyes of a person are similar and mirror images of each other, this phenomenon is called enantiomorphism. This is useful to decide whether a cornea is normal or not, by comparing it with contralateral eye.

Elevation Maps

Various points measured on corneal surface are compared against a reference plane and any point higher or elevated than this is presented with warm colors and points lower than reference are represented with cooler colors. Reference plane may be best fit sphere (BFS) or best fit toric ellipsoid (BFTE).

BFS is important for:
- To see the shape of cornea.
- To look for risk factors like isolated island or tongue like extension.
- To locate the cone in keratoconus.

BFTE is important for:
- To evaluate details of corneal surface
- To evaluate severity of the cone in keratoconus.

Pentacam shows following elevation map (Figs 7.13A and B)
- *Front elevation map*
  While interpreting, we look at the values within central 5 mm circle on map displayed in BFTE float mode. Clinical interpretation is as follows:
    - Normal ≤ +12 μ
    - Suspicious +13 μ to +15 μ
    - Risky > +15 μ
- *Back elevation map*
  Clinical interpretation is as follows.
    - Normal ≤ +17 μ
    - Suspicious +18 μ and +20 μ
    - Risky > +20 μ
    - Any isolated island on front or back surface in BFS float mode is suspicious even if values are within normal limits.

Corneal Thickness/Relative Thickness Map

Thickness of cornea at all points is calculated by the difference between front and back surface elevations as calculated by the software on elevation maps. *Clinical interpretation of corneal thickness map is as follows:*
- *S-I ratio:* At 5 mm circle, compare symmetric superior and inferior values. Difference >30 μ is suspicious
- Difference of pachy at thinnest location between two eyes should not be >30 μ
- Difference between pachy apex and pachy at thinnest location <10 μ
- If thinnest point is decentered from apex by > –500 μ (0.5 mm) it is suspicious of KC.

Other clinical interpretations for:
- Deciding about various procedures like LASIK, INTACs or corneal cross linking.
- Diagnosis of corneal ectatic disorders like keratoconus, PMD, iatrogenic ectasia, etc.
- Observing the progression of ectatic disorders.
- Confirming diagnosis of diseases like Fuchs dystrophy.

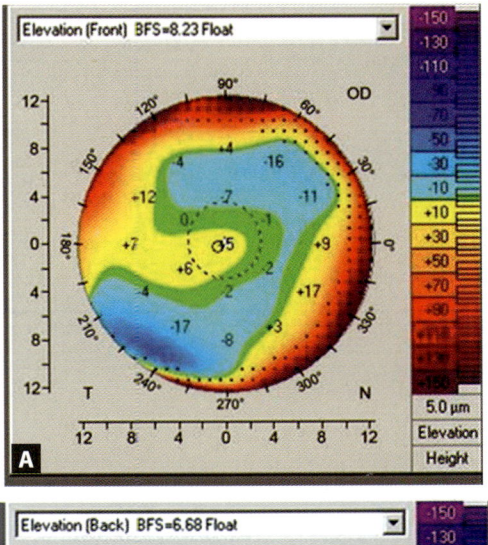

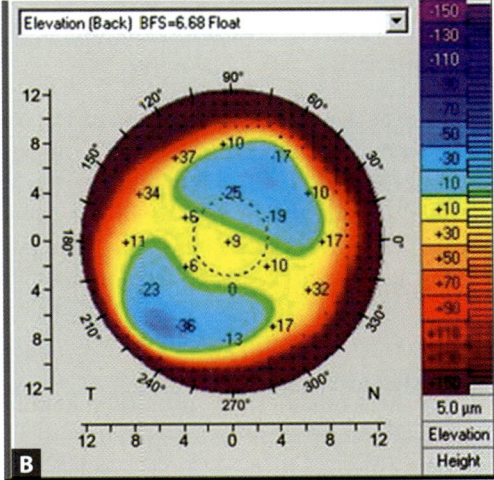

Figs 7.13A and B Front and back elevation maps

Asphericity

Asphericity of cornea is shown by Q value. Q value of normal cornea is about –0.26 to 0.35.

- When cornea is steeper in center, Q value is negative (Aspheric **Prolate**).
- When cornea is flatter in center but steeper in periphery, Q value is positive (Aspheric **Oblate**).
- When center equals periphery cornea is spheric.

Keratometry Power Deviation Map

The keratometry power deviation (KPD) map is calculated by excluding the effect of the anterior curvature power map from the true net power map, i.e. it

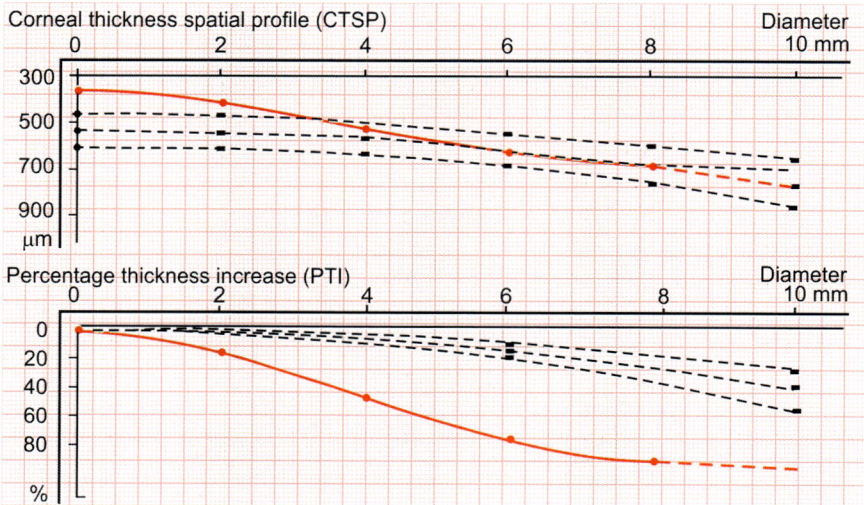

Fig. 7.14 Abnormal curve in a case of keratoconus

represents the effect of the back surface of the cornea on the true net power map in every corneal point. The normal value at any point should be <+0.75. Any value falling between +0.75 and +1.5 is doubtful and borderline, but it is not considered significant unless there is a corresponding posterior elevation. Any value more than +1.5 is an abnormal value, especially if it is in the lower part of the map, or if there is a corresponding elevation at the back elevation map.

Progression Index

It is derived from the corneal thickness/location relationship and reflects the rapid change of thickness from the thinnest location to corneal periphery. More the progression higher the progression index and vice versa. Normal value is ≤1.1. High progression index >1.1 is usually seen in ectatic disorders of cornea like keratoconus.

Belin-Ambrosio Enhanced Ectasia Display

It is the first screening tool which represents height data of the anterior and posterior corneal surface in combination with a progression analysis of the corneal thickness. It is overall more precise and enables early keratoconus detection. The corneal thickness progression analysis is calculated using concentric rings of diameter 2, 4, 6, 8 and 10 mm, starting at the thinnest point and extending to the periphery.

The three black dashed lines show the result of the standard value study. The center line represents the average value of the corneal thickness of all corneas analyzed (Fig. 7.14). The upper or lower line represents the double standard deviation (95%) of the corneal thickness of all corneas measured. The computer gives red color to the curve of the examined cornea. The red curve should be within the normal range and the course of the red curve should be parallel to the normal range. If the red curve deviates at the 6 mm circle or after, it is normal. Otherwise, it is a risk factor because the quick downward deviation means that the corneal center is relatively thinned in relation to the periphery, which proved to be risky either with LASIK, or to some extent with PRK, whether the patient is hyperopic or myopic.

Pentacam has significantly improved the diagnostic and fitting success for fitting of contact lenses in irregular cornea. One of the most useful aspect is that these newer topographic systems can indicate where the cone displacement is located, the size of the cone, any significant astigmatism outside the cone as well as defining the initial diagnostic lens selection. Various contact lens fitting software in these systems can be used for virtual lens fitting and assessment.

CHAPTER **8**

Fitting Philosophies

Various experts have put forward different lens designs, fitting techniques and fitting philosophies, though with time these have changed. Over the last two decades, fitters have seen larger diameters being replaced by smaller and flatter alignment fitting replaced by steeper fitting.

Irrespective of the type of the lens and the fitting philosophy, a successful fitted lens must exhibit the following criteria:

- Eyes should look normal with contact lens.
- Contact lenses should be worn for at least 8–10 hours a day.
- Visual acuity should be better or as good as with spectacles.
- There should not be any short or long-term deleterious effect on the cornea.
- There should not be any undue discomfort.
- Lens weight must be distributed uniformly over the cornea.
- Lens should not move excessively.

The last three criteria are particularly important for proper physiological functioning of the cornea.

FITTING TECHNIQUE

Lenses are fitted by two methods:
1. Trial lens
2. Keratometric method.

The first method observes the behavior of a lens with known base curve, power, diameter, edge and thickness. *It has the added advantage that:*

- It gives an opportunity to the patient to feel the lens in his eye.
- The fitter can also judge the patient's reaction.
- The fitter can have a fairly good idea about corneal topography and its influence on lens behavior, vulnerable epithelium which may show staining even after a proper contact lens effect of the lids on the contact lens.
- An idea about the behavior of the contact lens of nearly exact specification over the cornea is thus obtained.

Keratometric method: This methodology finalizes the lens specification by measurement of eye dimension. Factors which influence the lens dimensions are corneal curvature, horizontal corneal diameter, pupil size, lid position, lid tension and the power of the lens. Values of parameters after a study of 4000 Indian patients are given in Table 8.1.

Table 8.1 Normal parameters in contact lens			
	Minimum	Maximum	Average
Spectacle RX	0	−24.00	−5.37
		+17.50	
Keratometry H	40.12D	49.00 D	44.75 D
V	40.50 D	50.25 D	44.62 D
Keratometric toricity	-	6.00	0.87
Corneal diameter	9.00 mm	13.50 mm	11.52 mm
Pupil diameter	3.00 mm	7.00 mm	5.012 mm
Palpebral aperture diameter	8.50 mm	16.50 mm	11.507 mm
Position of the lid	3.00 mm	2.00 mm	0.98 mm
Pachymetry central	0.501 mm	0.637 mm	0.573 mm
Pachymetry peripheral	0.591 mm	0.764 mm	0.670 mm
Difference between C and P	0.43 mm	−0.150 mm	0.97 mm
Change in central TC after 1 hour of contact lens wear	0.12 mm	0.015 mm	0.135 mm

The main objection to this method is that it cannot predict the exact relationship between the optical zone radius of the lens and the apical zone of the cornea.

Corneal diameter: It can be measured by calipers or by scale held over the cornea. For a 10.00 mm cornea the size of the lens used is 8.0 mm. For every 0.5 mm increase in corneal diameter, increase the lens diameter by 0.2 mm.

Palpebral aperture: It is measured by PD ruler. The average is 9 mm. For every 0.5 mm above or below this, increase or decrease the lens size by 0.2 mm.

Lid tension: It is judged by pinching the upper lid. Loose lid demands lens diameter bigger by 0.2 to 0.5 mm.

Pupillary diameter: It can be easily measured in dim room illumination by holding the PD ruler across and measuring with ophthalmoscope (+10.00 D lens) dim illumination with only a part of light falling over the eye, the remaining light is put over the PD ruler. This avoids pupillary constriction.

Optical zone: The diameter is always 1–2 mm larger than the pupil.

Power: Higher minus lens rises high on the cornea due to a base up prism. This demands a bigger lens diameter to avoid edge glare. Increase the OD by 0.5 mm if power is 5 D or higher.

Base curve (BC): A lens with diameter of 8.5 mm is fitted on K. For every 0.5 mm increase in the lens OD flatten the lens BC by 0.25 D.

Intermediate posterior curve (IPC): It is kept 5 D or 1.00 mm flatter than base curve. Its width is 0.25 mm for lenses of diameter between 8 mm and 9 mm.

Peripheral posterior curve (PPC): It is usually 3 mm flatter than the BC and 0.4 mm in width. The diameter of such lenses is usually between 8 mm and 9 mm.

Blend: Any two curves that is BC and IPC or IPC and PPC can be blended by choosing a curve which is average of the two, i.e. BC 45 IPC 40 so the blend would be 42.50. It is better to keep them unblended in trial lens to know their exact specification but the patient's definitive lens should have them thoroughly blended. If the blend is less than 0.2 mm width, it is called the touch blend.

Thickness: It depends upon the dimensions of the lens and quality of plastic used. It is not safe to go below 0.07 mm in thickness.

Edge: It is one of the most important factors for determining comfortable lens wear. It should be specified on order form and checked on receipt of the lens.

Front bevel: This is to reduce the thickness of the high minus lens in its periphery. This shaves off the plastic and thins the lens periphery which is basically thick due to base out construction of the minus lens. It is almost done away for lens above a power of –4.00 D.

Color: Light gray is the most popular tint. It helps in identification, but does not lower the transmission. Fancy colors like green, pink, blue, brown red and grey are available in light, medium and dark shades. They can only be used over light colored iris. Since majority of Indians have a brown or dark iris, these tints cannot be used over them. Their use over the dark iris gives the eye an artificial look.

Power Calculation

This is one of the most important factors which shows its effects as soon as one puts the lens on the cornea. Wrong calculation would mean a subnormal visual acuity. This can be calculated by any of the following three methods, though the first is the best.

Over-Refraction

Patient is refracted through a trial lens. If cylinder is detected in refraction (a) it may be dropped; if the patient is asymptomatic and if it is up to 0.50 (b) if the cylinder is more than 0.5 and vision does not improve beyond 6/9 without cylinder a spherical equivalent is given, i.e. for –1.0 cylindrical give –0.5 spherical or if the patient agrees, cylinder may be given in the form of spectacle cylinder over the contact lens (c) a cylinder may be prescribed in the form of spectacle cylinder over the contact lens, i.e. toric lens (Table 8.2).

Example: If trial lens is 3.00 D and refraction over the contact lens demands an additional power, then proceed as follows:

2.00D cyl can be dealt with according to the rules elaborated earlier. If the over-refraction is above ± 4.00, then the power of the trial spectacle is changed into power at corneal level with the help of effectivity tables or effectivity formula

$$(Fs)/(1 \pm Fsd)$$

Table 8.2 Final power of contact lens by over refraction	
Trial frame lens after refraction over CL of (–3.00 D)	Power of contact lens needed by the patient
–2.00 Dsph	–5.00 Dsph
+2.00 Dsph	–1.00 Dsph
–3.00 Dsph/.–2.00 Dcyl	–6.00 Dsph/–2.00 Dcyl

Fs is the spectacle power and 'd' is distance of spectacle lens from the surface of the cornea.

Example: If a patient demands + 9.00 and another demands –9.0 over the –3.00 contact lens at a vertex distance of 13.00 mm, the power of contact lens is:

$$-3.00 + (+ 10.19 \, D) = 7.19 \, D \text{ is effectivity of } +9.00 \text{ at 13 mm vertex distance}$$
$$-3.00 + (-8.06 \, D) = 11.06 \, D \text{ value of } -9.00 \text{ spectacle lens at corneal level}$$

Power calculation by this method may be wrong due to two reasons (a) the patient may accommodate to accept more minus (b) wrong calculation of effectivity if the additional trial frame lens is of higher power. This can be avoided by using a high plus or high minus trial frame lens approximate to the patient's prescription.

Short Method

If the lens is fitted on K and spectacle power is below ± 4.00, spectacle prescription is transposed into the minus cylinder and the cylinder is dropped.

Example

	Spectacle power	Contact lens power
1.	–3.50 – 1.00 × 180	–3.50 Dsph
2.	–2.00 + 0.75 × 90	–1.25 Dsph
3.	+3.00 + 0.25 × 180	+ 3.00 Dsph

For power higher than ± 4.00 Dsph or cylinder, consider effectivity. If the lens is not fitted on K, then the fluid lens power has to be considered.

Example I:

K = 42.00
Trial contact lens power –3.50
Contact lens BC 42.50
Final contact lens power –4.00

–0.50 Dsph is added to neutralize +0.50 fluid lens which is created by going steeper than K.

Example II:

K = 44.0
Spectacle power +2.00
Contact lens BC 44.25
Contact lens power +1.75

For every 0.25D where the contact lens BC is steeper than K, minus contact lens power is increased by 0.25D. This is due to the + 0.25D fluid lens. The short method is very good if the spectacle and corneal cylinder have the same axis but if they are 90° apart, cylinder gets exaggerated as will be evident in the long method of power calculation.

Long Method of Power Calculation

This method predicts the residual cylinder and considers the keratometric and the spectacle cylinder. *It can be calculated in steps:*
- Spectacle power is recorded at corneal plane.
- Corneal cylinder is taken as minus cylinder along the flatter meridian.
- If the spectacle and corneal cylinders are at 90°, the former transposed into plus form.
- Subtract the corneal cylinder from spectacle correction.

Example:
- When corneal and spectacle cylinder have the same power and axis—
  - corneal plane refraction –2.00 –1.00 cyl × 180
  - corneal cyl. 44.00 @ 180°:45.00@99° = 1.00 cyl × 180
  - not necessary
  Power of contact lens = 2.00 Dsph
- When corneal and spectacle cylinders are 90° apart—
  - corneal plane refraction –5.00 – 1.50 × 90°
  - cylinder 43.25 @ 180: 44.75 @ 90° = 1.50 × 180°
    –6.50 + 1.50 × 180°
    –(–1.50 × 180)/6.50 + 3.00 × 180° = Contact lens power.
- When corneal cylinder is more than in spectacle—
  - corneal plane refractions 2.50 – 1.50 × 180°
  - corneal cylinder 44.00 @ 180:47.00 @ 90° = –3.00 × 180
  - not necessary
  - –2.50 –1.50 × 180–(–3.00 × 180)
    Contact lens power –2.50 + 1.50 × 180
    or –1.00–1.50 × 90
- When cylinder is only in spectacles—
  - corneal plane refraction –4.00 = –3.00 × 180
  - corneal cylinder 44.00 × 180 44.00 90 = zero
  - not necessary
  - –4.00 –3.00 × 180
    –(nil)
    Contact lens power –4.00 –3.00 × 180

The residual cylinder so calculated may be verified by an over-refraction. The two may not be the same as discussed in the chapter on astigmatism. Residual cylinder is dealt with as described in over-refraction method for power calculation, i.e. spherical equivalent spectacle cylinders or toric lens.

INDICATION

The author examined 750 cases and reported indications for short, long and refraction through methods for power finalization. The indications are described below.

Short Method

- When keratometry and spectacle are spherical.
- When cylinder in cornea and spectacle is of the same power, axis and sign.
- When corneal and spectacle cylinders are of the same sign and axis but power difference is within 0.75D.
- When corneal and spectacle cylinder are of opposite sign and the difference is not more than 0.50D.

Long Method

- When difference between corneal and spectacle cylinder is more then 0.75D.
- When difference between corneal and spectacle cylinder is more then 0.5 and the signs are opposite.

Through Refraction

This is indicated in cases of corneal opacity, keratoconus, post-corneal graft, aphakia, high myopia and when the cylinder axis discrepancy is more than 20 degrees. 6/6 vision in these methods was 87% and 95.33% respectively.

Trial Lens Method of Fitting

- *Keratometry:* Corneal measurements are taken in stronger and weaker meridians in both eyes and toricity is noted.
- Choice of the trial lens BC A tabulated guide for choice of BC has been shown in Table 8.3. The author's experience shows that if the VKD, RAPCOS set is used, the following rules may be followed:
  - Toricity 0.0–1.00D, add 25% of the difference between steep and flat meridian, to the flat meridian.
    Example, Keratometry 44.00:45.00 trial lens is 44.25.
  - Toricity 1.00–2.00 D add 33% of the difference between the two meridians to the flat keratometry.
- *Trial set:* An ideal clinic should have trial sets with different diameters and different powers to suit ordinary myopic errors, high myopia and aphakia. Commonly used trial sets are detailed in tabular form in Table 8.4.
  In majority of cases the author uses his own trial set with diameters of 8.5 or 9.00 mm VKD RAPCOS.

VKD RAPCOS-I Set
This is universal set which can be tried in all cases, the author has fitted 90% of his cases with this set. *It has the following advantages:*
- Medium size

Table 8.3 Choice of base curve					
BC	OD	OZ	PPC/00	IPC/00	Power
40.00	9.00	7.7	–/0.25	12.55/04	–3.00
41.00	8.9 mm	7.6	–/0.25	12.25/01	–3.00
42.00					
42.12 to 44.00	8.8 mm	7.5	–/0.25		–3.00
44.12	8.6 mm	7.4	–/0.25	11.25/0.4	–3.00
46.00					
46.12	–8.6 mm	7.3			
48.00					
48.12	–8.5 mm	7.2	–/0.25	12.25/0.4	–3.00

Abbreviations: BC, base curve; OD, right eye; OZ, optic zone; IPC, intermediate posterior curve; PPC, peripheral posterior curve.

Table 8.4 Trial sets	
Number of lenses in a trial set: It is best to have the following steps in choosing the base curves. A total of 25 base curves should have the following break up:	
39.50–42.00 in 0.50 D steps	6 lenses
42.25–45.00 in 0.25 D steps	12 lenses
45.50–48.00 in 0.50 D steps	5 lenses
49.00 and 50.00 in 1.00 steps	2 lenses

- Lesser edge flare
- Lesser edge discomfort
- Lesser blinking problem
- Lesser metabolic problem
- Lesser losses
- Easy to handle
- Easy to modify
- Lesser changes in physical characteristics
- Lesser flare in decentered corneal cap
- More variations possible for a good fit
- Can be used in all types of cases

Small Lens Set
It is similar to VKD RAPCOS-I system but the diameter varies between 8 mm and 9 mm.

Other Trial Sets
Apical 7.5–8.4 mm. It is a set with a very small OD (Table 8.5). It is indicated in (1) Narrow lids aperture, (2) over-sensitive lids, (3) when large lens does not centre, (4) highly irregular peripheral cornea, (5) cornea abrades easily, (6) in hot and humid climate, (7) when a very large lens is otherwise necessary,

Table 8.5 VKD RAPCOS II trial set

Base curve	Diameters		
39.00	8.2		
39.50	8.2		
40.00	8.2		
40.50	8.2	8.7	9.2
41.00	8.2	8.7	9.2
42.00	8.2	8.7	9.2
42.25	8.2	8.7	9.2
42.50	8.2	8.7	9.2
42.75	8.2		
43.00	8.2	8.7	
43.25	8.2		
43.50	8.2	8.7	
43.75	8.2	8.7	
44.00	8.2		
44.25	8.2	8.7	
44.50	8.2		
44.75	8.2		
45.00	8.2		
45.25	8.2		
45.25	8.2		
45.50	8.2		
45.75	8.2		
46.00	8.2		
46.50	8.2		
46.50	8.2		
47.00	8.2		
	PPC 0.35 wide and 1.5 mm flatter than BC	IPC 0.35 wide 1.5 flatter than BC, PPC 0.4 wide and 1.3 mm flatter than IPC	IPC 0.35 mm wide and 1.5 flatter than BC, PPC 0.4 wide and 1.3 mm flatter then IPC

(8) backward head tilt with conventional lenses, (9) in some cases of grafted cornea and keratoconus. *This set has certain problems as follows:*

- Being small, lenses are difficult to handle
- Edges need more precise finish
- Less variations possible for a good fit
- Lot of edge flare if apical cap is decentered.
- Flare problem is very common
- Modifications are difficult
- Shows more physical changes than a larger lens
- Losses are greater
- More lid discomfort

Contour Set
9.00 to 9.8 mm. It is of a bigger diameter. It is used (1) in some cases of keratoconus, (2) Eccentric apical cap, (3) In cases with edge flare, (4) Upriding lens, (5) Sensitive lid, (6) Patient used to a bigger lens, (7) Lenses which are used to change the color of iris, and other cosmetic lenses where almost the entire cornea needs coverage, (8) Very wide pupil, (9) Wide palpebral aperture, (10) Prominent eyes and (11) Large corneas.

Following problems are seen more often with the contour set:
- Metabolic problems
- Corneal distortions
- Spectacle blur
- Limbal irritation

Keratoconus Set
This set has diameters from 7.5 to 8.2 mm and base curve 48.00D–60.00D. This is used in keratoconus and ectatic cornea.

Fluorescein Evaluation

Orbing in 1935 introduced fluorescein evaluation to evaluate corneal lens relationship. After the tearing has stopped with the trial lens, wet fluorescein strip is touched over the contact lens and the pattern is studied with ultraviolet light of high intensity and wavelength 300–400 µ with a peak at 350 µ. This light is provided either by Burton lamp (Fig. 8.1) which has +5.00D observation lens or by the slit lamp.

Fluorescein is an organic compound (resorcinol-phthalein) which is nontoxic to tissue. It fluoresces in ultraviolet (350 µ) light from yellow to opaque yellowish green. It gets easily contaminated with *Pseudomonas aeruginosa* which is

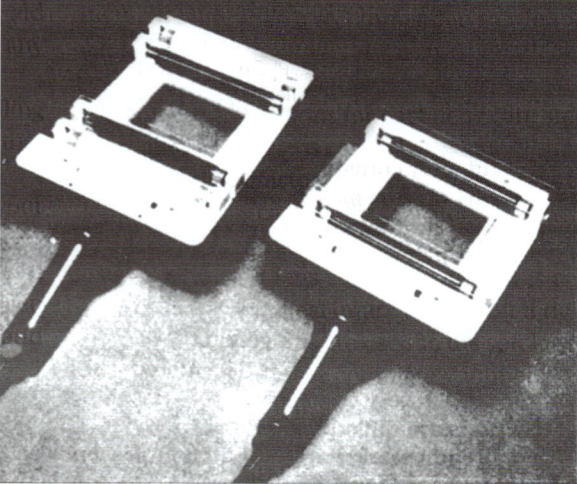

Fig. 8.1 Burton lamp

normally found in skin, stool, sometimes in tap water, well water and conjunctiva. It is best to use fluorescein strips which are individually packed and rinsed with sterile saline solution before use. Author uses blotting paper strips dipped in 20% fluorescein solution and sterilized by autoclaving with glass ware.

Pattern of fluorescein depends upon:
- Corneal shape
- Contact lens back surface
- Amount and quality of tears
- Contact angle of contact lens
- Corneal surface wettability
- Gravity
- Eye movements
- Lid movements
- Amount of light and fluorescein

Pattern of fluorescein between lens and cornea can be judged accurately only if lacrimation has become normal, front surface of lens does not have fluorescein and when pattern remains unchanged after deliberate pushing for fluorescein behind the lens by pressing the lower limbus at 6 o'clock.

Fluorescein Patterns

The following are the common fluorescein patterns (Fig. 8.2). Basically fluorescein is observed with an ultraviolet light in which touch or bearing is indicated by blue, and area of pooling by green.

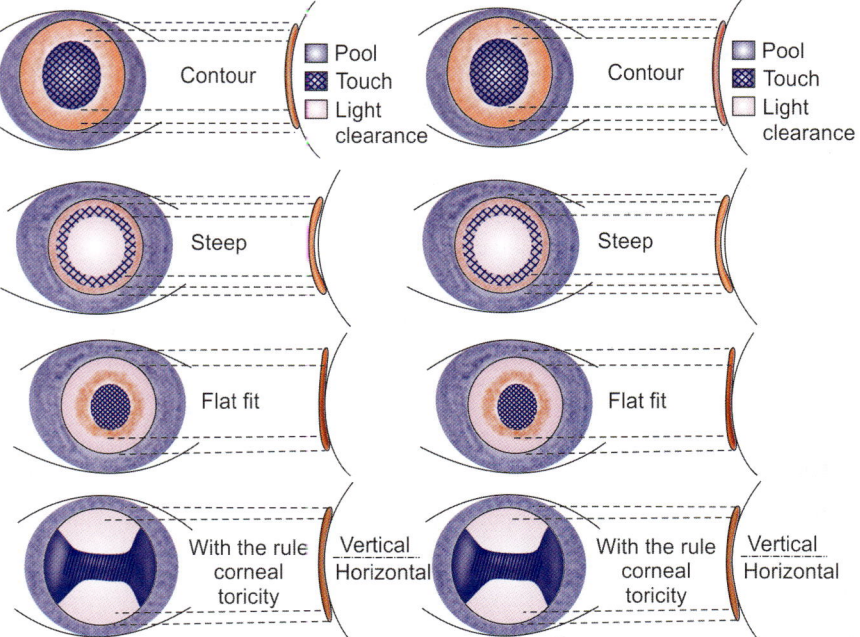

Fig. 8.2 Fluorescein patterns

- *Ideal fluorescein pattern:* There should be a uniform thin layer of fluorescein under the entire back surface of the contact lens.
- *Flat fit:* With ultraviolet light it appears as a blue center and a green film around.
- *Steep fit:* There is central green pool with circular blue touch in the periphery
- *With the rule corneal toricity and a steep lens:* There is a green vertical dumbbell.
  - With-the-rule cornea, fitted slightly flatter than flattest K will show a band of touch in the horizontal meridian.
- Against-the-rule-cornea, fitted slightly steep lens. There is a green horizontal dumbbell.
- *Keratoconus:* There is a central touch and peripheral ring touch with ring of green pool between the two areas of touch.
- *Decentered lens:* There are two areas to touch (a) Corneal apex against lens periphery and (b) lens periphery against the corneal periphery. In between these two areas of touch there is a pool or even bubble because the center of the base curve domes over the intermediate zone of the cornea.

Slit Lamp

Besides the study of corneal-lens relationship by fluorescein under ultraviolet light, it is used to see the lens dynamics under high magnification by various methods (a) direct visualization, (b) tear movements, (c) bubble position, (d) cornea-lens relationship, and (e) staining areas. The movement of tears, debris or bubble under the periphery and center indicate a flat and a steep fit respectively. Slit is used to know (a) thickness of fluorescein layer, (b) cornea-lens relationship (flat or steep), (c) edge bumping. Bumping is seen by noting the movements of the lens as it slides down against the lower lid or seeing the movement of the upper lid as it comes down against the edge after retraction.

Normal lens movements: During blinking, lens slides down a little then rises up the lid and falls back due to gravity. A well-fitted lens falls by 1–2 mm after a blink or after retraction of the upper lid. It lags behind by 1–2 mm as the eyes look to the right or the left. A lens should never reach the limbus.

Tear exchange: Depending upon the cornea-lens relationship, the fluid exchange takes place during the blink continuously. A lens may look immobile but may rock and exchange during the blink. Sometimes bubbles or debris can be seen to enter behind the lens.

Choice of Base Curve

If the previous lens is flat or steep a new trial lens is tried to give it an ideal fit.

Refraction

Refraction is done through the trial lens, and power is finalized as detailed earlier.

Final Order

The trial lens and refraction give the (1) base curve, (2) power, (3) overall diameter, (4) optic zone diameter, (5) peripheral curve, their radius and width, (6) edge, and (7) thickness.

Most of the trial lens specifications such as base curve, overall diameter, optic zone diameter, peripheral curve specifications and edge are mentioned in the final order.

A GUIDE FOR LENS FITTING

See Table 8.6.

Rapid Gas Permeable Fitting

- This is done on the general principles of PMMA fitting.
- *Trial lens which is larger than the PMMA by 1–1.5 mm is chosen on the basis of:*
  – Corneal radius
  – Corneal diameter
  – Lid characteristics
    • Vertical palpebral aperture
    • Position of lid margins
    • Lid tonus
  – Pupil diameter
  – Spectacle prescription
- *Trial lens fitting assessment is done seeing the behavior of static lens and moving lens:*
  – Dynamic
  – Contraction
  – Movement
  – Static
  – Central fit
  – Contact zone
  – Peripheral fit
  – Tear layer thickness.

  The above fit should be optimal and it should be neither tight nor loose.

The rapid gas permeable (RGP) lens should not disturb the:
- Vision
- Comfort
- Corneal integrity

The vision will be good, if:
- Lens is centered well
- Lens is moving within 1 mm
- Lens is not flexible on blinking
- Optic zone is not small.

Table 8.6 Lens fitting guide

	Modified contour		*Small lens*		*Optic cap*		
1.	*Lens diameter and optic zone diameter*							
	Palpebral Aperture	*Flat K*	*Dia mm*	*OZD mm*	*Diam mm*	*OZD mm*	*Diam mm*	*OZD mm*
	13.0 mm	39.00	9.8	8.0	9.0	7.7	8.5	7.3
	11.0 mm	41.00	9.6	7.8	8.8	7.5	8.3	7.1
	9.5 mm	43.00	9.4	7.6	8.6	7.3	8.1	6.9
	8.0 mm	46.00	9.0	7.3	8.3	7.0	7.8	6.6
	6.0 mm	48.00			8.0	6.8	7.5	6.3
2.	*Base curve*							
	Corneal toricity (-K)	*OZD mm*	*BC*	*OZD mm*	*BC*	*OZD mm*	*BC*	
	0	8.0	K–0.50	7.7	K	7.3	K + 0.12	
	0.25	7.8	K–0.25	7.5	K + 0.12	7.1	K + 0.25	
	0.50–1.00	7.6	K	7.3	K + 0.25	6.9	K + 0.37	
	1.25–2.00	7.3	K + 0.25	7.0	K + 0.37	6.6	K + 0.50	
	2.00	7.0	K + K/4	6.8	K + K/4	6.3	K + K/4	
3.	*Second curve radius*							
	Base curve	*OZR+*	*OZR+*	*OZR+*				
	42.00 DK	1.0 mm	1.0 mm	1.0 mm				
	42.00–45.00	0.8 mm	0.8 mm	0.8 mm				
	45.00 DK	0.6 mm	0.6 mm	0.6 mm				
4.	*Peripheral curve radius and width*							
	Base curve mm	*Rad mm*	*Width mm*	*Rad mm*	*Width mm*	*Rad mm*	*Width mm*	
	42.00 DK	11.0	0.5	11.0	0.4	11.0	0.4	
	42.00–45.00	10.5	0.5	10.5	0.4	10.0	0.4	
	45.00 DK	10.0	0.5	10.0	0.4	10.0	0.4	
5.	*Lens thickness*							
	Lens diam	*C.*	Minus lenses; t = C + F/100					
	10.0 mm	0.24	Minimum t = 0.10 mm					
	9.5 mm	0.22	Plus lenses:					
	9.0 mm	0.20	0 to + 5.00 D t = C + 2F/100					
	8.5 mm	0.18						
	8.0 mm	0.17	Plus lenses					
	7.5 mm	0.16	+ 5.00 to + 8.00 D t = C + 3F/100					

"F" is the back vertex power and "K" refer to flatter meridian of the cornea.

The lens will be comfortable, if:

- Movements of lens are within 1 mm
- Edge of the lens is rounded and not sharp
- Edge is located either in the middle or at the back and not towards the front.

- If diameter of the lens is bigger, corneal integrity should be maintained. And disturbance will be noted by staining of cornea or distortion and warpage of the cornea.

The key elements to be considered in RGP fitting are documented by Brain Holden of cornea and contact lens research unit (CCLRU) as follows.
- Centration and movements
  - Lens centration
    - Position and stability
  - Lens movements
    - Amount of post-blink movement
    - Speed (slow, medium, fast)
    - Direction (vertical, nasal, temporal)
    - Type (smooth, apical, rotation, rocky)
  Ideal post-blink movement of the lens should be 1–1.5 mm, smooth, medium to fast and vertical.
  - Lens interaction, with the upper lid, superior edge of the lens should preferably rest under the upper lid to give comfort.
- Lens back surface relationship with cornea
  - Central tear layer thickness (ideal 5–10 μm).
  - Pressure on mid peripheral cornea (minimal).
  - Edge clearance (60–90 μm).
  - Width of the peripheral zone (0.25–0.5 mm).
- Lens characteristics
  - Edge profile
    - Shape rounded
    - Position of apex-central
    - Thickness
  - Central thickness (manufacturer's responsibility)
  - Oxygen transmission (DK/L)
    - Above 30 for daily wear
    - Above 90 for extended wear.

FITTING ASSESSMENT OF RAPID GAS PERMEABLE

- *Centration:* The lens should remain well-centered to ensure better vision, movements, lid action on lens metabolic pump. Centering is dependent on (1) lens corneal relationship, (2) lens diameter, (3) peripheral lens design, (4) upper lid interaction, it should ride up or down and should never be on conjunctiva. Following options may be practiced to center the lens.
  - Increase or decrease diameter
  - Fatten or steepen the base curve
- *Movements:* It should be smooth and in vertical direction without apical rotation. Limbus should not be crossed at any time. If movement is excessive, make the fit tighter by steepening the base curve.

If movement are inadequate i.e. less than one mm then the lens should be loosened by flattening the base curve or reducing the diameter.

- *Central fit:* There should be a very thin layer of tears in the center (5 μm), avoid touch or defined pool. Central touch and pool are treated by steepening and flattening the base curve respectively.

  Alignment fit and moderate apical clearance will have 1.5 μm and 10–15 μm thick tear layer.

- *Mid-peripheral fit:* There should be a very light touch in the mid-periphery. Avoid a well-defined touch and avoid its continuity with the edge.

  In a well-defined touch or when it is too tight, flatten the base curve or reduce the diameter

  If the mid-periphery fit or when it is too loose, steepen the base curve or increase the diameter.

- *Edge fit:* In daily wear, RGP lens edge should be 0.25 mm wide and should be 50 μm away from cornea (clearance).

  In an extended wear RGP lens edge fit should show width of 0.4–0.5 mm and clearance of 75 μm.

  Try to avoid bubble under the edge, try smaller width and clearance.

  Too tight or too loose edge fit is dealt by flattening or steepening the base curve by modifying the lens periphery.

Excessive edge clearance results in:
- Decentration
- Dislocation
- Pops out of the eye
- Bubble at the edge
- Epithelial dessication

Too little edge clearance results in:
- Poor exchange
- Poor movements
- Corneal indentation
- Difficulty in removal

There are six pearls for improving the initial comfort of the RGP lenses:

No. 1   Use anesthetic drop during trial lens fitting but never prescribe them for routine use.

No. 2   Improve the edge quality, i.e. edges should be rounded, smooth and located either posteriorly towards the cornea or towards the center. It should never be located interiorly. Junctional thickness should be 0.12–0.18 mm.

No. 3   Avoid decentration

No. 4   Blend the junctions.

No. 5   Keep the edge clearance uniform.

No. 6   Present RGP realistically

Rapid Gas Permeable Benefits

- Crisp visual acuity
- Keeps good ocular health
- No limbal compression
- Excellent oxygen transmission
- Excellent durability
- Easy to handle
- Good for orthokeratology
- More profitable.

Modifications

Following modifications can be done in a lens after it has been finally fabricated.
- Reduction in overall diameter
- Reduction in optic zone diameter
- Increase in peripheral curve radius
- Increase in peripheral curve width
- Increase in radius and width of blend
- Increase in the bevel
- Surface polishing
- Power change up to – 1.00 D

VKD RAPCCOS methodology of contact lens fitting: It is trial lens method of lens finalization which basically divides fitting procedure into 3 stages:
- Physical stage-first 2 to 15 days
- Physiological stage
- Psychological stage

Lens finalization involves the following steps:
- Keratometry
- Measurement of diameters of pupil, cornea and pelpebral aperture.
- Choice of trial lens depending on toricity.

The trial is VKD RAPCOS-I table set:

Toricity	Percentage of toricity added to 'K'
0–1	25%
1–2	33–50%
Above 2	33%

Example: If keratometry is 45.00: 46.00, then toricity is 1.00 D and trial lens is 45.33 or 45.50.
- *Fluorescein pattern:* Tearing stops in about 15 minutes. An ideal fluorescein pattern is attained. This may involve trial of one or more than one trial lens on the cornea.
- *Refraction:* Final power is known by refracting through finalized trial lens.
- *Variations suggested in the final lens:* On the basis of trial lens fit, variations may be suggested in:
  - Overall diameter

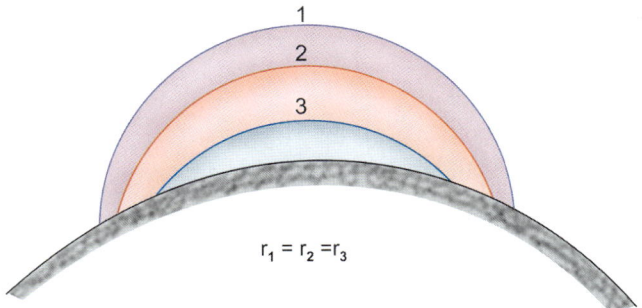

Fig. 8.3 Vaulting effect due to change in overall diameter of lens

- – Optic zone diameter
- – Peripheral curve radius and width
- – Edge
- – Blend
- – Bevel

- *Final diameter ordered is bigger than the trial lens by 0.5 mm if:* (This may be tried by the beginner by using various diameters of VKD RAPCOS II trial set)
  - – Trial lens riding high
  - – Trial lens edge reaches the pupil due to large pupillary diameter.
  - – Corneal diameter is more than 10.50 mm
  - – Palpebral aperture is wider than 10.00 mm
  - – Upper lid is loose
  - – Eyes are prominent
  - – Power is above –4.00 D
  - – Lens has a tendency to sag down
  - – Patient is used to bigger diameter
  - – The trial lens is eccentric in position
  - – Purpose is specific like cosmetic, occlusion, sports and tinted lenses.
    An increase in OD by 0.5 mm calls for a flattening of base curve by 0.25 D (Fig. 8.3)
- Peripheral curve radius and width. If the fluorescein under these curves of the trial lens is minimal, it indicates a need for an increase in radius of the peripheral curve. If the fluorescein is too much and lens is standing off in the periphery, the peripheral curve radius should be decreased. The width can also be varied. An increase in width is at the cost of optic zone diameter.
- *Edge:* If trial lens edge is irritating, order a rolled edge.
- Blend is given if the unblended peripheral curves of the trial lens cause a stain over the cornea, or impair the exchange of tears.
- *Anterior bevel:* Peripheral edge thickness is reduced in high minus lenses, i.e. after –4.00 D by specifying a flatter anterior bevel.

To summarize VKD RAPCOS-I, steps are:
- Keratometry
- Trial lens is chosen on the basis of toricity
- Lens is finalized by fluorescein pattern.
- Power is finalized by refracting through the trial lens.
- Peripheral curve radii and width are changed, if indicated by fluorescein pattern.
- Overall diameter is varied according to the parameters discussed earlier and by judging the behavior of the trial lens.

A duplicate pair should be prescribed in cases when patients are helplessly dependent on contact lenses like cases of keratoconus, corneal opacities, aphakia, high refractive error, cosmetic lenses also for patients living at distant places. Both pairs should be kept in use by weekly alternation.

Design Considerations

- Lens diameter varies between 8.6 mm and 9.6 mm. Larger diameter lens indents cornea. Adherence is similar in smaller and larger lenses.
- Optic zone is 7.1–8.1 mm
- Multicurve lenses are better because of better vision and patients preferred them in the long run.
- *Periphery:* When aspheric was compared with multicurve the former is expected to be better because it shows:
  - Less limbal staining
  - Better initial comfort
  - Better tear exchange

Tear exchange is governed by the following main factors:
- Movements
- Centering
- Mid-peripheral fitting
- Edge fitting

If the above four factors are optimized, then the effect of peripheral design on tear exchange is negligible.

Stability of lens: Lens is more stable in there is a large area of thin tear film underneath.

3–9 o'clock Staining is least with larger diameter when 9.96 and 10.1 mm OD lenses were compared.

Lens Adherence and Edge Fitting

There is no difference in adherence when tight and loose edge fitting are compared.

As a general rule 0.4–0.5 mm width and about 70 µ clearance is preferred.

PHYSICAL STAGE

(Patient is taught lens hygiene, insertion and removal and the instruction booklet of the author is given for further clarification).

- He wears the lens for an hour on the first day and increases the duration by an hour every day for four days.
- Patient is called to the clinic on the 4th day.
- His reactions in respect of tearing, lid swelling corneal staining are noted objectively and subjectively.

    This stage gives a good idea about the physical inconvenience of the contact lens to the patient. Physical inconveniences are experienced by every patient but least in those with high motivation. They get used to them within a week or two though some complaints persist along as the lens is kept on the eye. They are:

- *Foreign body sensation:* Basically methylmethacrylate is hard and patient keeps on feeling as a foreign body. This may cause (a) altered blinking, (b) tearing, (c) difficult in looking up, (d) feeling of itching in eyes (dry lens), (e) minor discomfort, and (f) irritation. This sensation usually stops bothering the patients within a week or two.
- *Patient may complain of:* (a) lenses off-center, (b) edge reflection, (c) lens movements in the first few days. These symptoms are sometimes persistent: the patient soon learns to live with them without getting bothered.
- The patient may complain of foggy vision with the lens. This may due to lipoid secretion over the lens. Removal, cleaning and reinsertion treats this lipoidal secretion. Haze after removal even with spectacle for half an hour is normal for the first few weeks. Persistence of haze after removal for more than 30 minutes calls for consultation with an ophthalmologist.
- Sharp pain due to the displacement of the lens on the eye becomes an infrequent symptom as patients get used to lenses.
- Morning wear is usually difficult and should be avoided for first few weeks.
- Burning sensation is usually caused by the residual cleaning soaking solution. The lens should be thoroughly rinsed with saline before use.

    Mild hot sensation for the first few weeks is noted especially in a crowded atmosphere.

    The fitter notes the physical reactions of the patient with care and sympathy.

PHYSIOLOGICAL STAGE

This is a stage of metabolic adaptation to the corneal insult. Patient will not show any symptoms or signs if tear exchange is adequate enough to create an oxygen tension of 12–20 mm Hg at corneal surface.

    If the patient does not show any odd reaction in the form of tearing, corneal staining or lid edema, he is given the above lens and asked to wear the lens according to a milder schedule. Milder schedule means increase in wearing time by 4 hours in a week to ten days. The patient is called on 1st, 7th, 15th, 30th and 45th day and the following symptoms and signs are noted.

Does the patient have any of the following complaints and if so what is their relation to the wearing time?

- Burning associated with watering
- Inability to open eye completely
- Severe irritation and redness
- Blurred vision which lasts for more than one hour after removal of lenses
- Pain with and without lenses
- Colored halos around light

Examination includes a check for:

- Edema (edema is judged by scleral scatter, keratometry and pachymetry): Edema that changes K by more than 0.50 D is abnormal. Cases which show edema more than 6% do not behave well.
- Staining or abrasion (by fluorescein)

This indicates a metabolic or a physical insult:

- Relation of the lens edge to the pupil
- Almost all the above symptoms and signs call for a new lens, which will be modified symptomatically. This is detailed in the chapter on post-fitting care.

This new or the modified lens is given to the patient and follow-up is continued till the above symptoms are relieved.

A final design is a physically and physiological well-tolerated lens.

PSYCHOLOGICAL

After physical and physiological adaption, the complaint which persists without any accompanying sign is psychological. It is dealt with by psychotherapy. Some patients may show failure due to psychological reasons though the lens may be very well-adapted physically and physiologically.

CHAPTER 9

Handling Instructions

A proper instruction to the patients is the key to the success of contact lens fitting. Teaching the patient regarding insertion, removal and care and maintenance of the contact lens is of utmost importance to achieve optimal outcome and patient satisfaction with contact lens.

INSERTION BY PRACTITIONER

The initial insertion should be done by the practitioner rather than by an assistant to maintain the confidence of the patient. The patient should be instructed to fixate on an object in his lower field of view preferably his own left thumb. The practitioner then balances the contact lens on the index finger and places it on the patient's cornea. Care should be taken to avoid blocking the patient's vision until the lens is placed on the cornea. This is possible if the practitioner approaches the cornea either from the side or above. The lens should be allowed to remain on the eye for twenty minutes for the patient to adapt to the initial sensation. The symptoms will gradually subside and the patient will find the lenses reasonably comfortable. He may then be allowed to remove the lenses himself; removal is usually easier than insertion for the new wearer. By being allowed to remove his lenses the patient gains confidence in his ability to handle them. If he has extreme difficulty in removing his lenses, the fitter should remove them before the patient damages his eyes.

REMOVAL BY PRACTITIONER

The patient should be told to open his eyes widely. The contact lens is then removed by placing the index fingers at the outer canthus of the eye. The lower lid should be manipulated into a scissors position by gently pulling the outer canthus. The lens will be caught and ejected by lid margins.

After the patient is able to remove his lenses he may be taught insertion procedures. Various procedures may be used.

Instruction for Lens Insertion by Patient (Figs 9.1A to F)

- Wash and dry hands.
- Using the forefinger and the thumb, distribute wetting solution evenly on both surfaces on the lens.

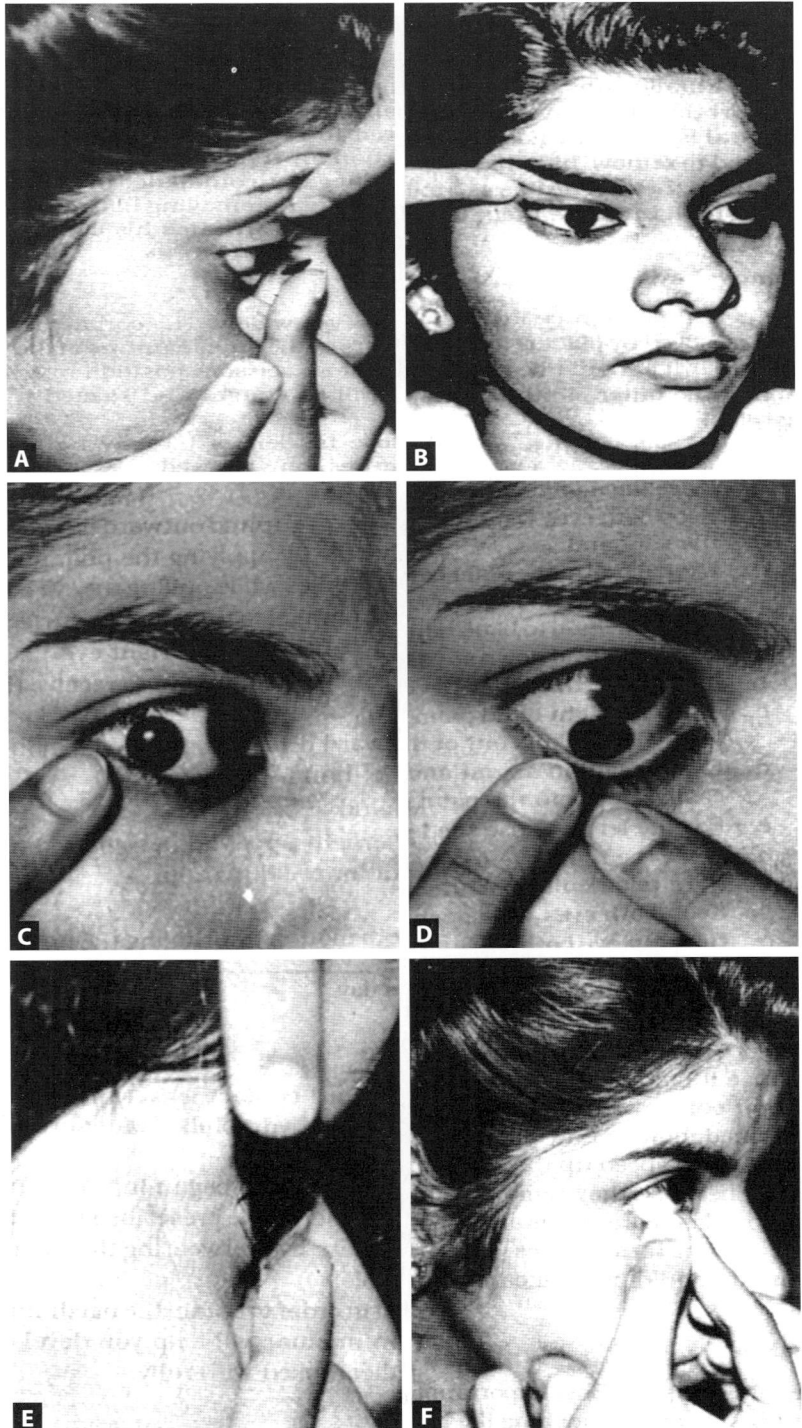

Figs 9.1A to F Steps for lens insertion

- Rinse the lens with cold or lukewarm water (but never with hot water)—keep the lens moist.
- Moisten the forefinger of the right hand and place the clean, moist lens concave surface upward on the tip of that finger.
- Bend the head down so that the eyes will be fixating straight down and looking at the working surface (table surface for example).
- Keep both eyes open all the time during insertion.
- Place the left middle finger at the margin of the upper right eyelid; grasp the lashes and pull the lid up. (This should be done in such a way that the lens will not touch the lashes during the insertion).
- Place the right middle finger at the margin of the lower lid and pull it down.
- Slowly bring the right forefinger with the lens which can be seen as a blurred circle. It is important to keep the eyes straight.
- Gently place the lens on the cornea and release the lower lid first, and then upper lid slowly.
- Straighten the head down, and blink several times.
- Repeat the same procedure for the left eye.

Some alternative methods of insertion are listed below:
- Place the lens on the tip of right middle finger.
  - Hold the right upper lid with the left middle finger and the lower lid with the right forefinger.
  - The rest of the procedure is the same as above.
- Place the lens on the top of the right forefinger.
  - Place the left forefinger at the right upper lid margin, and the left thumb on the lower lid margin and pull the lids apart.
  - The rest of the procedure is the same as above.
- If it is impossible to look through the lens as it approaches the eye, put a mirror on working surface in front of the face, and place the lens right on the cornea by looking into the mirror.
  - Learn not to use the mirror as soon as possible.

Recentering the lens: If not inserted correctly, the lens may be off-center. In this case any of the following methods may be used to recenter the lens.
- One finger method
  - Locate the lens by closing the eye and feeling over the lid by the right forefinger.
  - When located, massage gently towards the center, looking at the direction of the lens until it slips back into proper position.
- Instead of the forefinger, all five fingers may be paced over the lid
  - Locate the lens first and then gently massage it back to the centre, looking towards the direction of the lens.
- Mirror method
  - Place the left middle finger on the margin of the upper lid and the right middle finger on the margin of the lower lid, and pull the lids apart.
  - Looking into the mirror locate the lens; it may be necessary to move the eye around slowly.

- When the lens is located slide the lens back to the center by pushing it with lower or upper lid margin.
- Locate the lens first by using a mirror or by feeling with the fingers.
  - When located open the eye and move the eyeball horizontally away from the lens position. Thus, the lens is now at the central region of the lid opening.
  - Place the left middle finger on the upper lid margin and the right middle finger on the lower lid margin and gently squeeze the lids so that the lens is kept in this central position.
  - Now move the eyeball to the straight ahead position. The lens should slip back to the center of the eye.

Removal of the lens: Remember that removal is easier if the lens is on the center of the eye; therefore, recenter the lens before removal if it is off-center.
- Bend the head down so that it is parallel to the working surface.
  - Place the left hand, palm up beneath the lens which is being removed, so that the lens is caught as soon as it falls out of the eye.
  - Place the right middle finger at the outer canthus of the right eye.
  - Keep both eyes wide open and look straight ahead at the palm of the left hand.
  - Exert a pull at the outer canthus in the up and outward direction.
  - The lens should slip out easily only by applying the up pull, but it may be helpful to blink hard a few times while pulling the eyes lids.
- Bend the head down so that it is parallel to the working surface.
  - Place right thumb at the outer canthus of the right eye.
  - Open the right hand palm in front of the right eye to receive the lens when it falls out of the eye.
  - Exert a pull in an out and upward direction. The lens should easily drop into the palm of the hand.
  - For the left eye use the left hand.
- Place the right forefinger at the right upper lid margin and the right middle finger at the right lower lid margin.
  - Keep both eye wide open.
  - Gently move both lids in scissors motion by bringing the fingers together and then apart.
  - The lens should drop into the palm of the left hand which has been placed beneath that eye.

ADAPTIVE SYMPTOMS

During the first few days of contact lens wear the patient experiences a number of subjective symptoms which are normal reactions to the lenses. A contact lens is a foreign body. These adaptation symptoms normally diminish greatly in a few hours and are nearly gone by the time the patient has reached full wearing time. Persistence of the symptoms usually indicates improper fit.

Tearing: The first time contact lenses are placed on the eye profuse tearing usually results, which subsides greatly after about ten minutes. As the wearing time is increased, the amount of tearing rapidly decreases to a nearly normal amount. It may be noted, however, that a slightly greater than normal tearing persists for several weeks. Tearing is increased by any factor which tends to irritate the lids. Tearing which persists beyond the normal time may be caused by a bad lens edge or by a flat fitting lens. If the tearing subsides in a normal manner but later recurs, the cornea has probably been irritated by the lens or by the presence of a foreign body.

Lid irritation: One of the most sensitive areas stimulated by the contact lens is the lid margin. A tickling sensation is often evoked, but this can usually be eliminated by holding back the patient's lids, so that they do not touch the lens.

Difficulty in looking up: It may happen that when the patient attempts to look up the lens will be drawn upward and will drop and strike the lower lid, initiating a blink reaction and tearing. This can be observed by watching the patient closely and noting whether a blink is instigated when the lens touches the lower lid. By directing the gaze downward; the lens is moved less by the upper lid and less sensation is felt.

Intermittent visual blurring: The patient may note when the contact lenses are first worn he is able to see very well initially but then periods occur when his vision blurs or becomes misty. Part of this problem is caused by the excessive tears under the lens which cause a pooling effect and do not present an even optical surface. A second contributing factor is that, due to the large amount of tearing the lens has a tendency to move around on the cornea, and very often the optical zone is displaced from the front of the pupil.

Difficulty in moving eyes: Some patients fear losing the lens and they attempt to move the eyes as little as possible. This fear is usually unwarranted, and the patient's apprehension can be relieved by purposely directing him to roll his eyes.

Reflections: In the early stages of wear, the patient may report that he is bothered by the shimmering appearance of objects. This is caused by the pooling of excessive tears on the lens and at the lens edge. It will subside after the patient has adapted to the lens.

Head tilt: In an effort to reduce lens movement and the resultant lid sensation the patient may tilt his head backward and appear to be in a rather awkward position. A few patients continue to do this even after the period of adaptation simply due to their habit, and they will stop if a conscious effort is made to keep the head in the normal position.

Excessive blinking: An increased blink rate is caused by the lens irritation of the lid margins. Blinking which persists after the normal period of adaptation usually indicates a lens with a bad edge or a loose fit.

Photophobia: In the initial period of contact lens wear photophobia can be considered a normal symptoms, resulting from lens irritation of the cornea and lids. Bailey demonstrated the anesthetizing the corneas of contact lens wearers relieved the photophobia. With normal adaptation the photophobia will diminish.

It is recommended that the patient wear spectacle sunglasses for the outdoors during the adaptation period. Lightly tinted contact lenses usually are not absorptive enough to be effective against photophobia and darker shades are inconvenient for night wear. The spectacle sunglasses must be dark shades. Tinted spectacles also offer some protection against wind and dust.

Since, it is normal for the patient to experience a number of adaptive symptoms, he should be forewarned of their probable occurrence. Written instructions are often helpful in this regard.

Instructions for the Care and Wearing of Contact Lenses

One of the primary requisites for a successful contact lens fitting is a cooperative and well informed patient. There are many things that must be learned about wearing contact lenses. You will be instructed by student clinicians. These printed instructions will supplement his verbal instructions. They are result to many years of experience and careful observations. Study them in a detail and pay careful attention to them.

The following is a list of "do's" and "don'ts" normal and abnormal symptoms. This list will help you learn about wearing contact lenses. The "do's" and "don'ts" should be followed implicitly. The normal symptoms in general, will subside with time and patience. The normal symptoms may indicate a need for further attention to the lenses or further instructions on proper wearing habits. When in doubt about procedures or symptoms do not hesitate to contact your clinician for advice or instructions.

Do's

- Do follow the instruction given to you. These instructions are the result of long experience and must not be disregarded. Adherence to them will aid us in obtaining an optimum lens fit and will keep you from experiencing any unnecessary discomfort.
- Do be sensible about proper hygiene. Wash your hands well before handling the lenses. Use the contact lens wetting agent to wet the lenses each time that insert them.
- Do clean your lenses after each day's wear and prior to placing them in your soaking case. A germicidal contact lens cleaning agent is recommended.
- Do keep your lenses wet at all times. When not wearing the lenses they should be kept in a "soaking case" containing a contact lens soaking solution. Keep this case clean by washing it occasionally with a household detergent and rinsing thoroughly with tap water.
- Do wear the lenses according to the wearing schedule given to you. This is a maximum schedule. You must not exceed the assigned wearing time. If you miss wearing the lenses one day, or wear them less than scheduled, reduce your wearing time the next day and bring it back up to schedule gradually over the next few days.

- Do consult the fitter regularly even after you have adapted to your lenses so that one can be certain that your eyes are continuing to respond to the lenses in a normal manner.
- Do be careful with your lenses. They are easily lost, easily scratched, and costly to replace and refit. If they become scratched or nicked, they must be returned for refinishing.
- Do remove, wet and reinsert the lenses at least once a day after about seven or eight hours of wear.
- Do carry you contact lens identification card in your wallet for removal of lenses by a doctor in case of emergency.

Don'ts

- Don't be foolish about your endurance. We want you to adapt to the lenses gracefully: we don't want you to be a hero. If the lenses are uncomfortable, remove, wet, and reinsert them. If still uncomfortable, remove them and report to the clinic for instructions.
- Don't wet your lenses by placing them in your mouth. Not only is it unhygienic but an easy way to spread infection.
- Don't rub your lenses with tissue. There should never be a need to wipe them in this manner.
- Don't sleep with your lenses on. This is unnecessary and undesirable. Give your eyes a rest too. If you take a short nap while wearing them, upon waking remove, wet and reinsert them.
- Don't wash lenses in hot water as they could possibly warp.
- Don't insert lenses over a sink. Many lenses have been lost down the drain.
- Don't engage in sports with your lenses on until well adapted to wearing them. For field sports one can wear a soft contact lens.
- If you drop a lens don't scrape it across the surface. Pick it up by having it stick to a wet finger.
- Don't undertake rapid eye movements in the beginning. This will become much easier in time.

NORMAL SYMPTOMS

- *Lenses off center:* Often the lenses will not remain centered on the corneas, but will ride a little on to one side due to the physical construction of the eyes.
- *Lens movement:* Lenses are designed to have a small amount of movement at all time to permit a normal fluid flow beneath the lenses. This movement may be excessive at first due to the amount of fluid present and to increased lid tension.
- *Edge reflection:* May be aware of the lens edges under certain conditions during the first few weeks.
- *Tearing:* When a foreign body, regardless of how smooth it is placed on the eye, tearing results. This tearing generally subsides quickly as you adapt.
- *Minor irritation or discomfort:* At first you will be aware of the lenses upon your eyes and in contact with your lids. This sensation will gradually disappear.

- *Light sensitivity:* Almost all contact lens wearers in the beginning are bothered by bright light. The use of a good pair of plain sun glasses is recommended for outdoor wear.
- *Burning:* You may experience mild burning or warm sensation when reading, watching TV or movies, or when in a closed room.
- *Morning wear:* Morning wear is generally more difficult and should be avoided during the first few weeks.
- *Blurring:* Some of the natural oily secretions by the lid glands may accumulate on the lenses and cause the vision to blur. Remove, wet, and reinsert the lenses. Use a contact lens cleaner occasionally.
- *Spectacle blur:* You may experience a blur with your spectacle lenses after wearing your contact lenses. This should clear within about an hour in most cases.
- *Foreign body reaction:* A sudden sharp pain is usually caused by a bit of dirt being trapped under the edge of the lens. Remove, wet, and reinsert lens.
- *Looking up:* This may be difficult during the early weeks of wear until the lids adapt to the presence of the lenses.
- *Lens becoming dislodged:* During the first weeks the lenses may have a tendency to move off centre or even to fall out due to excessive tearing and lid tension.
- *Blinking:* Excessive blinking during the early weeks of wear is not uncommon. This is preferred over inadequate blinking.
- *Itching:* The eyes may itch after removing the lenses. Do not rub them. Use a cold cloth or cold water to soothe them.
- *Dizziness or headache:* You may experience lightheadedness or a slight headache for a few days especially if you wear a complex spectacle prescription.
- *Haze or foggy:* Vision may fog towards the end of the wearing period until the eyes develop a tolerance for the lenses and adjust to the fluid exchange rate. If this fog persists or reoccurs after removing and rewetting the lenses, discontinue wear and report for instruction.

ABNORMAL SYMPTOMS

- Pain when placing the lenses on the eyes, while wearing the lenses or after removing them.
- Burning or hot feeling causing excessive watering of the eyes.
- Inability to keep eyes open.
- Severe or persisting haze, fog or halo.
- Long lasting spectacle blurs.
- Severe irritation or redness.

If any of the above symptoms occur, discontinue wear and contact your clinician for instructions.

Abrasions and infections: If the lenses becomes less comfortable to the wearer than when they were first placed on the wearer's corneas, this may indicate the presence of a foreign body. The lens should be removed immediately and the patient examined. If any eye abrasion, ulceration, irritation or infection is present, a physician should be consulted immediately

Wearing restrictions: Soft contact lenses should be removed before sleeping or swimming and in the presence of noxious and irritating vapors.

Visual blurring: When visual blurring occurs the lens must be removed until the condition subsides.

Lens sanitation: Patients who would not or could not adhere to recommended daily sanitary care of soft lenses should not be provided with them.

Precautions

Storage

Soft contact lenses must be stored in normal saline solution or in the solution recommended. If left exposed to air, the lenses will dehydrate, become brittle, and break readily. If a lens dehydrates, it should be soaked in normal saline solution until it returns to a soft, supple state.

Cleaning and Asepticizing

Soft contact lenses must be both cleaned and asepticized daily. One procedure does not replace the other. Cleaning is necessary to remove mucus and film from the lens surface. Asepticizing with the soft lens Aseptor-Patient Unit has been shown to prevent the growth of certain organisms, namely *Staphylococcus aureus, Pseudomonas aeruginosa, Bacillus subtilis, Candida albicans* and Herpes simplex, on the lens and in the soft lens carrying case.

Fresh normal saline must be prepared daily for cleaning and storing the lenses. The carrying case must be emptied and refilled with fresh normal saline solution just before asepticizing the lenses.

If a soft lens Aseptor-Patient Units is not available for asepticizing the lenses, the lenses must be boiled in their carrying case in a pan of water for 15 minutes.

Hygiene: Hands must be washed, rinsed thoroughly, and dried with a lint-free towel before handling the lenses.

Cosmetics, lotions, soaps and creams must not come in contact with the lenses since eye irritation may result. If hair spray is used while the lenses are being worn, the eyes must be kept closed until the hair spray has settled.

Adverse reactions: Serious corneal damage may result from wearing a lens which has been soaked in a conventional contact lens solution containing preservatives.

Eye irritation may occur within a short time after putting on a hypertonic lens. Removal of the lens will relieve the irritation.

Very rarely a lens may adhere to an eye as a result of the patient sleeping with the lens or on wearing a hypotonic lens. If a lens adheres for any reason, apply normal saline and wait until the lens moves freely before removing it.

Soft Lenses: Dosage and Administration

Conventional methods of fitting contact lenses do not apply to soft contact lenses.
There may be a tendency for the patient to over-wear the lenses initially. Therefore, the importance to adhering to the following initial daily wearing schedule should be stressed to the patient.

Lens Wear and Replacement Schedules

The wearing and replacement schedule should be determined by the eye care professional.

Daily Wear (<24 hours, While Awake)

- To avoid tendency of the daily wear patient to overwear the lenses initially, stress the importance of adhering to a proper, initial wearing schedule. Normal daily wear of lenses assumes a minimum of 6 hours of non-lens wear per 24 hours period.
- It may be advisable for patients who have never worn contact lenses previously to be given a wearing schedule that gradually increases wearing time over a few days. This allows more gradual adaptation of the ocular tissues to contact lens wear (Table 9.1).
- *Extended wear (>24 hours, including while asleep):*
  - The eye care professional should establish an extended wear period up to 6 continuous nights that is appropriate for each patient. Once the lens is removed, the patient's eyes should have a rest period with no lens wear of overnight or longer, as recommended by the eyecare professional.

Table 9.1 Initial wearing schedule of contact lens					
Day	Wear time (hours)	Rest period (hours)	Wear time (hours)	Rest period (hours)	Wear time (hours)
1	3	1	3	1	3
2	3	1	3	1	3
3	4	1	4	1	4
4	4	1	4	1	4
5	6	1	6	1	4
6	6	1	6	1	4
7	8	1	8		
8	8	1	8		
9	8	1	8		
10	10	1	balance of the waking hours*		
11	12	1	balance of the waking hours*		
12	14	1	balance of the waking hours*		
* Lenses should never be worn 24 hours a day					

– It is suggested that new contact lens wearers first be evaluated on a daily wear schedule. If the patient is judged to be an acceptable extended wear candidate, the eyecare professional may determine an extended wear schedule based upon the response of the patient.

Lens Replacement

The replacement schedule is determined by the eyecare professional based upon the patient's individual needs and physiological conditions.

Hygiene

Cleanliness is the most important rule of contact lens care. Always wash your hand before touching the lenses. Then rinse them thoroughly and dry them with a lint-free towel. Before putting on the lenses, avoid handling oily substances such as hand creams, lotions, and cosmetics.

Putting on the Soft Lenses

Wash hands thoroughly, making certain that all soap residue has been washed away. Work with the right lens first in order to avoid confusing the lenses. After removing the lens from the case, examine it to be sure that it is moist clean and clear. Be careful not to touch the inside surfaces of the lens. Then check to see that the lens has not been turned inside-out. This may be done simply by flexing the lens between the thumb and index finger. If upon position the edge is erect and pointing slightly inward, it is in its correct position. If the edge turns outward, folding back on the fingers, it is inside-out and must be reversed.

- Place the lens on the outer edge of the index finger of your dominant hand.
- With your head erect and gazing straight ahead, retract the lower lid with your middle finger.
- Look up and fix your gaze on a point above you. Then roll the lens on the white part of the eye.
- Remove your index finger and slowly release the lid.
- Close your eyes momentarily and lightly massage the lid to help center the lens. This removes the air bubble also if it is under the lens.

Removing the Lenses

- Never probe about on the eye in search of a lens. Always be sure the lens is in the correct position on your eye before attempting to remove it. A simple checking of your vision with each eye separately will tell if a lens is in the correct position. If vision is poor it is likely that the lens has been lost from the eye. If vision is poor, yet you feel certain that the lens is still in your eye, you should obtain professional assistance for its removal.
- Having washed your hands and rinsed them thoroughly, begin the removal procedure by holding your head erect and turning your eyes upward. Retract

the lower lid with the middle finger and place the index finger tip on the lower edge of the lens. Slide the lens down to the white part of the eye.

- Compress the lens lightly between the thumb and index finger. Rolling the thumb and index finger together causes the lens to double up between the finger, allowing air underneath. Remove the lens from the eye.
- Clean the lens with normal saline solution and replace it on the cap of the carrying case.

Cleaning the Lenses

Place the lens in the palm of your hand, concave side up. Wet it with normal saline solution. Rub the lens gently but thoroughly with your fingertip; be careful not to touch the lens with your fingernail.

With the availability of good quality multipurpose solutions in the market, the soft lens is mostly cleaned with these solutions.

Other Important Information

- Be sure you have read the package insert at the beginning of this chapter, particularly the sections entitled "warnings" and "precautions".
- If a lens becomes less comfortable than it was when it was first placed on your eye, remove the lens immediately. Clean and asepticize the lens before returning it to the eye. If the condition persists remove the lens immediately and your eye should be re-examined. If any abrasion, ulceration or infection is present a physician should be consulted immediately.
- Never sleep with the lenses on. If you forget, however, check to see, immediately upon awakening, if the lenses move on the eyes. If they do not move readily, do not attempt to remove them. Place several drops of lubricants or normal saline solution in the eye every few minutes and try moving them again. If after several applications of normal saline solution, the lenses still do not move, you should obtain professional assistance for removal of the lenses.
- If by chance, the lenses dry out completely, they will shrivel and become brittle. Handle them carefully. Drop them into a small container of normal saline solution and let them soak until they return to their soft supple state. After asepticizing they will again be ready for wear.
- If, after placing a lens on your eye, you do not see clearly through it, massage the closed lid to center the lens. If you still do not see clearly, check to see if you have put on the wrong lens, or if the lens is inside-out.
- If a lens becomes irritating and you suspect that it may have become contaminated with cosmetics, lotions, soaps, or creams, clean the lens very carefully.
- Always close your eyes before applying hair spray as it cannot be removed from the soft contact lens. Keep in mind that the spray mist lingers in the air after application.
- If a lens adheres to its carrying case mount, wet the lens with normal saline solution, close the case, and shake it. Let the lens soak until it moves freely.

- If a lens floats off the cap, close the case, turn it upside-down, and tap it in the palm of your hand. This should return the lens to its mount. If not, empty the case, catching the lens in the palm of your hand.

Wearing Schedule

Follow the schedule set up for you. Do not vary the wearing schedule especially during the adaptation period.

Basic instructions for lens cleaning and disinfection: When lenses are dispensed, the eyecare professional should recommend an appropriate system of lenscare and provide the patient with instructions according to the package labeling.

The eyecare professional should review the following instructions with the patient:
- Lenses must be cleaned, rinsed, and disinfected each time they are removed, for any reason. If removed while the patient is away from the lens care products, the lenses may not be reinserted, but should be stored until they can be cleaned, rinsed, and disinfected.
- Cleaning is necessary to remove mucus, film, and contamination from the lens surface. Rinsing removes all traces of the cleaner and loosened debris. Disinfecting is necessary to destroy remaining microorganisms.
- Lenses must be cleaned, rinsed, disinfected, and stored in accordance with the package labeling of the lens care products recommended by the eyecare professional.
- Heat disinfection has not been tested and is not recommended.
- To help avoid serious eye injury from contamination:
- Always wash, rinse and dry hands before handling the lenses.
- Use only fresh sterile solutions recommended for use with soft (hydrophilic) contact lenses. When opened, sterile non-preserved solutions must be discarded after the time specified in the label directions.
- Do not use saliva, tap water, homemade saline solution, distilled water, or anything other than a recommended sterile solution indicated for the care of soft lenses.
- Do not reuse solutions.
- Use only fresh solutions for each lens care step. Never add fresh solution to old solution in the lens case.
- Follow the manufacturer's instructions for care of the lens case.
- Replace the lens case at regular intervals to help prevent case contamination by microorganisms that can cause eye infection.
- Never use a rigid lens solution unless it is also indicated for use with soft contact lenses. Corneal injury may result if rigid lens solutions not indicated for use with soft lenses are used in the soft lens care regimen.
- Always keep the lenses completely immersed in the recommended storage solution when the lenses are not being worn to avoid lens dehydration.

10

Follow-up
Post-fitting Problems

INTRODUCTION

Post-fitting problem may be physical, physiological or psychological. These factors overlap, e.g. physical factors may lead to physiological change.

Physical problem are due to the lens and can be correlated with a physical cause.

Physiological problems are more serious, due to the effect of the lens on the functions of the eye.

Psychological: This may have no physical or physiological basis being purely due to the mental make-up of the patient. It may come up immediately or sometime after contact lens wear.

Post-wear problems can be solved and their causes found easily, if a systematic examination is conducted.

- *History:* This decides between adaptive and abnormal symptoms the former tend to disappear after a fortnight or so; the latter may persist and rarely may continue insidiously. The time of occurrence of a symptom may be noted and its relation to the time of wear. The patient is further asked whether the symptoms (immediate or delayed), fluctuate or remain constant or become worse as wearing of lenses is continued.

This elucidation often helps in differential diagnosis of the complaints. Further examination is just a correlation of physical findings with the complaint.

The following tests may be done in each case for reaching a precise conclusion.

- *Visual acuity:* Record the visual acuity in each eye separately. If, it is below 6/5, perform over-refraction through the lens.
- Refraction through the lens with — sphere
                                              — cylinder.

  Note the best visual acuity with sphere, cylinder or spherocylinder.
- *Orthoptic check-up:* This may include movements, convergence, accommodation, muscle balance for near and distance, binocularity.
- *Examination:* Following parameters may be carefully looked for posture:
    - (a) Face turn
    - (b) Head tilt
    - (a) Infrequent blinking
    - (b) Complete lack of blinking
    - (c) Squeezing the eyelids
    - (d) Unilateral or bilateral ptosis
    - (e) Increased frequency in blinking.

- (a) Abnormal eye movement during blinking
  (b) Swelling of the lids.
  (c) Deposit of white secretion at the angle of the eye.
  (d) Congestion or redness of the bulbar conjunctiva.
  (e) *Movements of the lens:* It should not normally move more than 2 mm with each blink. It should never touch the limbus or sclera.
  (f) Position of the lens.
  Note the lens position over the eyeball whether it is central, eccentric to the right or left and whether up or low riding.
  Note the movements of the lens by holding the upper lid. A normal lens should not gravitate more than 1 mm.
- *Biomicroscopy with white light to look for:*
  – Topography of lens
  a. Movement of the lens, positioning of the lens.
  b. Surface of the lens for scratches, deposits and their position.
  c. Edge of the lens for chipping.
  – Corneal-lens relationship is judged by debris movement. If it moves under the lens periphery, it is a flat fit. Movement or collection of debris in the central pool under the lens indicates a steep corneal lens relationship.
  – *Edema:* By focusing a broad slit at the limbus (scleral scatter), edema of cornea stands out as a central, circular clouding, it may be diffuse or irregularly shaped. The latter has always an epithelial pathology over it either stippling or abrasion.
  – Corneal stippling can be seen through the lens as white pin head spots while abrasion appears as a clear area surrounded by white pin head spots located in a diffuse haze.
- *Biomicroscopy with fluorescein and white light:*
  – This examination helps to observe the corneal stippling and abrasion which take up a yellowish green strain.
  – *Corneal-lens relationship:* Pooling of the yellowish green tear fluid under the periphery, or at the center of the lens, indicates a flat and a steep fit, respectively.
- *Biomicroscopy with fluorescein and ultraviolet light:*
  – *Corneal-lens relationship:* The blue ultraviolet light is absorbed by the yellow fluorescein and emitted as green light. Location of the green lacrimal fluid under the periphery with a blue center indicates a flat lens. A central green pool and a peripheral blue ring indicates a steep corneal lens relationship.
  – Stippling and abrasion will take up stain and will appear as green pin head spots (stippling) and green areas (abrasion). These may be possibly due to steep or flat lens, foreign body, lash and eccentric lens.
- *Biomicroscopy of the cornea without the lens and with white and ultraviolet light:*
  This examination helps to confirm
  – Edema of the cornea
  – Stippling and abrasion.
  – Other details of the cornea, anterior chamber, iris and the lens.

- Lens inspection is detailed in the chapter on lens inspection and verification.
- Keratometry indicates changes caused by lens wear. Comparison with initial records helps to decide about steepening or flattening of the cornea. Corneal irregularities are indicated by blurred and distorted mires.
- *Ophthalmoscopy:* Observation of the fundus should form a part of the prefitting and follow-up regimes.
- *Retinoscopy:* For assessment of a change in sphere or cylinder.
- *Record:* The findings may be recorded, and drawings made of corneal-lens relationship, lens position, movements and fluorescein pattern.

POST-FITTING PROBLEMS

A lens may be worn satisfactorily even though it may not satisfy the criteria of a good physical fit. It is common experience that the flat as also the steep lens may be well tolerated, physically and physiologically. Gross deviations from the physical requisites are likely to cause unwanted symptoms and signs. Some signs like pressure on the limbal vessels by the upriding lens need immediate treatment, even before its effects are seen.

Every eye must be given an appropriate trial lens; a careful note must be made about the physical, physiological and optical effects of the contact lens on the eye.

The effects are best judged if a trial lens of the patient's exact specification is used and the patient is allowed to wear it for four hours daily for a few days or a week.

Common post-wear problems may be physical and physiological. Physical problems may be:
- Faulty insertion
- Faulty removal
- Improper storage
- Switched lens
- Lens edge in the pupillary area
- Lid irritation
- Low riding lens
- Upriding lens
- Foreign bodies
- Cetavlon injury

Faulty Insertion

Patient may insert the lens so poorly that an abrasion is caused.

Complaints

Abrasion is noted by the sudden occurrence of a pain, irritation, lacrimation and blepharospasm.

Signs

There is usually a crescentic abrasion which is stained green with fluorescein.

Treatment

- *Prophylactic:* Every patient should be taught the insertion technique properly and he should be asked to demonstrate the insertion technique before the lenses are delivered
- Abrasion is treated by bandaging the eye with an antibiotic eye drop and use of topical preservative free lubricants.

Faulty Removal

Complaints

The patient takes more time to remove than to insert lenses. He may have to have the assistance of another person or a doctor to remove his lens. It is usually the left lens which presents this difficulty.

Signs

The eye is usually red, when repeated attempts have failed to remove the lens. This may be associated with tearing.

Treatment

- *Prophylactic:* Teach the removal technique and ask the patient to demonstrate it. It should not take more than 2 blinks to remove the lens.
- Very rarely, a rubber suction cup may be given to an intelligent patient who fails to remove the lens because of loose lid skin or to the patients with operated detachments; for retinal tears are likely to recur after faulty removal.

Caution

Patient may keep on applying suction cup on cornea to create corneal abrasion.

Improper Storage

A dirty lens with mucus or lipid (oil) sticking on the surface may be stored as such.

Complaints

Such lenses usually do not clean well and result in blurred vision. A dried secretion may even abrade the cornea.

Signs

There may be a subnormal visual acuity. On slit lamp examination, the lens looks dirty and there may be thick dried mucus on its surface. Lenses may show an odd fit due to the pull of the dried mucus.

Treatment

- *Prophylactic:* Demonstrate to the patient the methodology of cleaning and storing, and ask him to demonstrate them once in your presence.
- *Proper:* A dirty lens is cleaned in the laboratory by carbon tetrachloride or buffing.

Switched Lenses

While storing the lenses in the lens case, the patient may put the right lens in the left case and *vice versa*, with the result that the right lens gets in the left eye and the left lens in the right eye.

Complaints

If the difference in the powers of the two lenses is significant, the patient immediately complaints of blurred vision. He may start complaining of physical symptoms if the base curves of the two lenses are significantly different.

Signs

Visual acuity may be abnormal. Lens with the 'R' mark may be over the left eye. Fluorescein pattern may demonstrate an odd fit.

Treatment

- *Prophylactic:* During training in handling techniques, the patient should be demonstrated the proper methodology of storage. The 'R' mark may be clearly shown to the patient, and he should be asked to see it before the lens is put in the right eye.
- *Proper:* Mixed lenses are sorted out by studying the lens specifications.

Edge in the Pupil

This is disturbing to the patient due to irregular refraction through a non-optical area the edge. The patient complains of increased flare due to irregular refraction of light by the prism of the lens edge, and the fluid prism at the edge. There is a drop in visual acuity which keeps fluctuating due to edge coming and going out of the papillary area. The lens edge is found in front of the pupil on examination.
- *Treatment:* It is treated by preventing the edge coming nearer to the pupil. The following steps may be helpful to avoid edge coming in the papillary area.
  - Increase the overall diameter.
  - Increase the optic zone diameter.
  - Steepen the base curve.
  - Steepen the peripheral curves.
  - Increase the thickness of the lens.
  - Decrease the thickness of the lens.

Lid Irritation (Scratchy Feeling)

The patient feels uncomfortable as soon as the lenses are worn and there is immediate relief as soon as the lenses are removed. *This may be due to:*
- Excessive movements
- Bad finish of the edge
- A low riding lens which strikes the lower lid.
  On examination there may be an excessive movement of the lens which shows more than 2 mm of excursion or the lens may sag to touch the lower lid. A badly finished edge is judged by feeling it with the tip of index finger or over the front of the forearm.
- *Correction:* Excessive movement can be dealt by any of the following methods as required.
  – Steepen the base curve.
  – Steepen the peripheral curves.
  – Increase the overall diameter.
  – Increase the optic zone diameter.
  – Reduce the edge thickness.
  – Reduce the central thickness.
  – Proper blending of the peripheral curves.
  A low riding lens with resultant lower lid touch may be avoided by:
  – Steepening the base curve.
  – Steepening the peripheral curves.
  – Reducing the overall diameter.
  – Reducing the central thickness.
  – Putting a minus carrier at the edge.
  – Increase the overall diameter to allow a better action of the upper lid over the lens.
  A poor edge is treated by refinishing or re-edging.
  The author has reported an odd lateral version of the eye before each blink to avoid lid irritation.

Low Riding Lens

This is a common problem especially with heavier lenses or lenses of higher plus powers.

Complaints

The patient complains of a fluctuating or jumping visual acuity—there may be lid irritation; after a few hours of wear the patient may complain of discomfort, stinging, burning, hazy vision.

Signs

The lens is riding low after a blink. It may remain below and may not ride up again or the edge of the lens might encroach on the pupil. There may be circular patch of diffuse corneal edema below the center of the cornea as seen by sclerotic scatter. Fluorescein shows decentered pool over the area of corneal edema.

Treatment

A low riding lens is treated by:
- Flattening the base curve.
- Steepening the peripheral curve.
- Reducing the overall diameter.
- Reducing the central thickness.
- Putting a minus carrier at the edge.
- Rarely increasing the overall diameter.

   Putting a flange and increasing the overall diameter are the best solutions in the author's experience.

Upriding Lens

This is more common than low riding lenses. It is also physiologically more compatible than a low riding lens (Figs 10.1A and B).

Complaints

The patient complains of blurred and fluctuating vision and more glare due to the edge coming in the papillary areas. There may be an edge sensation at the upper limbus. Rarely though, the patient may feel discomfort and stinging after few hours of wear.

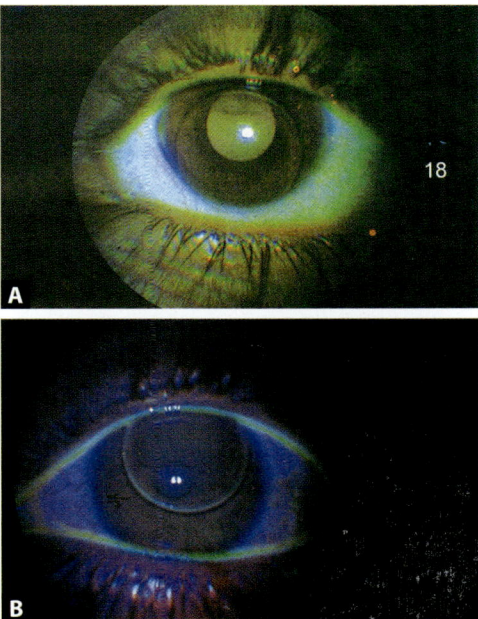

Figs 10.1A and B Low riding and up riding contact lens. (A) Low riding corneal lens; (B) Up riding corneal lens

Signs

The center of the lens is placed higher than the center of the cornea. The edge of the lens is usually found in the pupil. A fluorescein pool is found over the upper 1/3 of the cornea under the lens. There might be some staining under the center and edge of the lens.

Treatment

An upriding lens is treated by one of the following:
- Increase the overall diameter.
- Increase the optic zone diameter.
- Steepen the peripheral curves.
- Steepen the base curve.
- Reduce the edge thickness to reduce the lid action.
- Increase the central thickness to enhance the action of gravity.
- Decrease the central thickness to avoid the action of the lid.
  Increasing the overall diameter and steepening the base curve are the best in the author's experience.

Foreign Body

This may be solid, fluid, or gas. A particle on the eye behind the contact lens is felt much more than a particle in the eye while wearing spectacles.

Complaints

This varies from slight discomfort to severe irritation causing profuse watering, pain, photophobia and blepharospasm.

Signs

A solid foreign body due to its movements with the lens causes a zig-zag stain. Staining becomes more apparent when it is examined with fluorescein. It may sometimes get embedded in the cornea to cause a localized stain.

The effect of liquid and gases may vary from small superficial staining to complete sloughing of the cornea.

Treatment Prophylactic

Protective glasses should be used in areas where gas, liquid or solid is likely to enter into the eye.

The contact lens is removed, the eye washed and the lens put in again.
- If irritation persists with the immediate use of the lens, an overnight (6–12 hours) rest is given to the eye.
- If there is severe irritation, pain, photophobia and blepharospasm, the lesion should be treated as a corneal abrasion—The eye is padded and bandaged

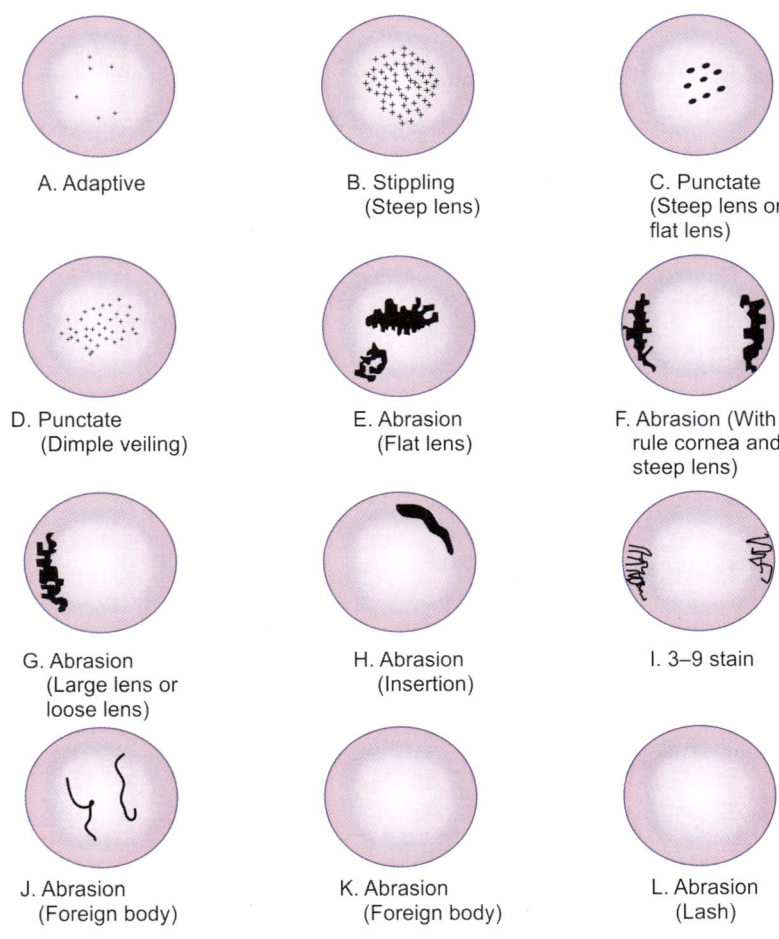

A. Adaptive

B. Stippling
(Steep lens)

C. Punctate
(Steep lens or
flat lens)

D. Punctate
(Dimple veiling)

E. Abrasion
(Flat lens)

F. Abrasion (With
rule cornea and
steep lens)

G. Abrasion
(Large lens or
loose lens)

H. Abrasion
(Insertion)

I. 3–9 stain

J. Abrasion
(Foreign body)

K. Abrasion
(Foreign body)

L. Abrasion
(Lash)

Fig. 10.2 Staining patterns in various corneal lesions

with terramycin ophthalmic ointment for 12 hours. Continuation of the bandage is indicated if corneal staining persists. Lenses are not worn on cornea for seven days even after the abrasion has healed (Fig. 10.2).

- For severe corneal insults with acid, alkali or other chemicals, the lens should be removed, a thorough lavage of the eye should be done with clean water and patient should be referred to the hospital with pad and bandage.

Cetavlon Injury

Cetavlon is a common contact lens cleaning agent in India and England.

Complaints

If the lens is not properly washed, patients start having immediate irritation, watering, pain, photophobia and blepharospasm.

Signs

Cornea shows varying extent of staining which is more apparent after fluorescein staining.

Treatment Prophylactic

- Demonstrate to the patient the cleaning technique properly.
- Never keep the cetavlon powder near the tap and never use a powder for cleaning.
- Put a red level on the cetavlon 2% solution and label it "for external use only and not to be used in the eye".

Proper

The eye is thoroughly washed with saline, terramycin ointment applied and bandage given.

PHYSIOLOGICAL PROBLEMS

Faulty Exchange

Tear exchange is essential to wash away the residual tears and debris from the fluid lens and to supply fresh nutrients with oxygen to the cornea covered with the contact lens.

Cause

Faulty exchange is usually caused by:
- Steep lens
- Flush fitting lens
- Thin lens
- Partial blinking
- Upper lid pressing on the lens as in upriding lens, lower position of the upper lid and tight upper lid

Complaints

The patient feels hot, dry a deep ache in the eye burning, smarting, stinging, colored halos around light and misty vision with glasses which persist for more than half an hour after contact lens removal. The complaints build up after some hours of wear and are seldom immediate.

Signs

The lens may show slow movements. This may be compatible with good exchange as the lens may rock during a blink to have sufficient exchange. On the contrary a lens may move considerably without permitting adequate exchanges. This may be seen in certain cases of upriding, low riding and eccentrically placed lenses.

Slit lamp examination may also show stippling which may be bigger in size and called punctate staining. Both stippling and punctate staining appear as white pin points which become more apparent when observed with fluorescein stain. Small bubbles may be seen under the lens and the cornea may show dimples in place of the bubbles after lens removal.

Slight corneal edema is normal in the first few days of contact lens wear. If the corneal edema persists for more than half an hour after lens removal, if it is more than 0.50 D (keratometry) if it involves the stroma, if it shows bubble formation, or if edema is more than 6% on pachymetry, it is usually indicative of a poor exchange and is abnormal.

Treatment

A steep lens is the most common cause of faulty exchange and is dealt with in one of the following ways.

- Reduce the overall diameter
- Reduce the optic zone
- Flatten the peripheral curves
- Blend the peripheral curves
- Order a new lens with flat base curve.

A thin lens should be replaced by a thicker lens or a lens with a larger diameter to promote lid action and thus tear exchange. No lens should have a thickness less than 0.10 mm. A flush fitting lens should be steepened by at least 0.37 diopters to achieve good exchange.

A steep lens, a thin lens and a flush fitting lens cause disturbances which are localized to the center of the cornea—upriding and low riding lens have already been dealt with under physical factors. An eccentrically placed lens is dealt with by one of the following methods, in order of preference.

- Increase the overall diameter
- Increase the optic zone diameter
- Steepen the base curve
- Steepen the peripheral curves
- Use of a small thick lens.

Undue Pressure Over the Cornea

This may be caused in the center of the cornea by a flat lens or at the periphery of the cornea by a steep lens. It may also be caused by a spherical lens over the astigmatic cornea.

Complaints

The patient feels the lens awareness more than normal. This feeling starts immediately after insertion and persists as long as the lens is worn. After a few hours, the patient develops tearing, burning and stinging.

Signs

A flat lens moves and the weight of the lens is borne by the central cornea which serves as a fulcrum. This area suffers metabolically by pressure, causing edema.

Characteristics of edema due to pressure are (1) Exactly 2.5 mm in diameter. (2) margins are clear cut (3) corresponds to the area of lens bearing (4) punctate staining, erosion and abrasion occur in the area over the edema.

Edema due to faulty exchange caused by a steep lens is characterized by:
- An area of 2.5–4 mm
- Blurred or hazy margins
- May contain a few bubbles of air
- May show stippling and punctate staining.

Fluorescein pattern of a flat lens may be difficult to make out due to excessive tearing. However, it is characterized by a central area of touch and peripheral pooling all around, under the area of lens lift. Later an abrasion may occur which will take up the fluorescein stain.

Treatment

Such a flat lens moves more and exerts more weight over a particular corneal area. *Excessive movement is avoided by:*
- Steepening the base curve
- Steepening the peripheral curve
- Increasing the overall diameter
- Increasing the optic zone diameter
- Decreasing the central thickness of the lens
- Decreasing the edge thickness of the lens
- Blending the peripheral curves.

Of the above steps, only blending and reduction in thickness can be done in same lens, the remaining require a new lens. Steepening the base curve and increasing the overall and optic zone diameters are better methods than others. Steepening by 0.37 diopter changes minimally flat fluorescein pattern into a steep fluorescein pattern.

Wearing Schedule Changes

Patient may gradually increase the wearing time in the beginning and restart, after discontinuation for a few days.
- One hour on the first day and one hour increase daily.
- One hour in the morning and one hour in the evening with one hour increase in both every day.
- One hour in the morning, one hour in the afternoon and one hour in the evening with one hour increase at each shift are better schedules than quick jumps by 2 or 4 hour increases at each shift.

The restart should never be more than 6 hours a day.

Complaints are noted when:
- If the routine schedule is not followed and lenses are overworn for an hour or so. There may be more irritation in the evening which is completely all right by morning.
- If lenses are overworn for several hours, restart is for several hours on the first day or there is a quick build-up in wearing hours say 2–4 hours increase every day, the patient may have irritation, watering, pain, photophobia and blepharospasm, usually one to two hours after lens removal.

Signs

In milder episodes there is a central edema with some stippling over it. In severe cases there is an area of diffuse central edema which is studded with multiple punctate spots which take the form of a uniform green carpet in the center when stained with fluorescein.

Treatment Prophylactic

Follow the wearing instructions and schedule religiously. Give a proper fit of contact lens.

Proper

The affected eye or eyes in severe cases are padded and bandaged with terramycin ophthalmic ointment. Analgesics and sedatives are given orally for relief of pain, proper rest advised.

Optical Problems

The most common denominator of optical complaints is the blurred vision. This can be caused by a wide variety of causes, discussed below:

Blurred Vision

This is a common complaint. It may start immediately after insertion or may be start after some time of wearing on the same day or after a few weeks or months.

Cause

It can be commonly caused by:
- Under correction
- Over correction
- Residual astigmatism
- Edge in the pupil
- Secretions over the lens surface
- A steep or a flat lens
- Warped lens

- Development of astigmatism in the cornea due to contact lens
- Increase in myopia
- Inconsistency of image due to presence of contact lens fluid in front of contact lens.

Complaints

Blur due to under or over correction, residual astigmatism and edge in the pupil starts immediately after insertion. Over correction is more common than under correction and the latter is less tolerated than the former. Secretions over the lens-surface cause symptoms immediately or sometimes later. A warped lens induced corneal astigmatism and increase in myopia are other causes of blurred vision which manifest immediately after insertion. Except for the warpage which may develop on any day, the other two set in after a few months of lens usage.

Blurred vision due to flat or steep lens starts, after some time of wear and is accompanied by symptoms, explained earlier.

Examination

- Edge may be found in the pupil; this has been dealt with earlier.
- By a refraction through the contact lens, under and over correction, residual astigmatism induced astigmatism and increase in myopia are detected.
- On fluorescein examination under a slit lamp, a flat and a steep lens is apparent, by a central and peripheral touch respectively. A warped lens is indicated by lack of simultaneous focus of all parts of the target by radioscope and focimeter.

Treatment

Having estimated the under correction, over correction, residual astigmatism, induced astigmatism and increased myopia by retinoscopy, spherical power directly ground over the lens. *The cylinder is prescribed as follows:*

- Half of the cylinder is given with the sphere.
- Full cylinder is given in the spectacles over the contact lens.
- Bitoric lens is given.
- Small cylinder may be ignored if vision is normal.

  Edge in the pupil has been dealt with earlier. Secretions over the surface of the lens are treated symptomatically. They may be due to (1) Constitutional factors, when a person secretes more of lipoid from the Meibomian glands, (2) Meibomian gland infection, (3) Staphylococcal infections of the lid margins (4) Allergic conjunctivitis, (5) Partial blinking and (6) Lens factors like a flat lens, steep lens, thick lens, thin lens, eccentric lens, bad edge and excessive movements. Secretions are treated by removing the cause and washing the face and the lens 4–5 times a day.

  Steep and flat lenses, their symptomatology and treatment have been dealt with earlier.

- *Ghost images:* This is an additional experience in comparison to spectacles. They are due to peripheral curve, especially when optical zone is small. This is due to difference in focus of center and periphery. The lens should be stabilized better in increase of the optic zone. Those who do not get over this difficulty might revert back to spectacles.
- Halos are formed by imperfections in the optical media or by edema of the epithelium and stroma.
  – Colored halos around white lights are due to edema of the cornea.
  – White halo seen as a white flare or a semicircle around objects is due to upriding lens. It is treated by better centration.
  – Halos due to of the surface tear film are always associated with radiation image scatter. A proper wetting solution corrects this.
- *Polyopia:* This is due to variable peripheral curves and rapid movements.
  Diplopia can be due to displacement of lens relative to the two eyes. This is like ghost images and is most disturbing at night particularly while driving. Contact lens users should not drive at night in the first 3 months, as edema will exaggerate complaints.
  This is treated with better lens form, i.e. the use of an aspheric front surface.
- *Spectacle blur:* Blurred vision occurs with spectacles when contact lenses are removed after having been worn for several hours. This is due to corneal edema. It should last for less than an hour only in the initial adaptation but in certain ill fitted patients, blur may last for a few hours to a few days.
  If the cornea is permanently warped the blur will be persistent. This is treated by getting better contact lens fitting which ensures proper tear circulation and this lens has the latest spectacle power.
- *Veiling:* A very common cause of early intolerance is depression or bubbles under contact lens due to edema caused by a bad fit. When the bubble is in the center, the dimming of vision is called "Dimple veiling".
- *Photophobia:* This may be produced by one or more of other following causes.
  – Contact lenses are closer to the eye. It collects more light compared to spectacles.
  – More transmission of short-wavelength light as compared to spectacles.
  – Irritation of the epithelium. It causes reflex photophobia along with mucus, lacrimation and hypotonic tear.
  – Glare is due to diffraction of light.
  – Edema remaining even after removal of the lens.
  – Decentered lens can produce this more often.
  – The spherical front curve of the lens tends to brighten the image, which produces photophobia.
- *Prismatic effect:* This is due to decentered lens, usually similar in both eyes, or if dissimilar it is usually compensated. Diplopia due to this factor is very rare.
- *Binocular single vision:* Visual discomfort due to underlying binocular imbalance may be caused by:
  – Contact lens induced aniseikonia.
  – Poor convergence in myopes with contact lenses.

- Accommodation/convergence as also accommodational imbalance can be troublesome.
- In unilateral aphakia (magnification discrepancy)
- It may be more of a problem due to prismatic imbalance for those who switch from spectacle to contact lens and therefore do not get adjusted to contact lenses.
- It can be noted by orthoptic and aniseikonic check up and treated by:
  - ♦ Orthoptic exercise
  - ♦ Aniseikonic glasses.
  - ♦ Advice to use contact lenses or glasses, whichever gives better orthoptic and functional results.

Accommodation Considerations

Accommodation plays an important part in contact lens practice (a) A patient may be over corrected due to stimulation of accommodation during refraction. The author has noted over correction in 96% of his cases when the power is calculated by refracting through the contact lens. It is ideal of assess the power under relaxed accommodation. For example, by making the patient watch an object at infinity, or under cycloplegia. (b) A myope in the presbyopic age group may precipitate his need for near add with contact lenses. This is due to change in powers of accommodation through spectacles compared to their values which calculated at the corneal level. A myope in the presbyopic age group should be educated about this difficulty before starting contact lenses.

- Every new patient for contact lenses should be refracted under relaxed accommodation to verify prescription. The patient should also be refracted through the contact lenses to rule out any discrepancy in power calculated theoretically and by refraction. This refraction through the contact lens excludes the possibility of over correction and is the best method to judge the residual cylinder.
- Accommodation of every myope in the presbyopic age should be assessed with glasses with trial contact lenses and if accommodation is weak with contact lenses, the impending difficulty of a near addition should be explained to him.

Differential Diagnosis and Solution of Common Problems

Burning

This is common symptom and may be immediate or delayed (after few hours). Immediate is due to dirty lens, allergy to solution or entry of a cleaning solution in the eye which is meant for external use only. There might be some stippling or stain which is confirmed by fluorescein.

Treatment

Use a proper solution. If the solution for external use goes into the eye, wash the eye thoroughly with saline and give pad and bandage with terramycin ointment (if it shows staining).

Delayed

Burning, which comes after some hours of wearing is usually due to faulty exchange, which has been dealt with earlier.

Deep Ache in the Eye

This usually comes after some hours of wearing. The lens is steep as confirmed by fluorescein.

Treatment

It is dealt with under faulty exchange.

Red Eyes

Conjunctivitis may occur due to contaminated lenses. Besides, iritis has been seen, in one out of 5000 cases. Redness may be immediate or delayed.

Immediate redness is caused by insertion, dirty lenses, bad edge flat lens or allergy to solution. Signs and treatment of above conditions have been dealt with earlier. A change of solution might help the patient if the solution does not suit him.

Delayed Redness

It is most often caused by a faulty exchange as detailed earlier.

Difficulty in Upgaze

This is normal during adaptation. Later it may be causes by a flat lens or a bad edge, which have been dealt with earlier.

Lid Swelling

Some degree of swelling is common in adaptation. A moderate degree is common in bad edge or flat lens, which irritate the lids. A severe lid swelling is caused by over wear and corneal abrasions.

Lens Displacement

This is commonly caused by a too flat or too small lens and is corrected by steepening the base curve and increasing the overall diameter by at least 0.5 mm respectively.

Oily secretion over the lens has been dealt with earlier.

Sudden acute pain like stabbing or cutting is usually due to a sharp lens edge striking against sclera or cornea. This might cause an abrasion on the eye which will be apparent by fluorescein stain.

Treatment

- *Prophylactic:* Do not dispense a lens with sharp edge
- *Proper:* If an abrasion has developed, treat it by pad and bandage after instillation of antibiotic eye drops.

Three and Nine O'clock staining

This is common occurrence. This is within the limbus at 3–9 O'clock positions. This can lead to chronic redness of the eye and opacification of the cornea and may be due to any of the following factors:

- Lids are held away by a thick lens and so do not wet that part of the cornea
- Sharp edge of lens rubs against the cornea
- Incomplete and poor blinking
- General dehydration
- Birth control pills
- Use of diuretics.

Treatment

The following treatment is recommended:
- Reduce the edge thickness.
- Provide good edge, i.e. flatter peripheral curves.
- Use of the ointment at night.
- Use of wetting solution three to four times a day.
- Increase the lens overall diameter to promote proper blinking.
- Patient should blink properly.
- Reduce the wearing time.

PSYCHOLOGICAL PROBLEMS

If the symptoms do not follow any definite pattern and are unaccompanied by correlative signs, the phenomenon is due to psychological reasons and is better attended to by giving psychotherapy rather than lens modification or change.

Blinking is the most important factor for proper tear exchange which the patient can control. It frequently decides between success and failure. Proper

Table 10.1 Pathologic reaction to contact lens wear

Complaint	Probable cause	Treatment
Excessive lacrimation	(Normal in adaptation)	Refit the contact lenses check edge
	Rough edge, improper and loose fit	
Lid swelling	Over wearing or imperfect fit adjust fit	Reduce wearing time decongestant eye drops
Difficulty in looking-up	Improper edge (normal in adaptation)	Recheck thickness and edge
Photophobia	Tight lens or too flat	Loosen if tight, refit in flat
Fluctuating vision	Excessive lacrimation too flat a lens (early stages normal)	Tighten lens
Fogging (Late)	Tight lens dirty lens	Loosen lens, clean wet and soak properly
Distortion	Tilting of lens (too small or too flat)	Make larger or steeper lens
Ring flare	OZ inadequately covering pupil	Make larger lens increase OZ
Visual acuity less than spectacles	Residual astigmatism improper lens power	Toric lens or change power
Reduced acuity	Warped lens, switched (late) or wrong lens	If warped better to replace, mark lenses
Hazing, halos fogging	Inadequate exchange of tears	Reduce OZ/flatter BC wider PC reduce lens size
Reading blur	Refractive problem poor blinking	Refraction through lens teach correct blinking
Pain after removal	Corneal edema	Flatter-wider BC
	Too tight lens	Make lens smaller or flatter or reduce OZ
Can't look up	Improper edge or sensitive lids if persistent	Check edge motivate patient to look up
Burning (hotness)	Tight lens corneal periphery flat	Reblend periphery
		Flatten lens clean the lens with wetting solution
Sharp cutting pain	Cracked, chipped or tight lens foreign body behind lens	Inspect lens carefully clean lens with wetting solution

Contd...

Contd...

Complaint	Probable cause	Treatment
Ache (Deep)	Tight lens	Loosen lens-flatter BC/reduce OZ
Itching	Allergic conjunctivitis	Treat conjunctivitis
Central touch	Lens flat	New lens steeper BC
Central pool with touch inside PC	Lens too steep Flatter PC	New lens flatter BC
Edge stands off	Flat PC	Make new lens with steeper PC
Lens shows off	Excessive corneal much rocking astigmatism	Toric secondary curve
Fine corneal stippling	Insufficient tear circulation width/ smaller lens	Loosen lens reduce OZ/increase PC
Zig-zag corneal staining	Foreign body under lens	Clean lens
Stain 12 or 6 O'clock position	Improper finish flat lens causing rocking steepen lens	Check lens edge give better blend and edge
Deep corneal stain with pain	Tight lens or too long wearing	Stop wearing lenses Loosen lens, Institute medical care
Unusual change in refraction	Lens too flat or tight	Take 'K' again after a week, refit
Mucus on lens	Conjunctivitis or scratched lens Polish lens	Treat conjunctivitis
Lens falls out	Too small or too flat	Larger or steeper lens
Lens rides to side	Astigmatism against rule	Make steep lens and reduce OZ or make toric secondary curve
Lens rides high	Too thick edge, pulled up by lid. Lens of flat	Small steep lens or lenticular lens (if tight upper lid high minus)
Conjunctival injection	Conjunctivitis or improper edge	Treat conjunctivitis check edge
Excessive movement of lens excessive lacrimation	Lens too loose	Tighten lens. Check corneal sensation
Insufficient movement of lens (No LAG)	Lens too tight dry eyes smaller lens. Check for hypothyroidism.	Flatter BC/reduced OZ
Displacement by lid	Edge too thick, lens too flat	CN bevel the edge, steep BC larger OZ
Bubbles under lens	Lens too steep	New lens flatter BC Flatter PC

Table 10.2 Pathological response to contact lens wear

Tissue	Causes	Effect
Epithelium	Pressure	Squamous cell membrane breakdown
	Hypoxia	Cells separation and edema cysts
	Desiccation	Basal cell flattening, cell loss, ulceration, infection
Basement membrane	Trauma	Recurrent erosion of basement membrane
Stroma	Water retention	Edema and collagen separation
	2° hypoxia	Keratocyte degeneration
	Immune response	Infiltration : white cells,
	Inflammatory response	fibroblasts
	Desiccation	Collagen lysis
Endothelium	pH imbalance	Cell vacuolation
and Descemets	2° to hypoxia	Cell separation
membrane	Cell morphology changes	
Lids	Trauma	Squamous blepharitis
	Infection	Exudative Blepharitis
	Immune response	Meibomianitis
	Papillary and follicular	
	Conjunctivitis	
Anterior chamber	Inflammatory	Anterior uveitis and cells

blinking can be achieved with proper exercise, the steps of which are: (1) Relax for a moment, (2) Close your eyes all the way shut, (3) Say pause-pause-pause, (4) Open the eyes and (5) Say pause again. These are five steps which are done 15 times a day and each time this blink cycle is repeated 10 times. This is done for 3–8 weeks and afterwards at a reduced level.

Pathological reactions due to contact lenses may be due to physical hypoxic, infective, allergic, toxic and due to tear film disturbances (Tables 10.1 and 10.2).

CHAPTER 11

Astigmatism

INTRODUCTION

Successfully fitting a contact lens over a cornea depends on its topography and the factors responsible for total astigmatism. The keratometer picks up approximately the central 3 mm, and the periphery of the cornea is totally ignored. Keratometer also determines the toricity: the physical property of cornea indicating the difference in the power of its two meridians. Astigmatism in contrast to toricity is the overall representation of the difference in the power of the two meridians of the eye.

It has been clearly demonstrated that:
- Fitting an alignment fit over a spherical cornea was physiologically unacceptable.
- Slight toricity (0.50 D) was best for successful physiological fit.
- Excessive toricity (over 2–3.00 D) caused problems and render the lens totally unacceptable, physically, physiologically and optically.

Although 3.00 D is the maximum tolerable toricity for a spherical contact lens fitting, the author has fitted corneas with 7.00 D of regular toricity and has failed to get a successful fit in certain spherical corneas due to marked peripheral corneal toricity.

CONSIDERATIONS ON CORRECTION OF ASTIGMATISM WITH RIGID GAS PERMEABLE LENSES

Factors which govern the correction of astigmatism with rigid gas permeable (RGP) are:
- Axis of astigmatism
- Relationship of corneal and spectacle astigmatism
- Amount of corneal astigmatism
- Lens thickness/material flexibility
- Fitting relation.
  1. *Axis of astigmatism:* With the rule astigmatism is easy to fit, against the rule is difficult to fit and may require a toric lens, the oblique gives variable results.
  2. *Relation of corneal to spectacle astigmatism:* Best results are obtained in fitting if both are with the rule and the difference in amount is nil or within ± 0.50 D.

     If direction is opposite or the difference between the corneal and spectacle astigmatism is more than ± 0.50 D, residual astigmatism occurs and toric lens may be required.

3. *Amount of astigmatism:* It is possible to correct 2.50 D astigmatism with most RGP lenses especially when it is with the rule.

Higher astigmatism, i.e. over 2.50 D if corneal, require toric lenses for better centration. Higher refractive/spectacle astigmatism may require toric lens for optical reason (to correct residual astigmatism).

4. *Lens thickness/material flexure:* For every RGP lens there is a critical thickness at which flexure is minimized and oxygen, transmissibility is maximized. More thickness will not assist in correcting the astigmatism and will decrease oxygen transmissibility. Thickness less than critical increases the flexure therapy and reduces the amount of astigmatism that can be corrected.

5. *Fitting relationship:* A flat fit corrects more astigmatism than the steep or aligned fit.

A steep fit results in greater flexure and therefore, a variable vision with each blink.

RESIDUAL ASTIGMATISM

This is the astigmatism which remains after the contact lens has been placed over the cornea to correct the ametropia. It may be physiological or contact lens induced. *The former can be due to:*
- Anterior corneal cylinder left neutralized by the tear fluid
- Posterior surface of cornea may be a factor
- Tilt of the crystalline lens of the eye
- Difference in the curvature of the meridians at lens interfaces
- Variations in the refractive indices of cornea, lens and vitreous
- Oblique incidence of light
- Eccentric position of the fovea
- Misalignment of optical constituents of the eye
- Irregularity in the shape of the macular area.

Lens induced residual astigmatism (RA) may be due to:
- Tilt of the contact lens
- Lag or sag of the contact lens
- Warpage
- Bitoric lens
- Change in the corneal toricity due to lens wear.

Prefitting Assessment of Residual Astigmatism

By subtracting the keratometric cylinder from the spectacle cylinder (at corneal level) residual astigmatism can be predicted. Keratometer cylinder (K) is taken as a minus cylinder along flat 'K.'

Example: Keratometry 43.00 at 180° and 44.00 at 90°
Spectacle Rx –2.00 D sphere –0.50 cylinder 180°
Residual astigmatism = spectacle Rx – K
–0.50 cylinder at 180°
K = – (–1.00 D cylinder, axis 180°/+0.50 D cylinder axis 180)

This theoretical value usually does not tally with the measured value, obtained by retinoscopy through the fitted contact lens. *The discrepancy may be due to any one of the following factors:*

- Cornea being aspheric
- Incident ray not at right angles to the cornea
- Incident ray not at right angles to the contact lens
- Error in keratometry
- Error in manufacture of the contact lens.

It has been the author's experience that the retinoscopic value of residual cylinder is usually half to one-third of the predicted value.

It is best to assess the RA by retinoscopy when the difference in axis of the retinoscopic and keratometric cylinder is more than 20°.

The author made a detailed analysis of 132 eyes. It was observed that the average residual astigmatism (RA) was 0.66 D (range 0–1.75 D). *Further, the following interesting features were noted:*

- *Type*
  Residual astigmatism against the rule 78 (59.09%)
  Residual astigmatism with the rule 30 (22.73%)
  No residual astigmatism 24 (18.18%)
- *Difference between theoretical or predicted and retinoscopic residual astigmatism:*
  - Retinoscopic RA tallies with theoretical 30 (22.73%)
  - Retinoscopic RA tallies with theoretical 102 (77.30%)
    - (b-1) Retinoscopic RA less than theoretical 78 (59.09%)
    - (b-2) Retinoscopic RA more than theoretical 24 (19.18%).
- *Other observations during the study were:*
  - Spectacle cylinder is almost always more than keratometric cylinder in against the rule cylindrical spectacle prescription.
  - When spectacle and keratometric cylinder are of opposite sing that is one with and the other against the rule, the spectacle cylinder is more than keratometric cylinder, and the former is usually against the rule.
  - Residual astigmatism is against the rule when spectacle and keratometric cylinder are of opposite signs.
  - Residual cylinder is against the rule when spectacle and keratometric cylinder are against the rule.

The author has documented the importance of contact lens trial in 20% of the astigmatic cases, which did not improve with spectacles. Amongst this group, 64% improved with contact lenses. This will reduce the number of astigmatic amblyopes with spectacles.

Fitting Techniques

Toric cornea can be fitted by:
- Spheric base curve
- Toric base curve and spheric front
- Toric base curve and toric front.

Spheric Base Curve and Spheric Front Curve

This is the most common solution for corneal toricity. The author chooses the base curve (BC) which gives a dumb bell-shaped fluorescein pattern. However, factors like physical comfort, positioning of the lens, residual astigmatism and physiological results after few hours of wear have also to be considered.

Choice of the Spheric Base Curve

Various methods have been advocated:
- Split the K (BC is in-between the keratometric readings)
- Use an ultra thin lens on 'k' (7.5–9.00 mm)
- Large lens on 'k' (9.5–10.5 mm)
- Double truncation
- Toric peripheral curves.

The authors think that split method is a good method for choice of BC. If the rule of finalization of BC is to get a dumb bell fluorescein pattern, then the authors' rule of adding 1/4 or 1/3 of the difference between the two keratometric reading to the flat 'K' may not be rigidly followed.

Residual cylinder with a spheric BC can be tackled by:
- Giving spherical equivalent in contact lens, if patient does not want glasses over the contact lens or if complex lens construction is not possible.
- Giving a cylinder on the anterior lens surface which has to be kept oriented by one of the following.
  – Prism-ballast (for a high lower lid). This lens is physically, physiological and visually unsatisfactory.
  – Single truncation (for high upper and high lower lid).
  – Double truncation for small palpebral aperture below 9.00 mm and against the rule toricity.
  – Scleral flange.
  – Toric peripheral curve (when corneal periphery is more toric) and center is moderately toric.
  – Bitoric contact lens.
  – Dynamic stabilization.

Toric Base Curve and Spheric Front Curve

Spheric front and toric back curve are used to obtain a good physical fit over a toric cornea where spheric base curve gives an unsatisfactory fit. Certain optical properties need consideration here.

- If there is an against the rule residual astigmatism with a spheric base curve lens and the cornea has against the rule toricity, there will be reduction or elimination of the residual astigmatism if a toric base curve is used over such a lens. This is due to correction of residual minus cylinder 90° by the induced minus cylinder at 90° to the toric base curve.
- If there is an against the rule residual astigmatism with a spheric BC lens and with the rule toricity, there will be an exaggeration of the residual astigmatism.

The induced cylinder of the toric lens over a with-the-rule cornea will be a minus cylinder at 180° or a plus cylinder at 90°. The meridian is made more myopic; so residual astigmatism is increased.

- If a spheric lens shows no residual astigmatism the toric lens will induce astigmatism equal to half of the keratometric difference between the two meridians of the toric base curve.

Bitoric Lens

Has a front and a back cylinder and is indicated:
- To avoid rocking, eccentricity and prism effect on the lens
- To avoid irritation of the upper lid
- To avoid residual astigmatism
- To avoid bigger lens without loosening the fit
- To avoid rotation of the anterior surface cylinder
- To avoid loose fit in aphakia.

Such a lens is best physically, physiologically and optically if:
- It is fitted flatter on both meridians than the keratometric readings
- Smaller sized lens (8–9 mm) is used
- Optic zone diameter is bigger than the pupillary diameter.

TORIC LENSES

Optical Principles

Toric BC induces cylindrical effect, which may exaggerate or diminish the residual cylinder.

The cylinder power of a toric back surface lens of refractive index 1.49 can be summarized as follows.
- Cylinder power of a toric back surface lens in air is equal to $\Delta KCl \times 1.452$,
- Cylinder power of a toric lens surface on the eye is $\Delta KCl \times 0.452$.

ΔKCl is a minus cylinder with axis along flat meridian as measured by keratometer.

It may be summarized as follows:

To convert from	to	multiply by
Contact lens surface power in air	contact lens surface power in fluid	0.314
K reading on contact lens surface	Contact lens surface power in air	1.452
K reading of contact lens surface	Contact lens surface power in fluid	0.452

a = 1.336–1.490/1–1.490 = 0.314
b = 1–1.490/1–1.3375 = 1.452
c 1.336–1.491/1–1.3375 = 0.452

If keratometric reading are 43.00 D and 45.00 D, Δ K is 2.00, cylinder power on lensometer is given 2 × 1.452 = 2.90 D: When the above lens is kept over the cornea, the value of cylinder is 2 × 0.452 = 0.90 D.

STEPS IN FITTING TORIC SOFT LENSES

Trial Set Fit

- *The trial lenses:*
  - *Base curve:* It should be slightly flatter than the flatter keratometric (K) reading.
  - *Diameter:* The lens should be 2.0–2.5 mm larger than the visible iris diameter.
  - *Sphere power:* The sphere power closest to the patient's Rx. Adjust the vertex distance for Rx > –4.00
  - *Cylinder power:* Should be less or equal to the patient's Rx.
  - *Cylinder axis:* Should be the closest to the patient's Rx.
- Place the trial lens for at least 20 minutes before evaluation.
- Check for comfort.
- *Check for the fit:*
  - Adequate movement
  - Good centration
  - Stable and consistent orientation (no more than 10 seconds for the lens to return to its initial stable orientation).
- *Verify the base curve:*
  - If too much movement, steepen the base curve.
  - If too little movement, flatten the base curve.
- *Check the lens rotation:* Check the lens rotation by means of laser marks at 3 and 9 O'clock or at 6 O'clock. Record the amount of rotation and the direction of the rotation. If the lens rotates to the practitioner's left direction, the amount of deviation in degrees is added to the spectacle axis (forget about the axis of the trial lens and take into consideration the prescription's axis to use in adding or subtracting). If the rotation is to the practitioner's right, the amount of deviation in degrees is subtracted from spectacle axis (LARS rule: Left add, Right subtract).
  PS: One clock hour = 30°.
- Over refract with sphere if all the other parameters are acceptable. The order lens should orient itself on the eye like the trial lens did the final position, rotation on blinking should be less than 5°.
- *Final lens selection:*
  - *Base curve:* Same as the trial lens.
  - *Lens diameter:* 2.0–2.5 mm larger than the visible iris diameter (VID)
  - *Sphere power:* Add spherical over refraction to sphere power of trial lens; correct for vertex distance.
  - *Cylinder power:* Same as trial lens cylinder.
  - *Cylinder axis:* Use "LARS = Left add; Right subtract".

- If rotation is to the left, add the amount of trial lens rotation to the axis from the spectacle refraction (Do not add it to the trial lens axis).
- If rotation is to the right, subtract the amount of rotation from the axis obtained in the spectacle refraction. For example, Spectacle Rx at the plane of the cornea: $-2.00 - 2.50 \times 10°$

  Contact lens (trial set): $-2.00 - 1.50 \times 10°$

  Lens rotation: 20° to the left

  Appropriate lens power for the patient: $-2.00 - 1.50 \times 30°$

The LARS technique is a viable way to compensate for on-eye lens rotation. However, it is important to remember that this technique does not correct for residual errors that may be present secondary to:

- Cylinder masking
- Vertex distance error.
- Tear effects flatter add plus (FAP), steeper add minus (SAM).
- Lens flexure effect.

  Resultant: Cross cylinder effect.

  Requires: Spherocylinder over refraction. Therefore, to identify both lens rotation and lens power requirements, the use of the sphero-cylinder over-refraction (SCOR) and LARS technique is important. The SCOR technique is used when the cylinder is higher than 3.00/4.00 D.

DISPENSING THE LENS

- Place the lens on the patient's eyes
- Allow to equilibrate (20 minutes)
- Record visual acuity
- Verify the lens fit and orientation with a slit lamp. *Fitting criteria should demonstrate:*
  - Acceptable visual acuity
  - Corneal coverage with 0.5–1 mm of movement with straight-ahead gaze
  - Stable orientation of laser mark.
- Allow patient to wear the lens for one week if visual acuity and fit are acceptable.

Presently due to presence of a high range of lenses available in the inventory, the fitting of toric soft contact lens has become simple and not as cumbersome as done before. The toric soft contact lens of the nearest power is placed on the eye and the rotation is checked and the axis is refined. There is no need to do the earlier 10 step procedure.

CHAPTER 12

Keratoconus

DEFINITION

It is an ectatic condition of the central cornea becoming manifest at puberty and resulting in visual impairment due to development of irregular astigmatism. It is always eccentrically displaced.

EPIDEMIOLOGY

Onset of keratoconus occurs immediately after puberty with mean age of onset being 16 years; however, onset has been reported to occur as early as 6 years of age. Keratoconus rarely develops after 30 years of age. Keratoconus shows no gender predilection and is bilateral in over 90% of cases. In general, the disease develops asymmetrically, diagnosis of the disease in the second eye lags about five years after diagnosis in the first.

PATHOLOGY

The process starts as fibrillation and fragmentation of the basement membrane of the epithelium followed by progressive thinning and scarring of the stroma. Deposits of inter lamellar granular material indicate altered activity of corneal cells (keratocytes).

Course

Usually the process may progress for four to five years and then remain arrested, or it may restart after remaining stationary or it may be acute in progression, it is milder in unilateral cases. In bilateral cases, it is milder in the eye involved later. Author has documented dioptric changes in well-fitted keratoconus patients over a period of 7 years. Of these, 70% of the cases showed an increase, 7% showed a decrease and 13% remained stationary in dioptric power as assessed by over refraction.

Symptoms

The patient presents with defective vision that fails to improve with spectacles despite repeated astigmatic refractive correction demanded by the eye. The patient may be slightly photophobic and keeps the lids partially closed. There

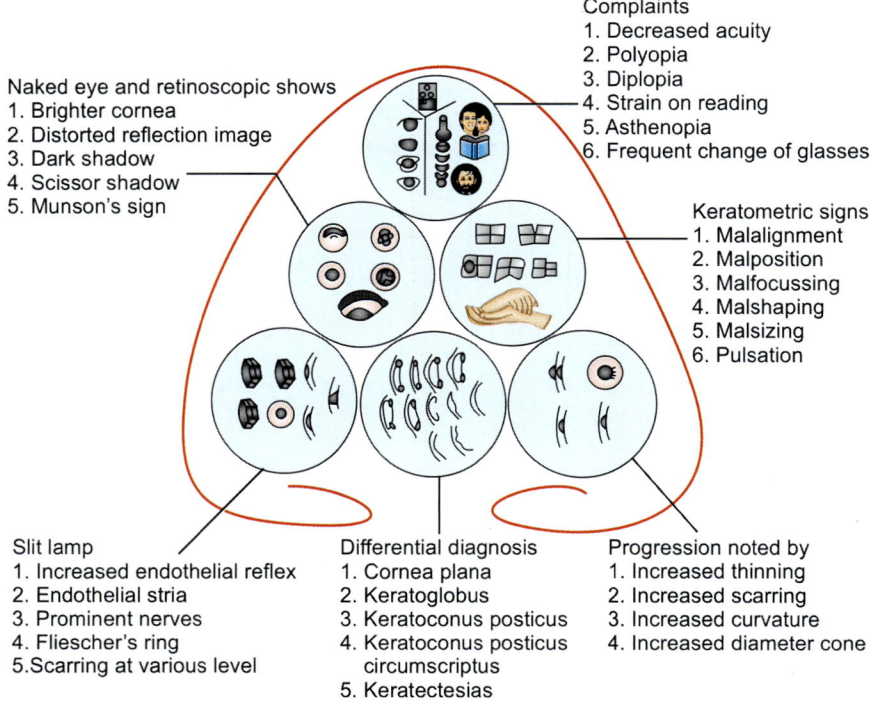

Complaints
1. Decreased acuity
2. Polyopia
3. Diplopia
4. Strain on reading
5. Asthenopia
6. Frequent change of glasses

Naked eye and retinoscopic shows
1. Brighter cornea
2. Distorted reflection image
3. Dark shadow
4. Scissor shadow
5. Munson's sign

Keratometric signs
1. Malalignment
2. Malposition
3. Malfocussing
4. Malshaping
5. Malsizing
6. Pulsation

Slit lamp
1. Increased endothelial reflex
2. Endothelial stria
3. Prominent nerves
4. Fliescher's ring
5. Scarring at various level

Differential diagnosis
1. Cornea plana
2. Keratoglobus
3. Keratoconus posticus
4. Keratoconus posticus circumscriptus
5. Keratectesias

Progression noted by
1. Increased thinning
2. Increased scarring
3. Increased curvature
4. Increased diameter cone

Fig. 12.1 Diagrammatic representation of features of keratoconus

may be diplopia or polyopia. Sudden diminution of vision may occur due to acute hydration, accompanied by pain lacrymation, photophobia and whiteness of the cornea. Figure 12.1 gives complete information about keratoconus diagrammatically.

Signs

On oblique illumination the cornea is usually bright. It may show opacification at the apex and pigmentation around the base. It may deform the lower lid during downgaze (Munson's sign) (Fig. 12.2). On scleral scatter, a sharply focused light illuminates the opposite limbus. On close follow-up thinning usually starts in inferior side, it progresses temporally and goes around and superior nasal is usually left uninvolved.

Slit Lamp Examination Reveals

- Thinning of cornea in center
- Bright endothelial reflex
- Fleischer ring "A yellow or olive green line forming a complete or incomplete ring around the base of the cone at the level Bowman's membrane". This is better seen under UV light

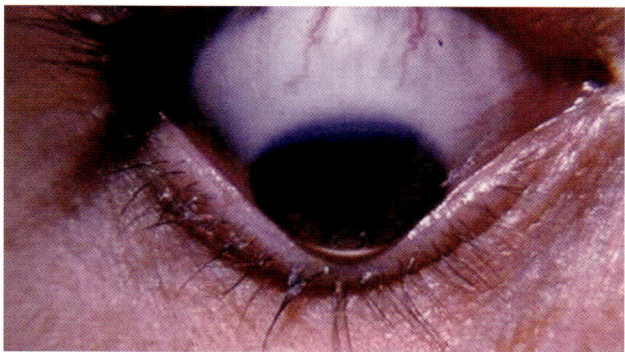

Fig. 12.2 Munson's sign

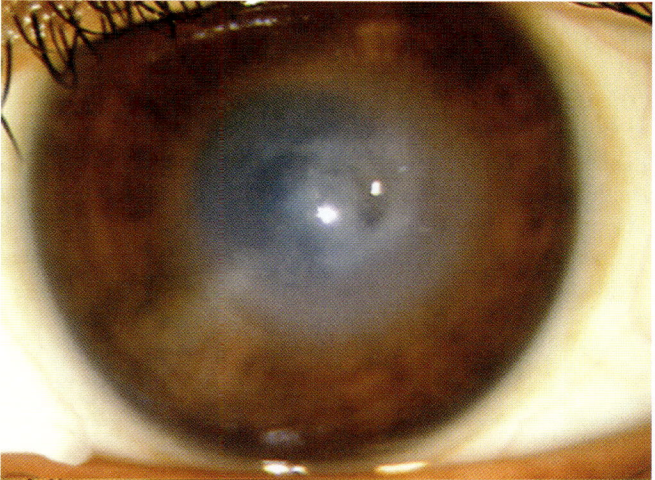

Fig. 12.3 Acute hydrops

- Prominent corneal nerves
- Vogt stripes or striae in deep stroma
- Corneal scarring
- Descemet's rupture and acute water logging of cornea (Fig. 12.3).

Retinoscopy

It shows a dark reflex against red background, yawning reflex or irregular shadows. Keratoconus is suspected in high astigmatic error. This dark reflex is called "oily droplet" reflex.

Keratometry

Keratometry may show malalignment, malapposition, malsizing malshaping, malfocussing, and pulsation of mires.

Corneal Topography

Corneal topographic maps are very useful tools for early detection of keratoconus and forme fruste keratoconus. The placido based topographic maps provide information about corneal curvature and details about the anterior corneal surface (Fig. 12.4). The slit scanning based Orbscan and the Scheimpflug image based pentacam provide information about both anterior and posterior surface (Figs 12.5 and 12.6).

Early Diagnosis

The author feels that retinoscopy and keratometry help in formulating a diagnosis at a very early stage. Nothing is in fact more diagnostic than a demonstrable keratometric steepening of the cornea. The author has seen keratoconic changes in highly myopic astigmatic errors. Munson's sign, placido disc, photokeratoscopy, Moiré keratometry, and small mire keratometry have been compared with differential pachymetry (comparing the thinnest cornea with the thickness at a point 35° outside). Though differential pachymetry is said to be the earliest diagnostic tool, the author does not agree to this, especially in stationary cases of keratoconus.

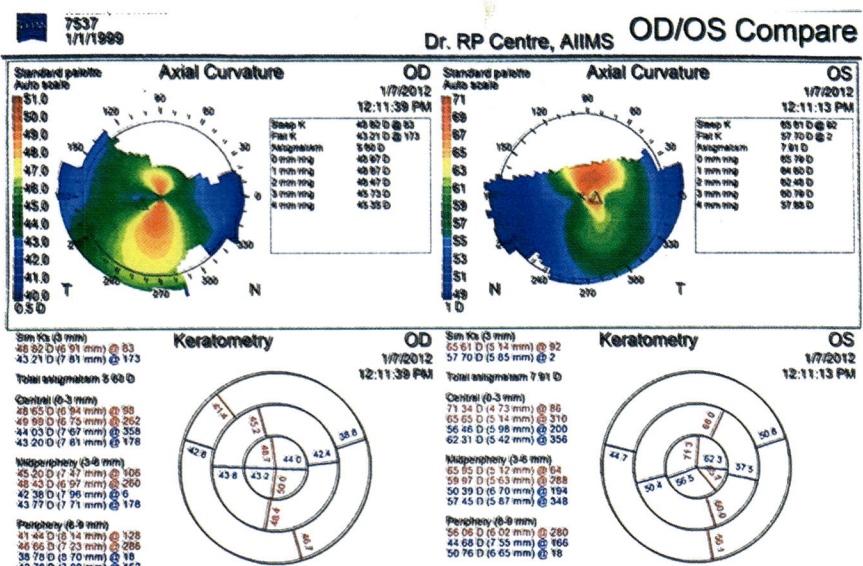

Fig. 12.4 Placido disc topography showing keratoconus

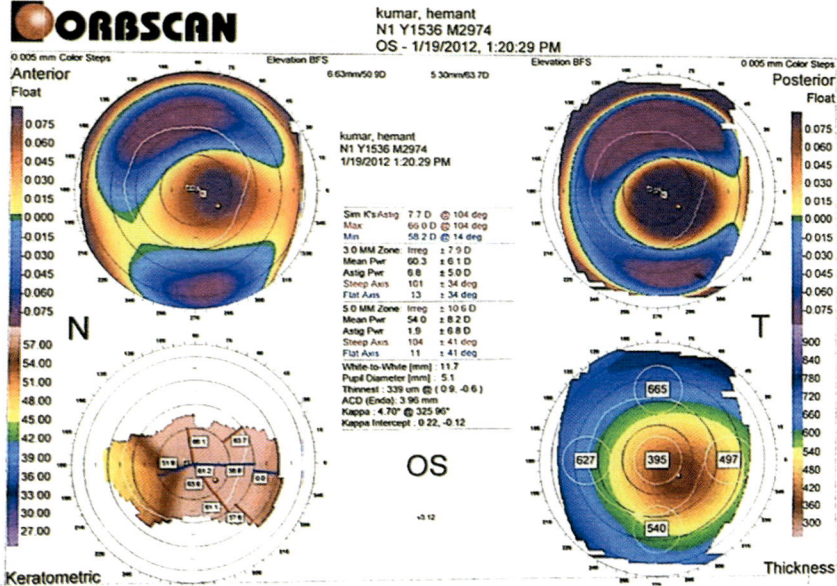

Fig. 12.5 Slit scanning topography showing evidence of keratoconus

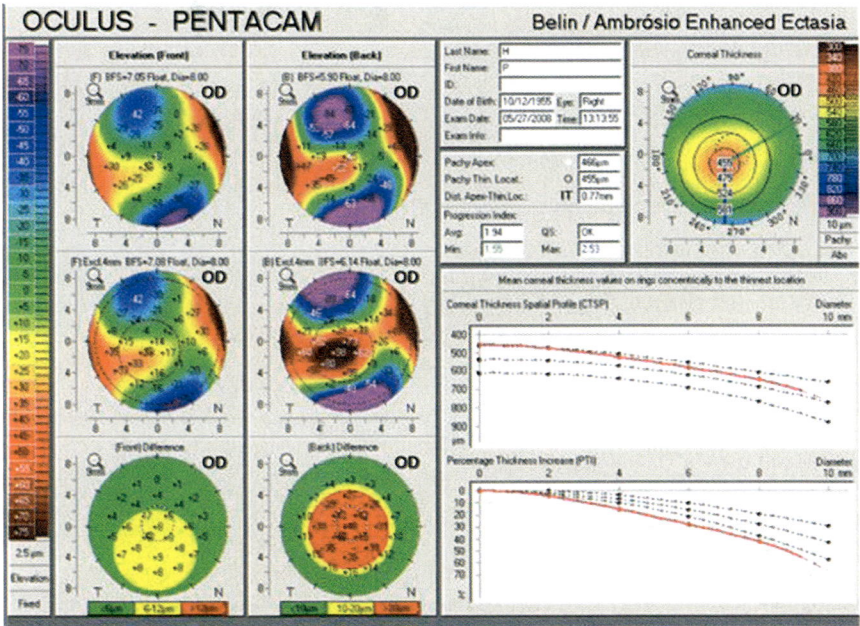

Fig. 12.6 Scheimpflug imaging showing evidence of keratoconus

Classification Systems

Keratoconus can be classified by cone shape, central keratometric reading, or progression. The simplest classification systems are based on keratometric reading or shape.

Based on Severity of Curvature

- Mild <45 D in both meridians
- Moderate 45–52 D in both meridians
- Advanced >52 D in both meridians
- Severe >62 D in both meridians

Based on Shape of Cone

- Nipple small diameter (<5 mm); round shape; easiest to fit with contact lenses
- Oval large diameter (>5 mm); often displaced inferiorly; more difficult to fit with lenses, most common by topography
- Globus largest diameter (>6 mm); 75% of cornea affected; most difficult to fit with lenses.

AMSLER KRUMEICH CLASSIFICATION

Stage I

- Eccentric steeping
- Myopia and astigmatism < 5.00 D
- Mean central K readings < 48.00 D

Stage II

- Myopia and astigmatism from 5.00 D to 8.00 D
- Mean central K readings < 53.00 D
- Absence of scarring
- Minimum corneal thickness >400 μm.

Stage III

- Myopia and astigmatism from 8.00 D to 10.00 D
- Mean central K readings >53.00 D
- Absence of scarring
- Minimum corneal thickness 300–400 μm.

Stage IV

- Refraction not measurable
- Mean central K readings >55.00 D

- Central corneal scarring
- Minimum corneal thickness 200 μm.

MANAGEMENT OF KERATOCONUS

The treatment approach to keratoconus follows an orderly progression from glasses to contact lenses to corneal transplantation. Keratoconus is initially managed conservatively with spectacles and contact lens. During the early stages of this disease, vision may still be correctable to 6/6 with glasses or contact lenses. However, as this disease progresses, there are situations when the patient cannot achieve optimum visual acuity with glasses or contact lens. Surgical management in the form of lamellar and penetrating keratoplasty are valid options in such situations. Over 90% of corneal transplants are successful with the majority of patients obtaining vision of 6/12 or better afterwards with either glasses or contact lenses.

Conservative management of keratoconus includes improvement by providing good optical aids. The mainstay of management remains use of rigid gas permeable contact lens. A gas permeable lens covers the irregular protrusion on the cornea and makes a new smooth surface for the light to bend through. Apart from these, management of other associated ocular and systemic problems should also be taken care off. Over the years there have been many different techniques advocated to fit contact lenses on patients of keratoconus. The goal of any contact lens is to provide adequate vision with maximum comfort over a prolonged period of time.

Contact Lens Options for Keratoconus

When a keratoconic patient is no longer able to obtain good visual acuity as a result of increasing levels of irregular astigmatism and higher-order aberrations, rigid contact lenses will be required, effectively to provide a new anterior surface to the eye. Contact lenses are considered when vision is not correctible to 6/9 by spectacles and patients become symptomatic. There are many lens designs for keratoconus and it is difficult to predict which design will be suitable for any particular patient.

Rigid Gas Permeable Lenses

Rigid gas permeable (RGP) corneal lenses are the lenses of first choice for correcting the irregular astigmatism, which occurs as the cornea changes shape. The aim is to provide the best vision possible with the maximum comfort so that the lenses can be worn for a long period of time. A mid to high Dk/t material is preferred as it provides the stability required for these high-powered lenses. A balance is required between a material, which is deposit resistant especially in patients who may be atopic, and providing sufficient oxygen flux. Keratoconic patients tend to have long wearing times and usually become long-term lens wearers. In some cases it may become necessary for the contact lens practitioner to try several different materials for a patient who has poor wettability.

Fitting Methods/Philosophies

Three-point-touch Design (Fig. 12.7)

The three-point-touch design is the most popular and the most widely fitted design for keratoconic patients. The aim is to distribute the weight of the contact lens as evenly as possible between the cone and the peripheral cornea. The ideal fit should show an apical contact area of 2–3 mm with mid-peripheral contact annulus. The area and shape of the contact zones may be more variable as a result of cone asymmetry; a crescent shaped mid-periphery is quite acceptable. Adequate edge clearance is required to ensure tear exchange. Three-point-touch actually refers to the area of apical central contact and two other areas of bearing or contact at the mid-periphery in the horizontal direction. This type of fitting philosophy works very well for small central cones.

Apical Clearance

In this type of fitting technique, the lens vaults the cone and clears the central cornea, resting on the paracentral cornea. This type of lens was suggested as it was argued that apical clearance would minimize trauma to the central cornea. These lenses tend to be small in diameter and have small optic zones; the small BOZD can result in glare problems. The potential advantages of reducing central corneal scarring are outweighed by the disadvantages of poor tear film, corneal edema, and poor visual acuity as a result of bubbles becoming trapped under the lens.

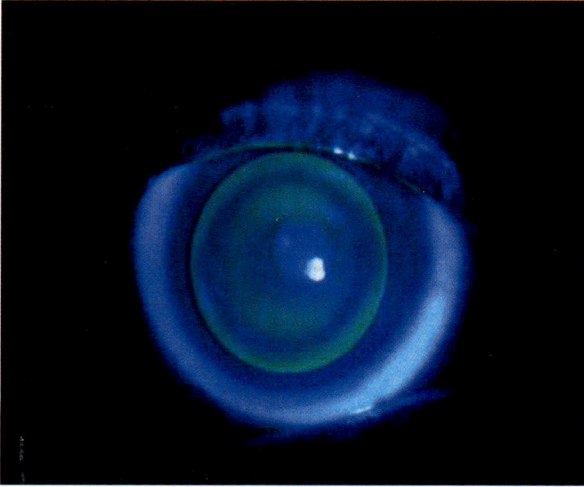

Fig. 12.7 RGP fitting in keratoconus—Three point touch

Flat Fitting

The flat fitting method places almost the entire weight of the lens on the cone. The lens tends to be held in position by the top lid. Good visual acuity is obtained as a result of apical touch. Wide edge stand-off cannot usually be eliminated. Alignment can be obtained in early keratoconus; however, flat fitting lenses can lead to progression/acceleration of apical changes and corneal abrasions. This type of fitting philosophy is useful where the apex of the cone is displaced.

Rigid Gas Permeable Lens Designs

There are numerous different designs available. A list follows of some of the designs commonly used. *Different types of RGP lens designs:*
- *Early keratoconus*
    - Aspherics or multicurve lenses
    - Kera I and II (No. 7)
    - Acuity K
    - Rose K
- *Moderate keratoconus*
    - Kera II
    - Quasar KNO7
    - Rose K
    - Woodward KC3
- *Moderate/advanced keratoconus*
    - Kera II/III
    - Rose K
    - Profile K
- *Advanced keratoconus*
    - Large diameter lenses
    - S-Lim
    - Dyna Intra-Limbal (No. 7)
    - Scleral lenses
    - PMMA
    - Gas permeable (innovative sclerals).

Aspheric Lenses

Aspheric lenses flatten in curvature from the center to the periphery. The eccentricity or 'e value' is independent of the base curve and determines the rate of flattening. Spherical lenses, on the other hand, have a constant radius of curvature in the optic zone and different curvatures cut into the lens in the peripheral areas. The average cornea has an 'e value' of 0.65. Decreasing the lens 'e value' decreases the rate of flattening; increasing the 'e value' increases the rate of flattening. The aim of aspheric lens fit should be good centration, central alignment or slight central bearing, good movement (1 mm), and peripheral clearance (0.5 mm). Useful for oval type cones are aspheric lenses, e.g. the Quasar

K (No. 7 Contact Lens Laboratory) or the Persecon Elliptical K (Ciba Vision) older design.

Multicurve Designs

All lens parameters are available from the manufacturers, which make these lenses easy to fit. The Woodward C3K is a specialist design, which can be used for moderate to advanced keratoconus.

McGuire Lens System

This lens system is based on the Soper lens system, which is no longer used in the UK. The McGuire system was first introduced in 1978 and consists of three diagnostic lens sets, nipple, oval or globus (see cone classification). The optic zone sizes vary from 6 mm for the nipple cone to 6.5 mm for the oval cone, and 7 mm for the Globus. The McGuire system has four peripheral curves; the secondary curve of the system is 0.5 mm flatter than the central base curve. The third curve is 1mm flatter than the secondary curve. The fourth and final peripheral curve is 2 mm flatter than the third curve.

Rose K

The Rose K is a unique keratoconus lens design with complex computer-generated peripheral curves based on data collected by Dr Paul Rose of Hamilton, New Zealand. The system (26 lens set) incorporates a triple peripheral curve system—standard, flat, steep—in order to achieve the ideal edge lift of 0.8 mm. The design starts with a standard 8.7 mm diameter and works by decreasing the optic zone diameter as the base curve gets steeper. It is available in base curves of 4.75–8.0 mm and diameters of 7.9–10.2 mm. Toric curves are available on the front and back surfaces as well as in the periphery. The practitioner has a choice of peripheral curves. Standard lift lenses should work 70% of the time. Peripheral curves can be configured to a toric design. Rose K lenses are very widely used.

Dyna Intra-Limbal

Dyna intra-limbal (DIL) lenses are useful when stability is required, especially in inferiorly displaced cones or in cases of pellucid marginal degeneration as well as post-graft. A range of diameters is available (10.8 mm to 12.5 mm). High DK materials are recommended.

Soft Lenses

These (hydrogels, silicone hydrogels) have a limited role in correcting corneal irregularity, as they tend to drape over the surface of the cornea and result in poor visual acuity. However, soft lenses designed specifically for keratoconus (e.g. Kerasoft) have a useful role in early keratoconus or where a patient may be intolerant of RGP. Soft lenses tend to be more comfortable compared with

RGPs. For example, Kerasoft lenses (Ultravision) (58% water content polymer), which are available in four series, A, B, C and D, and acuity K mark I and II (Acuity contact lenses).

Advantages

- They afford higher levels of comfort and longer wearing times, especially in patients intolerant of RGP corneal lenses or in monocular keratoconus.
- They are useful where the cone apex may be displaced, especially if it is very low.
- They are useful for certain groups of patients, for example, airline pilots.
- They are relatively simple to fit.

Disadvantages

- Visual acuity may be variable in cases of very high minus lenses.
- Low-powered diagnostic lenses may not provide an accurate guide to the fit of the final lens, which may be extremely high powered.
- There may be reduced oxygen transmissibility and the risk of neovascularization if the lenses are over worn.
- If the condition has progressed, it may be difficult to change to RGP's at a later stage.

Piggyback Lenses

Piggyback lenses are used for difficult cases, for instance in cases of RGP lens intolerance, presence of nebulae in keratoconus, or apical dimpling or where there are areas of recurrent epithelial erosion. The system consists of a rigid lens fitted on top of a soft lens. The aim is to maintain the same level of visual acuity as with a single lens. The RGP lens should be fitted first. Good centration is important and a slightly larger area of apical touch is usually acceptable, as the RGP lens will be cushioned by a soft lens (Fig. 12.8). A silicone hydrogel soft lens should be used where possible, with good movement and coverage/centration as in a normal soft lens fitting. Caring for the two types of lenses can be difficult long-term. Ideally, try to have the patient use the same care regime for the two lenses as this will make cleaning easier, or alternatively consider a disposable soft lens. The cornea should be observed carefully for dryness and neovascularization.

Hybrid Lens System

The Softperm lens (Ciba Vision) is a hybrid lens with a RGP center surrounded by a soft hydrophilic skirt. These lenses tend to be used in cases of RGP lens intolerance. There are many advantages to the Softperm lens as it provides better comfort than the rigid gas permeable (RGP) lenses, better centration and reasonable visual acuity. In the HES, these lenses tend to be used only in exceptional cases because of the risk of induced corneal edema and neovascularization. The

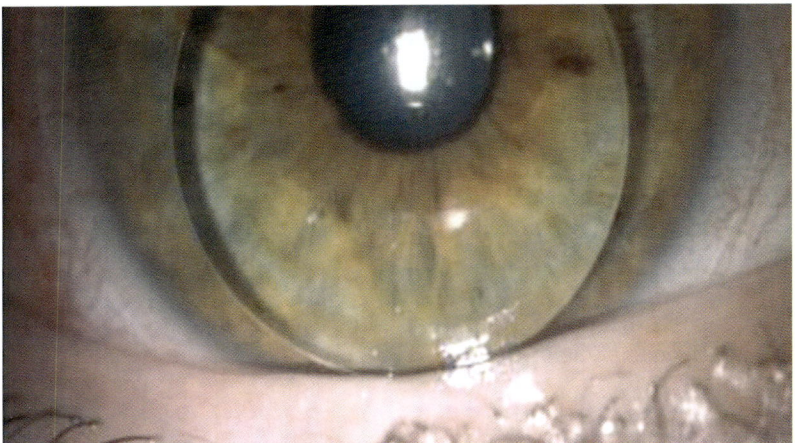

Fig. 12.8 Piggyback contact lens in keratoconus

main disadvantages of Softperm lenses are frequent breakage of the lens, giant papillary conjunctivitis and peripheral corneal neovascularization. It should be noted that the Softperm lens was not designed for keratoconus, but for a normal cornea. As it provides the comfort of a soft lens and visual acuity of a rigid lens it has been adopted by keratoconic patients who inevitably over-wear these lenses and end up with complications.

Scleral Lenses

Scleral lenses play a very significant role in cases of advanced keratoconus where corneal lenses do not work and corneal surgery is contraindicated. Scleral lenses completely neutralize any corneal irregularity and can help patients maintain a normal quality of life. These are of two types, i.e. sealed or those permitting tear exchange and can be used for moderate to advanced keratoconus. These are also being manufactured in India, e.g. Chandra Scleral Lens, a highly oxygen permeable rigid (120 DK) scleral contact lens. A PMMA lens can be used in cases of scleral toricity. PMMA scleral lenses are made by the impression method. This practice is confined to the HES. An impression is taken of the cornea, generally with alginate material (orthoprint) and a clear shell is made from polymethyl methacrylate material. Optic curves are ground on to the shell. This can be done in-house or the shell can be sent to Cantor and Nissel. The shell is fenestrated, adjusted, and ground until a desirable fit is obtained. Once an acceptable fit is obtained the lens can be sent for working to the required power.

Advantages

- Easy to insert and remove
- Any type of corneal irregularity is corrected

- Easy to store (dry)
- Long life

Disadvantages

- Much chair time is needed
- A very specialized fitting technique

Rigid Gas Permeable Sclerals

Ken Pullum (Innovative sclerals) confirms that these lenses are fitted from a preformed design and lathe cut. These lenses are filled with saline and inserted. The aim is to obtain overall central clearance. These lenses have many applications.

Mini-scleral Lenses

In very advanced cone, mini-scleral lenses are being fitted these days with good results (Fig. 12.9) Mini-scleral lenses function similar to scleral lenses; the smaller diameter results from a smaller peripheral or haptic zone. With a smaller peripheral zone, the distribution of the lens weights rests on a smaller area of the scleral surface, which may cause more scleral compression. Because scleral surfaces become more circumferentially uniform toward the limbus, a mini-scleral design, if not properly fit, may cause negative pressure to build up behind the lens with each blink, resulting in a plunger-like effect on the lens itself. This can result in limbal vascular engorgement and chemosis, and will eventually lead to corneal edema.

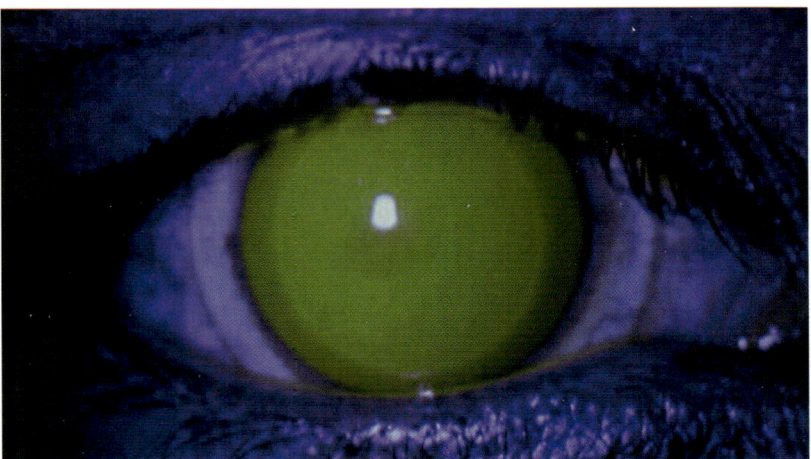

Fig. 12.9 Mini-scleral contact lens for keratoconus

KeraSoft Lens

KeraSoft IC lenses are soft lenses designed to fit irregular corneas, including keratoconus, pellucid marginal degeneration, and other corneal irregularities. Each lens can be fully customized to fit the shape of keratoconic cornea, and hence these lenses can offer increased wear time and improved comfort. KeraSoft IC lenses are a patented combination of the latest technologies in silicone hydrogel materials using geometries from complex mathematics to offer comfortable wear and excellent vision in irregular cornea.

Preliminary Examination

Many patients with keratoconus will be in their late teens or early twenties. They will need information and reassurance. They may present with concerns about the speed with which their vision has deteriorated. Quite often teenagers may be accompanied by their parents.

- It is important to explain the reason why the spectacle prescription has been changing rapidly over the past 12–24 months.
- The nature of the corneal thinning disorder and the reasons for corneal distortion should be explained. The advantages of contact lenses over spectacles should be emphasized.
- The progression of the condition and the prognosis should be discussed.
- An information leaflet explaining the condition, and information about the local keratoconus support group, should be provided.
- Any cost implications should be discussed.

Fitting Protocol

- After taking full history and symptoms, the preliminary examination should include age, occupation, and motivation. Any history of previous contact lens intolerance or allergies should be noted.
- Full slit lamp biomicroscopy is vital.
- Examine the keratometer readings. The mires may be very distorted, however they provide useful information at the initial stage.
- Choose the correct base curve; start with the base curve equivalent to the steeper of the two keratometer readings. Many variations on this philosophy exist.
- Allow the lens to settle for about 20 minutes before evaluating the fluorescein pattern.
- Examine the central area, the midperipheral area and the periphery.
- Evaluate the lens in the central position.
    Once you have judged the fit, alter the fit as necessary (for example flatten, if pooling) until you obtain gentle apical touch and the three-point-touch. Use the Guillon grading scale for assessing the fluorescein picture. There should be minimal bearing (touch) at the apex of the cone, as well as an area of bearing between the periphery of the lens and the intermediate zone of the cornea.

The lens should be ordered in mid-high DK material after an over-refraction has been undertaken. A collection appointment should be arranged. An aftercare appointment should follow four weeks after the collection appointment, when slight modifications may be necessary.

Normal Lens Fit Versus Keratoconic Fit

- *Normal lens fit*
  - Good centration
  - Alignment/slight pool on alignment
  - 0.75 mm movement
- *Keratoconic fit*
  A whole range of acceptable fits. It may not be possible to obtain the ideal fit. Ensure the cornea is observed carefully.

Cleaning Regime

Soft and corneal lenses for keratoconic patients do not require specialized regimes. Patients who suffer from GPC associated with keratoconus may need to use unpreserved solutions. Other eye drops may be necessary. RGP sclerals require a special cleaning protocol, which will be covered in a future series.

Fitting of KeraSoft IC Lens

The fit of a KeraSoft IC lens is assessed using movement, rotation, centration, comfort and VA which has the acronym *MoRoCCo VA*. This system assists the practitioner to easily distinguish between optimal and sub-optimal fits.

The Fit Assessment (Table 12.1) outlines the indications for an optimal fit (Green Characteristics), sub-optimal fits (Yellow characteristics) and fits that should be re-assessed (Red characteristics).

Post-fitting Care

- Wearing times should be increased very slowly (1/2 to 1 hour in four days).
- The total wearing time should be divided in two shifts with 1 or 2 hours interval of rest without lenses.
- Follow-up should be weekly for 2 months and every month for 6 months.
- A touch more than 4 mm should indicate a new steeper lens.
- Follow-up should include examination of the other members of the family.

Corneal Cross Linking and Contact Lenses

The introduction of corneal cross linking (CXL) treatment in routine clinical practice has changed the management of the corneal ectatic disorders. CXL is a minimally invasive surgical treatment used to increase corneal rigidity and stiffness and stabilize the ectatic cornea leading to inhibition of the keratoconus

Table 12.1 Fitting guidelines of KeraSoft IC contact lens

	Optimal fit (green)	Re-asses fit (yellow)	Incorrect fit (red)
Movement	1.0–2.0 mm vertical post-blink Up to 20 mm acceptable if patient is comfortable	<1.0 or >2.0 mm < 1.0 mm–try one step flatter > 2.0 mm–try one step steeper	Too mobile or immobile lens that moves with push-up, If lens too flat, try 0.4 mm base curve steeper, If lens too tight, try 0.40 mm base curve flatter
Rotation	Laser mark—vertical Up to 10° stable rotation is acceptable if fitting 0.20 mm base curve steeper or flatter does not reduce the angle	Up to 10° Erratic swing on blink—flat fit Limited swing on blink–tight fit	> 10° Erratic swing on blink—flat fit Limited swing on blink—tight fit
Centration	Central Minimal decentration is acceptable if visual acuity is good	Decenters on straight ahead gaze/ front optic zone drops to limbus on upward gaze Try lens 0.20 mm base curve steeper	Front optic zone edge drops below limbus on upward gaze Try lens at least 0.20 mm base curve steeper
Comfort	Comfortable Consistently good comfort	General discomfort Some edge aware-ness—flat fit Discomfort in one location—tight fit	Very uncomfortable Comfort does not improve with time
VA	No fluctuation Visual acuity should not fluctuate on blink	Fluctuation with blink Worse after blink—flat fit Clearer straight after blink—tight fit	Very poor vision Poor vision not improved by any over-refraction

progression. Reduction in K max, steep and flat keratometry and astigmatism has been reported following CXL in keratoconus. CXL treatment may also facilitate fit of contact lenses and these patients may not require penetrating keratoplasty after stabilization of progression of keratoconus following CXL.

CONCLUSION

- Patients with keratoconus are a challenge
- Keratoconic patients require ongoing care
- A wide range of contact lens designs and materials are available
- Excellent technical support is usually available
- Keratoconics can live a normal life with the help of a good contact lens practitioner.

CHAPTER 13

Aphakia

Contact lenses constitute the best optical treatment for aphakia. Since there are special problems in an aphakic patient, these deserve special mention.

PROBLEM WITH SPECTACLES IN APHAKIA

There are special problems, which particularly embarrass the function of an aphake.

- *Magnification:* An aphake shows 11–55% magnification with aphakic glasses (Fig. 13.1). This is responsible for problems of aniseikonia, phorias, fusion difficulty and diplopia, field restriction, false projection and false recording of visual acuity (6/6 instead of 6/9). In higher minus preaphakic eye magnification is same with contact lens and spectacles. In a hyperope of +6 (before cataract extraction) the image size with contact lens after operation will be same as before the operation.
- *Spherical aberration:* This causes a blurred peripheral field.
- *Marginal astigmatism:* This is responsible for a blurred image in oblique gaze.
- *Distortion:* Straight lines appear bowed inward due to unequal magnification of axial and marginal rays.
- *Jack-in-the-box phenomenon:* This scotoma (blind area) is due to the prismatic effect in the periphery and depends on the power, diameter and vertex distance. Scotoma is wider in higher power and in wider diameter spectacle lenses. It is reduced with increased vertex distance. An object in the periphery seems to come and go due to this scotoma.

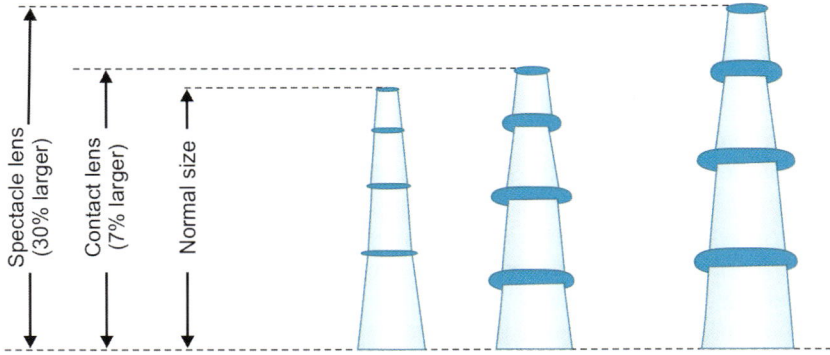

Fig. 13.1 Magnification with spectacles in an aphake

- *More convergence:* Uncorrected aphake demands more convergence due to base out effect of the spectacle glasses.
- *More glare:* This is due to more transmission caused by the absence of lens.
- *Period of adjustment:* The time usually taken by an aphake to become adapted to the abnormal imagery with aphakic spectacles is three to six weeks.
- *Irregular cornea:* These cases have blurred vision after early correction.
- *Heavier and ugly glasses:* The weight causes a shift in the position of the glasses and is responsible for blurred vision and frequent adjustment of glasses.
- *Dominance:* If the aphakic eye is dominant, will not tolerate occlusion.

COMPARISON OF CONTACT LENS AND GLASSES IN APHAKIA

The following are the advantages of a contact lens over a spectacle lens:
- *Lesser magnification (8–10%):* So more chances of fusion and binocularity.
- Decrease in peripheral aberrations.
- Disappearance of Jack-in-the-box phenomenon.
- Increase in visual fields.
- Reduction in marginal astigmatism.
- Lesser convergence.
- Better optical system because of correction being nearer the seat of error.

PRE-FITTING CONSIDERATIONS

For a successful contact lens fitting over an aphakic eye, it is imperative to asses the patient clinically. The following points deserve special mention as each plays a major role in determining success or failure.
- *Type of surgery:* Preferably do a round pupil extraction. Apply multiple sutures (6–8) over an outer limbal incision.
- *Times of fitting:* Usually, it is better to fit lenses 3 months after the surgery. For an early fitting it is essential that three keratometric readings taken at weekly intervals should be the same; the first reading being taken after three weeks of discharge from the hospital. Soft lenses can be given right after the operation.

PRE-FITTING EVALUATION

In the chapter on examination these procedures with their clinical relevance have been detailed. Here a mention of the relevant examinations with the special value on contact lens choice and fitting for aphakia will be listed.
- *Keratometry:* Corneal curvature, astigmatism, front surface irregularities, postoperative changes and their stabilization.
- *Refraction:* Refractive error, postoperative stabilization.
- *Slit lamp:* Magnified view up to anterior one-third of vitreous. It is of immense value for assessment of wound incarcerations, vitreous placement, corneal and tear film evaluation.
- *Pupil:* Size, shape, eccentricity and posterior synechiae.
- *Vitreous:* Placements, incarcerations, degenerations and inflammatory cells.
- *Iris:* Iritis, dystrophy and incarcerations.

- *Anterior chamber:* Lens matter, depth, synechiae, flare and pleomorphism.
- *Endothelium:* Appearance of mosaic, number of cells and pleomorphism.
- *Epithelium:* Sensations, edema, bullae, dystrophy, defects, staining, dry spots and down growth.
- *Conjunctiva:* Dryness.
- *Limbal anatomy:* Operation scar, ectasia, incarceration and bleb.
- Fields.
- *Tension:* Low and higher
- *Fundus examination:* Detachment, macular edema, and optic nerve lesions.

Preoperative Macular Function Tests

A good assessment can be made:
- Petit macular test (2-point discrimination).
- Entoptic phenomenon.
- Charting of acuity by laser interferometry (Rodenstock).
- Orthoptic check-up: This determines the associated problem of muscular imbalance and squint suppression, amblyopia and eccentric fixation that might demand a separate pleoptic, orthoptic or operative treatment even after the contact lens.
- *Fundus examination:* This informs about the condition of retina. It is very essential in cases of trauma and in cases of operated congenital cataract. The author has noted detachment of retina in cases of aphakia during the follow-up.

In cases fitted by the author, unilateral aphakes were 95% and bilateral were 5%. Male female ratio was 81.6%: 18.4%. Age of the fitted clients varied between 6 months to 75 years. Regarding the cause of cataract 67.2% were traumatic, 22% were senile, 8.9% complicated and 1.9% congenital. In study of corneal curvature of aphakes 8.5% were spherical and 91.5% were astigmatic. Astigmatism in these cases was with the rule in 44.5% against the rule in 30.4% and oblique in 16.6%. In spectacles 52.9% were spherical and 47.1% were astigmatic. Out of the 47.1% astigmats, 20% were against the rule, 19% were with the rule and 8.1% were oblique. The amount of cylinder varied from 0.12–8.00 diopters.

APHAKIA

Physiological Effect

- Reduced epithelial oxygen uptake
- Thinner epithelium
- Reduced corneal sensitivity
- Higher oxygen pressure at endothelium
- Reduced endothelial count
- Lower corneal edema response
- Decreased tear production

- Posterior segment changes such as macular edema, retinal detachment and capsular opacities.

Physical Aspects

- Increased astigmatism
- Decreased ultraviolet light absorption
- Lower lid tonus is decreased.

Contact Lens Considerations for the Correction

- Ocular factors
  – High power prescription
  – Astigmatism
  – Pupil size
  – Pupil shape
  – Lid position
  – Lid tonus
  – Blink quality
  – Blink quantity
  – Tear quality
  – Tear quantity
- Patient factors
  – Lens handling capability
  – Compliance
  – Assistance
- Prospects for success
  – 86% if age is less than 70 years
  – 27% if age is above 70 years
  – Extended wear has more complication rate than daily wear
  – Soft has more complication than rigid lens.
- Hydrogel lenses
  – Large optic zone available
  – High water contents are required for oxygen transmission
  – Thickness impairs oxygen
  – Vision is compromised
  – Deposit formation
  – Dry eye complaints
  – Risk of infection keratitis
- RGP lenses
  – Higher oxygen transmission lenses
  – Excellent tear pumps
  – Larger diameter over 10 mm possible.

Cornea in aphakia is compromized and demands more attention than a normal cornea. *The alterations in and around the cornea include:*

- Lid may show meibomitis
- Lids are lax, may lead to exposure and may not give support to the lens
- There may be altered blinking
- *Tears:* There is reduction in quantity and altered quality. Invariably show pathogens. Eye may show dryness
- Conjunctiva may show folds, scarring, and pinguecula
- Epithelium of the cornea show decreased and consequent barrier alteration. There is reduction in sensation resulting in alteration in mitosis, adhesion of basal cells, and defense mechanisms, poor healing, barrier disturbances. Contact lens further reduces the sensation
- Endothelium shows reduction in number, change in shape and size, shows more leakage, i.e. barrier dysfunction
- Shows less of glucose consumption
- Show less of oxygen consumption
- Shows less swelling on insult.

Contact Lens Fitting

Types of Lenses

An aphake can be fitted with various types of lenses (Fig. 13.2). These lenses with their indications are given below. Besides gas permeable lenses, soft lenses are also commonly used.

- *Single cut lens:* This has the usual lens construction and diameter; it is indicated in (a) steeper cornea with keratometry 45.0 D or more, (b) with the rule astigmatism and (c) irregular pupil like the keyhole, up drawn or widely dilated. It has a disadvantage of sagging due to its own weight. The lenticular lenses would cause more flare in aphakes with complete iridectomies or keyhole shaped pupils. It is best to see the behavior of such an aphakic trial lens on the eye.
- *Simple lenticular lens:* Lenticular lens has a central optic and peripheral level. Its usual diameter is 9.5 mm. It is indicated in round pupil. It has an advantage of lesser weight and lesser thickness but a firm upper lid may bump over the junction of bevel and optic zone. A lenticular design is indicated in (1) corneas flatter than 45.0 D, (2) Astigmatism 1.5 or more against the rule, (3) loose upper lid, (4) low lower lid, (5) high palpebral aperture, and (6) round pupil.
- *Tangent lenticular lens:* The above bumping is avoided in the lens by fabricating the bevel tangent to the optic zone radius.
- *Minus carrier lenticular lens:* The bevel in this lens has a curve to form a base out prism. It is indicated in low riding lens. The base up prism in the edge is picked up by the upper lid.

- *Single curve small lens:* It is 8–8.8 mm which is 1.5 or 3 mm smaller than the usual lens diameter. This lens is always steeper to the cornea and a toric base curve is indicated in toricity above 2.0 D.
- *Welsch's 7.5 mm lens:* This lens of + 14.5D and diameter of 7.5 mm is 40% lesser in weight as compared to the 8.5 mm lens of the same power. Peripheral curve is 12–13 mm radius and 0.2 mm width; blend is 0.1 mm. Welsch reports 100% success in cornea of 45.00 D and above.

Aphakic Trial Sets

- *Small lenticular:* Base curves between 40 and 46 D in 0.5 D steps, diameters 8.8 mm and 8.6 mm and power of +13.0 D, thickness between 0.35 and 0.33 mm.
- *Large lenticular:* Base curve 40 to 46 D in 0.50 D steps, diameter 8.9 mm and 9.4 mm, power of +13.0 D and thickness 0.39 and 0.37.
- *Single cut:* Base curves between 42 and 46 in 0.50 D steps, diameter 7.5 mm and 8.00 mm. +13.0 D and thickness 0.30 mm, 0.43 mm and 0.48 mm.

Choice of Trial Lenses

- Steeper cornea requires smaller lenses (smaller set above 45.0 D). The trial lens is fitted on K. For each diopter of toricity to 0.25 steeper than K. In the author series, 200 lenses were lenticular in type, ten were single cut and one was toric.
- *Base curve:* Having decided the type of lens, base curve is chosen on the basis of keratometric toricity and finalized on the basis of fluorescein pattern. Attempt to keep the base curve a shade steeper and it should allow free exchange to tears. Metabolic corneal insult is found to be more frequent with steeper and toric lenses. In the author series, the base curve varied between 38.0 D to 49.0 D, 80.5% were between 42 and 46 diopters. Average was 43.75 diopters.
- *Overall diameter:* It varies between 7.5 mm and 11.50 mm. Commonly, diameters between 9 and 10 mm are used, the average being 9.5 mm. Smaller diameters are used in steeper corneas and larger in flatter corneas. Smaller diameter causes more edge flare. In the author's series the diameter varied between 7.8 mm and 10.5 mm: 81.5% were fitted between 8.6 and 8.9 mm.
- *Optic zone diameter:* Varies between 7 and 8.5 mm but most commonly it is 7.5 mm. Larger diameters are used in larger, irregular and keyhole pupil.
- *Power:* Power is best calculated by refracting through an aphakic trial lens (+ 15.00 D). An alternative method is to calculate the effectivity of the spectacle lens for the corneal plane. Overplussing by + 0.50 in dominant and + 1.00 D in non-dominant eye gives latitude for intermediate distances, without affecting the distant visual acuity. It is only tolerated in round pupil. A separate correction is given for near in reading spectacles. In the author series the power of the fitted lenses ranged between –3 and +29.00 D, 87.7% between + 10 and 27.00 D 55% were between +13 and + 15 D.

- *Peripheral curves:* It is kept 7.00 D flatter than the base curve and is blended with the base curve by a curve 3.00 D flatter than the base curve. This blend should be smaller is width (0.2 mm). This ensures a contour fit.
- *Edge:* The edge should be well rounded. The thickness should be between 0.1 and 0.2 mm. Lesser than 0.1 mm elicits an unwanted lid sensation.
- *Tint:* Tinted lenses would avoid glare in bright light and minimize the transmission of the blue end of the spectrum (which was the normal function of the crystalline lens) Following points may be kept in mind.
  - Tinted lens should be light grey.
  - There should always be supplementary clear glasses along with tinted glasses.
  - Tinted glass lenses should not be used in the rain fog, evening or night or reduced illumination.

Special Handling Instructions

An aphake experiences lens-handling difficulties due to lack of dexterity, inability to see the lens and lowered sensation that makes him unaware of the lens position. Special procedures for handling are given below.

- *Insertion*
  - Index finger can be supported
  - Middle finger can be used for lens insertion and it can be supported by the index finger.
  - Use a +10.00 spectacle lens in front of the other eye to see the lens which is inserted through the empty frame aperture.
  - Use a rubber suction cup for holding the lens.
- *Removal*
  - Magnifying mirror can be used to see the lens.
  - Eye wash cup. The lens falls in the cup as soon as it touches water.

Other Considerations

- *Residual aniseikonia:* About 8–12% magnification remains even after fitting a contact lens in monocular aphakia. Minimizing the image of the aphakic eye by using an inverse telescope can solve this problem. Here aphakic lens is overplussed and it is neutralized by a minus lens in the spectacle: or the phakic eye is fitted with a minus contact lens and is neutralized by a plus glass in the spectacle. This telescope system magnifies. Each diopter of artificial error causes 3% difference in the image; therefore, 9% magnification can be minimized to normalcy by overplussing the aphakic lens by 3.00 diopters.
- *Duplicate lens:* Since the aphake is totally dependent on lens, he should start with two pairs, and they should be alternated every week to give adaptation to both. This ensures normal work during lens loss which is more in aphakes than the others.
- *Follow-up:* It should be more frequent due to lowered corneal sensation and more handling difficulties. It should be every week for the first month,

fortnightly for next 2 months, monthly for the next 6 months and then every 3 months, later on.

The author has noted the following interesting problems in aphakia during the follow-up.

- *Squint:* Every aphake should be given an orthoptic check up with trial contact lens.
  - Patients may show binocularity immediately after a contact lens or within a few hours.
  - Some may show a horizontal latent or manifest squint.
  - Some may show latent or manifest vertical deviation.
  - Some children may show eccentric fixation.
- *Posture:* Patient may show face turn or head tilt to coincide the optical center of the lens with the visual axis.
- *Subnormal visual acuity:* May be due to residual astigmatism and the vision may remain below 6/6 with corneal contact lens.
- *Bleb over the limbus:* May be increased in size due to contact lens wear. This may lead to opening up of the limbal bleb with the sharp edge of the lens.
- *Low riding lenses:* Sometimes replacement with larger (9.5 mm) or smaller (8.4 mm) aphakic lens helps. Behavior can be predicated by fitting a trial lens of the same type. This avoids error with a definitive lens.
- *Detachment:* Follow-up must include fundus examination as the author has noted detachment in 5 cases out of 100 fitted aphakes.
- *Faulty color judgment:* Colors look brighter to an aphake. This gets adjusted within a few months. Differential absorption of blue by the brown colored contact lens helps the patient out of the problem.
- *Hypotony:* A well fitted case of traumatic aphakia started showing repeated displacement. Examination revealed gross hypotony.

In a series of 201 cases fitted by the author, the following problems were noted. They were classified and mentioned in diminishing order of their occurrence.

Lens induced: Defective power –18, central edema –12, lack of near correction –10, low riding –7, edema with stain –6, upriding –6, eccentric lens –5, flare –5, diffuse staining –4, detachment –4, amblyopia –3 and eccentric fixation –2.

Incidental: Divergent squint 89.6% of traumatic cases –121, macular degeneration –18, delayed vitreous face opacification causing dropped visual acuity that required needling –4.

Aphakia in infancy: The author fits before 6 months of age. Keratometry, retinoscopy, corneal diameter and fundus are done under general anesthesia by turning the patient on one side and after detaching the frame for chin and head rest. Retinoscopy and contact lens trial may be done by putting the infant in the mother's lap. Fluorescein pattern is seen by Burton lamp. Average power in the author's series was +23 D. Both hard and soft lenses were well tolerated. The mother was asked to report every month. Watering and lid swelling should be taken as alarming symptoms and were fully explained to the mother. The author has also noted reduction of nystagmus in this age group.

Author's routine for a start or soft lens in infancy:
- Lens BC in 70% soft lenses is chosen 6.00 D flatter than 'K'.
- Power is effective power at the cornea. Add of +3.00 is done because infant activity is only at near.

  Add infants: 1 year + 3.0

  2 years + 1.0

  3 years nil
- Lens diameter is kept 1–1.5 mm larger than the corneal diameter.

  Example: K = 44 D,

  Corneal diameter = 11 mm

  Spectacle power = + 10.00 at 10 mm (+11.00 at cornea)

  Final prescription BC –38.00 Power + 14.00 OD 12 mm.

Silicone Hydrogel Lens

Soft lenses made of silicone hydrogel are commonly used these days for the visual rehabilitation of aphakia. They are well tolerated and easy to use. The fitting of these lenses is done as any other soft contact lens.

CHAPTER 14

Inspection and Verification

It is a common observation in contact lenses practice that quite a few misfits along with their adverse symptomatology could have been avoided, had the fitters taken the elementary procedure of inspecting and verifying the ordered prescriptions with the received specifications. Relaxation on the part of fitter encourages unacceptable relaxation by the workers of the laboratory as a consequences, grossly erroneous specifications occur.

The following characteristics should be checked:
- Base curve
- Power
- Overall diameter
- Optic zone diameter
- Peripheral curve width
- Blend
- Peripheral curve radius
- Central thickness
- Edge
- Surface quality
- Optical quality.

BASE CURVE

A keratometer is the most popular instrument with the contact lens fitter to check the base curve. Lens holder is attached to the keratometer. It has a platform to hold the lens in horizontal position. The image of the lens is seen vertically in a mirror inclined at 45° to the horizontal plane. The lens is placed over a cushion of water drop and reading is taken through the keratometer. Correction is applied from Table in Appendix (Page no. 161) to get real value for concave surface. The lens may be tested in different meridians. Variation of more than ± 0.12 indicates a warpage and calls for rejection.

There are other methods: (a) Radiuscope (Fig. 14.1) is a popular instrument with the manufacturers that is used for finding the base curve. The lens is kept with its concavity facing the objective. The microscope is moved up from the lowest position and two readings are taken for mires in the higher and lower position. The difference between the two gives the base curve, (b) In the R-C device, developed by Sarver and Kerr, the convex front surface of the unknown lens is placed over the concavity of the known lens. A drop of fluid is placed between the two lenses

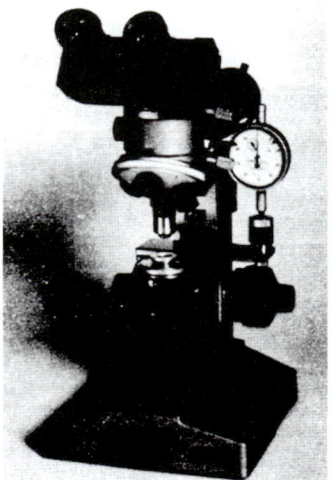

Fig. 14.1 Radiuscope to measure the radius of curvature of contact lens

(the fluid has same refractive index as the lenses). The back vertex power of the whole combination is read on the lensometer. Front surface, thickness, refractive index, back vertex power of the system being known, the back surface power, the radius can be ascertained from the Table in Appendix (Page no. 161), (c) Test spheres are also available in this, the unknown surface should conform to the surface of the known sphere. Conformity is judged by the Newton ring principle.

POWER

Lensometer furnishes a convenient method to find the power of the contact lens. It should be specified or understood whether front or back vertex power is being noted, back and front vertex difference being considerable in high powered lenses. Back vertex power is measured when back surface (concave) is placed over the stop of the instrument. Front vertex power is read when front or convex surface of the contact lens is placed over the stop.

It is assumed in the lensometer that the lens is placed against the stops, but the back surface arches away and the front surface dips in the stop. This discrepancy causes an increase in the back vertex power of the plus lenses and a decrease in the back vertex power of the minus lenses.

Two other factors influence the distance between the lens surface of the contact lens, and the stop of the lensometer or the lensometer attachment to make special aperture (a) lens surface is not in the place lens and decreases the back vertex power of the minus lens (b) the diameter of the contact lens; thereby the plus reads as more plus, and minus as less minus.

American optical: The latest models of AO have an attachment whose apertures do not affect the power of the lens because here the contact lens is in the same position as the original lensometer stop.

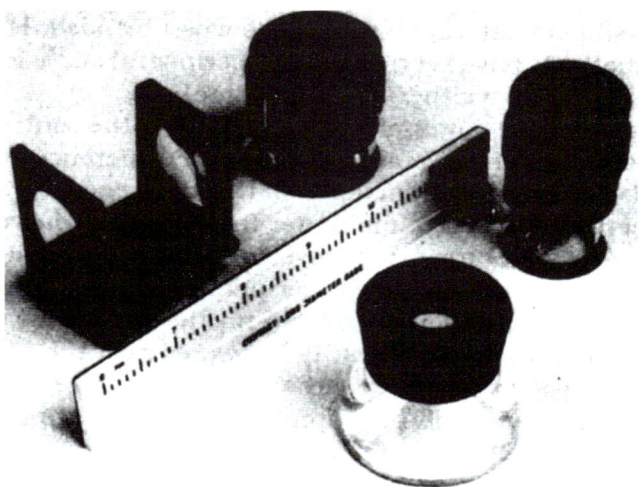

Fig. 14.2 Measuring magnifier to measure the total diameter

OVERALL DIAMETER

Total diameter and many other characteristics may be judged by measuring magnifier. It has a scale that is viewed through a magnifying lens (Fig. 14.2). The lens is placed with concavity on the scale, and a reading is taken. Two precautions need to be taken: (1) the lens should be perfectly dry otherwise the water at the edge would give a large reading than the actual (2), the lens may be rotated to verify that the dimensions are the same in various meridians.

Alternatively, total diameter can be checked by (1) V. Slot gauge: (a) progressively narrowing slot is calibrated in a plastic ruler. A dry lens is allowed to gently slip into the slot and reading noted. The accuracy to slot can be verified by measuring a button of the known diameter, (2) go or no go gauge, and (3) projection magnifier.

OPTIC ZONE DIAMETER

It can be measured by the measuring magnifier. A problem would arise, if the blend is greater and definition between the two adjacent zones, base curve and the peripheral curve, is not sharp. It is best seen by holding the lens against reflected light and by moving the magnifier from side to side when the zones of lens will appear as areas of different brightness. Alternatively, a projection magnifier may be used for the same purpose.

PERIPHERAL CURVE WIDTH

It is measured by a measuring magnifier as a ring different optical density, around the optic zone. The overall diameter minus the optic zone diameter gives the peripheral curve width.

BLEND

Appears as a bright or dark ring in the measuring magnifier. It is of importance because if its width is greater, it cuts down the effective diameter of the optic zone.

PERIPHERAL CURVE RADIUS

It is impossible to determine the radius when blended. However, the following methods have been used if the peripheral curve is unblended and of considerable width (0.7 mm or more).

- *Lensometer:* The power of the lens is read in the center and in the area of the peripheral curve. Every 0.75 D difference indicates 0.1 mm flattening approximately. If the difference is 3.50 D the peripheral curve is 0.5 mm flatter than the base curve.
- *Radiuscope:* The target is focused over the peripheral curve. This directly gives the value of the peripheral curve.
- *Polishing tool:* The lens is coated on the back with waterproof coating such as marks-a-lot. It is lowered over the polishing tool which has got approximately the same radius as expected for the peripheral curve. The area from which the coating is removed indicates the relationship between the tool and the peripheral curve. If the coating is removed from the area of the entire peripheral curve, the tool has approximately the same radius as the peripheral curve. If the coating is rubbed off from the inner or the outer edges of the area of the peripheral curve, it indicates that the tool is steeper or flatter than the peripheral curve.

CENTRAL THICKNESS

It is measured with thickness dial gauge (Fig. 14.3) which is goes up to one hundredth of a hundredth of a millimeter. An alternative method is to measure with a Geneva lens measure. The lens is placed on a flat glass piece and the thickness is read in terms of diopter. Each diopter approximately equals 0.10 mm of thickness. This is likely to scratch the lens until its points are blunted and polished.

EDGE

It is the most important, yet the most difficult to assess. It can be inspected by (1) stereomicroscope, (2) hand loupe, (3) projection magnifier, (4) rubbing on wrist or fingers, (5) wearing it on fitter's eye and (6) by moulding. The edge should not be very thick or thin. It should stand off slightly, i.e. 0.03 mm from the base line, apex of the edge should be more towards the posterior surface. The ideal edge should have a thickness of 0.08 mm, 0.14 mm and 0.16 mm at a distance of 0.05 mm, 0.2 mm and 0.5 mm from the edge respectively. Stereomicroscope gives a magnified view × 20 to × 40 times. The lens is rotated and the whole edge circumference is scanned. Hand Loupe × 7 and × 10 may be used to examine the

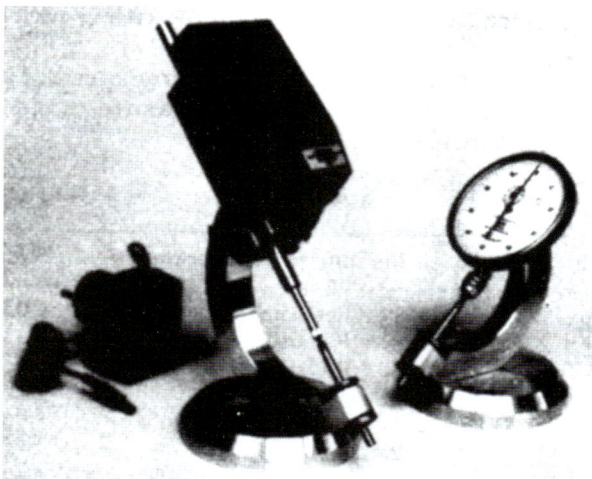

Fig. 14.3 Dial gauge to measure the thickness of contact lens

edge under magnification. Rubbing the edge over the wrist or the finger gives a fairly accurate idea about the edge quality. A fitter may use the lens in his eye to make subjective appraisal of the edge quality.

Moulding: A mould of the edge may be prepared, and sectioned to give an accurate idea about the edge shape.

SURFACE AND OPTICAL QUALITY

These can be studied (1) by observing transmitted light of a fluorescent tube with the naked eye. The tube should remain straight. This will detect any bubble or striae, (2) observation of the reflected light especially under magnification tells about the scratches, gouges and bumps on the lens surface (3) and (4) distortion of target in focimeter and the radioscope indicates a defective surface.

Color: It is confirmed by matching the unknown lens with a test lens of the laboratory.

The following appendix summarizes the parameters for inspection and verification, the instruments to measure them and the recommended tolerance.

Appendix		
Parameter	*Instruments for checking*	*Tolerance*
Base curve	Keratometer	± 0.03 mm
	Radiuscope	
	R-C device	
	Test spheres	
Overall diameter (OD)	Measuring magnifier	± 0.05 mm
	V slot gauge	
	Projection magnifier	
	Go or no go gauge	
Optic zone diameter (OZD)	Measuring magnifier	± 0.10 mm
	Projection magnifier	
Peripheral curve radius	Lensometer	± 0.10 mm
	Radioscope	
	Polishing tool	
Peripheral curve width	Measuring magnifier	± 0.12 mm
	OD minus OZD	
Power	Lensometer	± 0.12 D
Central thickness	Dial gauge	± 0.02 mm
	Geneva lens measure	
Edge	Stereomicroscope	± 0.20 mm
	Hand loupe	
	Projection magnifier	
	By feeling over the wrist to finger	
	Taking a mould	

15 Contact Lens Solutions

Various chemical solutions required to wet, soak (hydrate) and clean constitute contact lens solution. Since 1962, contact lens fitters have become more conscious of the eye mortality and morbidity due to contaminated contact lenses. Though the incidence of blindness or eyes removed is as low 14 in 50,000 patients yet it is a very serious problem. Workers have compared, the result of the lenses kept dry and soaked in an antiseptic solution. It was found that 5% of wet contact lens cases and 60% of the dry ones showed contamination. Low concentration of the preservatives and absorption of the same by the sponge rendered the preservatives less efficacious.

NORMAL FLORA OF CONJUNCTIVA IN INDIANS

In author's study at RP Centre, the following organisms were cultured from the conjunctival sac in order of prevalence.
- *Staph albus*
- *Aspergillus* species
- Penicillium
- *Strepto viridans*
- Pneumococci
- *Rhizopus*
- Mucor
- *Staph aureus*
- Diphtheroids
- Mima polymorpha.

As commensal, *Pseudomonas* is found in intestines, *Streptococcus* in tonsils and vagina and *Staphylococcus* in skin, nares and conjunctiva.

SOURCES OF THE CONTAMINATION IN CONTACT LENSES

The eye may get infected by:
- Dirty hands of the patients.
- Contaminated fluorescein solution.
- Infected water used to clean the lenses.
- From the normal florae of the skin or infected skin of eyelid.
- Infection from the lacrimal sac.
- Infection from the surrounding air.
- Saliva used as wetting solution.

Natural Factors for Eye Protection

Human eye is protected by a variety of mechanisms: (a) The projection of bony ridges around the eyes, the lids and the eye lashes protect the eye against foreign bodies, (b) Eyebrows protect from liquids flowing directly into eyes, (c) Low temperature due to continuous evaporation, (d) Lysozyme (an enzyme which kills bacteria), (e) Gammaglobulin (IgA), and (f) Barrier function of the corneal epithelium help to protect the eye against organisms.

WETTING

A solid is said to be properly wetted, if a fluid drop will spread into a uniform thin film over its surface. This wetting is dependent upon the relationship of the forces of cohesion (attraction of the molecules in the fluid for each other) and adhesion (attraction of the molecules of the fluid to the molecules of the solid).

Polymethylmethacrylate has special properties of ophthalmic interest. It has a transmission of 90%, refractive index of 1.49, hardness of 4.5 compared to 6.5 of glass and 10 of diamond. Its softness makes it more vulnerable to scratches. It has 1.5% water content after several days of immersion and remains relatively more hydrophobic due to higher concentration of methyl groups than carboxyester groups which determine the hydrophilic character. A hydrated lens wets more easily. Wettability of contact lens can be increased by giving it a thin coating of silicon tetrachloride.

Tears are constituted by protein, lipoids and traces of salts dissolved in water. Mucin of the tears is rubbed over the contact lens by blinking. In normal circumstances a lens should become wetted in 15 minutes due to mucin. Action of the mucin is disturbed, if the lens gets coated with lipoid secretion as in meibomitis.

Functions of Wetting

- A wetting solution changes a hydrophobic surface into a hydrophilic one and the effect lasts for about an hour.
- It allows cushioning by wetting solution between the lid and the lens, and the lens and the cornea.
- It stabilizes the lens over the fingertip.
- It does not allow oil of the fingertip on the lens.

Wetting solution is usually constituted by:
- Cushioning agents
- Preservatives
- Wetting agents.

Cushioning Agents

Cushioning agents or viscosity building agents, e.g. PVP, polyvinyl alcohol, gelatin and sodium alginate. Cellulose, methylcellulose, hydroxyethyl cellulose and hydroxypropyl cellulose are used as thickener, binder stabilizer, protective colloid and as suspending agent. It lubricates the lens and prevents contamination from the finger.

Preservatives

Benzalkonium chloride (Zephiran) has the following chemical formula.

Bzal + Nathim = Bz thim ppt + NaCl

It is the most commonly used preservative. Available as 100% powder and 17% solution form. It is active against both gram+ve and gram–ve organisms. It acts probably by interfering with respiration and glycolysis. It has a hydrophobic tail which is arranged away from the plastic surface. The effective hydrophobic tail makes it hydrophobic.

The usual concentration used varies from 0.004–0.01%. Higher concentrations cause superficial punctate keratopathy and degeneration of the conjunctiva. Concentration of 0.01% or more can be used safely in soaking solution provided, the lens is washed and wetted with wetting solution before insertion. It is used in 50% of the ophthalmic solutions.

Benzethonium chloride: It has the same properties as benzalkonium chloride.

Chlorobutanol: It has a synergistic action with benzalkonium chloride, and has the following chemical formula.

$$Cl_3C \quad OH$$
$$H_3C \qquad CH_3$$

Disadvantages:
- Being volatile its concentration falls when kept in solution.
- It dissolves at higher temperature.
- It breaks into hydrochloric and hydrocarbon with the pH is less than 6.
  It is used in 25% of ophthalmic solution.

Ethylene diamine tetra-acetic acid (EDTA): It is a chelating agent and inactivates metals in a solution. It disrupts the integrity of the cell wall and enhances the effect of benzalkonium chloride. It is used in 0.1–0.25% concentration. It has the following formula.

$$Cl^- \quad CH_3$$
$$CH_3 (CH_2)_{14} CH_2 \overset{+}{N} CH_2$$
$$CH_3$$

Benzalkonium chloride

It prevents discoloration due to trace metals.

Oxidation induced by trace metals is prevented by the sodium ethylmercurithiosalicylate (thiomersal or merthiolate). It is mercurial and is not very effective against *Pseudomonas* infection, sensitization is reported but it is not a serious problem. When used with benzalkonium chloride, it may form a precipitate as BZ thin ppt (Seen in zephiran).

Preservatives like benzalkonium chloride, benzethonium chloride, chlorobutanol, thiomersal, ethylene diamine tetra-acetic acid (EDTA), (propyl-p-hydroxybenzoate (propylparaben) and methyl p-hydroxybenzoate- Methyl paraben) are detailed under soaking solutions.

Wetting Agents

Wetting agents, e.g. polyvinylalcohol. Its chemical formula is

Poly(vinyl alcohol-*co*-vinyl acetate)

Its long chain makes it more absorptive and adhesive. This makes it a wetting and coating agent. Various wetting solutions differ in the concentration of the constituents, buffering system, self-sterilizing capacity and formulation methodology.

Soaking

If a lens is kept in a dry case after a day's wear, it not only causes higher prevalence of contamination through a dirty lens can put also makes it uncomfortable to wear due to haziness of its dirty surfaces and dried mucus which irritates the lids and the cornea. *A soaking solution:*
• Keep the lens in a permanent state of hydration.
• Maintain the sterility of the lens.
• Removes the mucus from the lens surface. It is safest to change the soaking solution daily.
A soaking solution is mainly constituted of preservatives.

Cleaning

A lens may become contaminated by oil, cosmetic or nicotine, transferred to it from the hand, dried mucus or a foreign body and may get badly attached to the lens surface. The contaminants lower the vision, irritate the eye and may serve as nidus for bacterial growth. Such a dirty lens may be cleaned by: (1) Friction rubbing, (2) Spray cleaning, (3) Hydraulic cleaning, (4) Ultrasonic cleaning.

A contact lens contaminated with cream, grease, paint, or nail polish can be cleaned with carbon tetrachloride, naptha or lighter fluid.

Caution

The following agents should be avoided because they spoil the surface of the lens, e.g. alcohol, acetone, chloroform, gasoline and saliva.

Friction Cleaning

This calls for rubbing the lens gently between the thumb and finger with a drop of wetting solution A piece of lint is usually used with a cleaning agent. This method of cleaning may result in scratching and warpage.

Spray Cleaning

This is done by placing contact lenses in a special container (Hydramat) that permits a back and fro pumping action through a liquid cleaner. *Titan:* This is a very efficient method of cleaning but the lens can warp or break, if vigorously used.

Ultrasonic Cleaning

This is the best method. The contact lens is placed in a liquid and ultra sound is passed through the fluid. High cost of the instrument allows its use only in manufacturing laboratories.

MULTIPURPOSE CONTACT LENS SOLUTIONS

The most popular type of care regime being prescribed today is the multipurpose solution. In the 70s and 80s when both rigid and soft contact lenses were gaining popularity, disinfection methods had several steps and adherence rates were low due to inconvenience. The disinfecting agents used at the time, such as benzalkonium chloride, thimerosal and chlorhexidine, which were extremely effective against microorganisms but also extremely toxic to the ocular surface. Newer contact lens multipurpose solutions use active agents of a higher molecular weight in very carefully balanced concentrations, such as polyhexamethylene biguanide (PHMB) and polyquaternium-1. These preservatives have shown a much lower incidence of solution toxicity and are becoming increasingly popular in modern multipurpose contact lens solutions, for both soft and rigid contact lenses.

Multipurpose solutions typically contain several components, one of which being preservatives or active ingredients. The main function of the active ingredient is to eliminate existing microbes from the contact lens as well as prevent further microbial contamination. Current ISO standards for microbial efficacy in contact lens solutions include activity against three strains of bacteria, *Pseudomonas aeruginosa*, *Serratia marsescens* and *Staphylococcus aureus*, and two strains of fungi, *Candida albicans* and *Fusarium solani*. The FDA is currently reviewing these standards to consider the possibility of extending this list and as well as adding Acanthamoeba to this list. Studies have shown that modern multipurpose contact lens solutions containing more than one active ingredient working synergistically (commonly referred to as multipurpose disinfecting solutions) are shown some efficacy against Acanthamoeba cysts. Although modern active ingredients are considerably less toxic to the ocular surface than those used previously, there is still a large percentage of the contact lens wearing population that do suffer from solution toxicity. The commonly used active ingredients in modern multipurpose solutions are 'detergent' type ingredients, which demonstrate antimicrobial activity by disrupting the cell membrane and causing cell lysis. Another method of disinfection is oxidation. Stabilized Oxy-Chloro (SOC) complex is an oxidative preservative with broad-spectrum microbial efficacy including both gram-positive and gram-negative bacteria as well as some fungi and viruses, which is currently being safely and effectively used in several ophthalmic preparations including eyedrops for the treatment of glaucoma and contact lens rewetting drops, however, has not been used in any other contact lens solutions that are commercially available in India. Oxidative preservatives are typically small molecules and restrict microbial activity by penetrating the cell membrane and interfering with cellular function. SOC has been shown to have low toxicity to mammalian cells. This is particularly relevant for those experiencing a toxic reaction to a contact lens solution, the toxic agent in most cases, as described by Holden, being the active ingredient. Signs of solution toxicity generally include diffuse punctate corneal epithelial staining and inflammation, which may present with bulbar and limbal injection and palpebral redness and roughness. Other components of multipurpose solutions include tonicity agents, chelating agents, buffers, viscosity agents and lubricating agents. Tonicity agents regulate the osmolarity of the solution, while buffers maintain the pH to match the pH of the tears to avoid discomfort. Chelating agents work synergistically with the preservative in disinfection and also have a role in removal of deposits, particularly calcium.

Multipurpose solutions have gained popularity over the years due the convenience of 'one bottle for everything'. In the mid-2000s, a wave of 'No-Rub' solutions entered the market. The manufacturers of these solutions claimed that the all-important 'rubbing and rinsing' step could be skipped. These solutions were recalled as quickly as they were introduced when there was an increase in contact lens complications associated with the introduction of 'No-Rub' solutions. Studies have shown that 'rubbing and rinsing' is a crucial step in contact lens hygiene as it is the most effective way of removing deposits off the contact lens surface. Deposits are bad news as they may be responsible for papillary conjunctivitis, resulting in discomfort and they also create an uneven contact lens surface, enabling bacteria to colonize on the surface of the contact lens.

Commonly used multipurpose solutions are as follows.

- *OPTI-FREE Contact Lens Solution (Alcon):* Opti-Free RepleniSH Contact Lens Solution is affordable, easy to use and effective multipurpose solution which does not require any scrubbing.

- *ReNu Fresh Multipurpose Solution (Bausch + Lomb):* ReNu Fresh Contact Lens Solution is one of those easy to use daily lens cleaners. It helps clean and disinfect contact lens and does it quick as well.
- *BioTrue Multipurpose Solution (Bausch + Lomb):* This multipurpose cleaning solution is pH balanced, and is good for people who have dry or sensitive eyes.
- *AQuify Multipurpose Solution (Boston):* AQuify is good for contact lens users who are constantly on the move. One can simply rub and rinse lenses for 5 minutes or so in this solution and use them again.
- *Moisture RICH multipurpose solution (Pharmasafe).*
- *Complete multipurpose solution (Abbott).*

HYDROGEN PEROXIDE BASED DISINFECTION

Multipurpose solutions are not the be all and end all in contact lens care regimes. Hydrogen peroxide systems are still the gold standard when it comes to efficacy against bacteria. Early hydrogen peroxide systems were two-step systems, where the initial step was an overnight soak in hydrogen peroxide and the second step was a 10 minute soak in a catalyst solution before wear. Modern peroxide systems only contain one step where the contact lens is soaked in 3% hydrogen peroxide (H_2O_2) alongside a catalyst, which over a period of six hours, breaks the hydrogen peroxide into water and oxygen (H_2O+O). Although two-step systems have become somewhat obsolete, they are more effective against acanthamoeba cysts than one-step systems. Hydrogen peroxide systems do not require additional preservatives due to the potency of the chemical and is therefore a good option for those suffering from solution toxicity with multipurpose solutions. However, unneutralized hydrogen peroxide is extremely toxic to the cornea where direct exposure can strip-off the corneal epithelium, making it a painful and traumatic experience for the patient. Therefore, when prescribing a hydrogen peroxide system, careful instruction and patient education may be required. Example of hydrogen peroxide based solution is *Clean Care No Rub Solution.* It is a hydrogen peroxide solution with a catalytic disk, which makes it the safest bet against acanthamoeba infections. A second wash with saline solution is required to remove the hydrogen peroxide completely and it works best with newer silicone hydrogel contacts. Using it on older lenses may cause unwanted chemical reactions, so caution should be practiced.

16

Special Lenses and Indications

CONTACT LENS AT EARLY AGE

Author's documented indication for contact lenses in infants and children were aphakia, high myopia, corneal scars, high astigmatism with amblyopia, anisometropia and cosmetic.

Infants should be seen at least once under anesthesia for assessment of fundus, cornea, keratometry, refraction and contact lens trial. As the fitter gains experience fundus remains the only important examination under anesthesia.

- Infants show quick healing. Lens should be fitted as quickly as possible to avoid amblyopia of arrest.
- Choice between gas permeable and hydrogel is fitter's decision.
- Follow-up after 1 day, 1 week for a month and then every 3 months.
- Spectacles may be given at two months of age in bilateral aphakes.

Orthokeratology: There is truth in the procedure, but who is going to benefit from this procedure cannot be predicted, and so the procedure does not have universal application. Author reported myopic reduction in 73%.

Anisometropia and contact lenses: Anisometropia of 2.00 D or more is mostly contributed by axial error. For the purposes of motor fusion contact lenses are a better device than spectacles.

Squint and contact lenses: Contact lens has special role in squint for
- Occlusion with opaque iris lenses
- Occlusion for intractable diplopia
- Over correction with 2.00 diopters in exotropia to stimulate convergence.

Color Defective and X-chrome (Red Contact Lens)

Red colored lens is worn in front of one eye. It is found more helpful on ishihara charts testing than on HRR plates. It is more helpful in green defective than in the red defective.

Colored Lenses

They may be in various tints like gray, green, blue, red brown and black. Each tint may have light, medium and dark shade. Tinted lenses are used for identification, cosmetic reasons and color defectives (red tint). Soft lenses of various iris color pattern are also available.

Sports Lenses

A large lens fitted tight to avoid displacement is called a sports lens. Scleral lens can serve the same purpose.

Guidelines to Fit Contact Lenses in Athletes

Fit extended wear lenses (EWL) as daily wear lens (DWL) to get maximum oxygen supply. Avoid thick low water content lenses. Disposable are ideal for occasional or part time use. The fit of lens should be such as to permit least movements in dynamic sports.

The correction of refractive error should be such as to give maximum visual acuity. Myopia should be corrected up to 0.25 D; anisometropia of 0.5 or more; correct significant hyperopia and astigmatism over 1.0 with toric soft or rigid gas permeable (RGP) lens.

Sports Lens

Sports lens should be soft with 55% water. It should have base curve of 8.9 and 9.2; overall diameter of 15 mm. It should be worn on daily wear basis.

Advantages of Contact Lenses

Contact lens increase usual stability eliminates chances of ocular injury due to frame and glasses, increases peripheral vision by 15%, gives better depth perception, reduces usual distortion (the object size is near normal). Contact lens also offers more comfort and permits the use of protective glasses over them. Contact lenses do not fog due to low atmospheric temperature and sweating as in spectacles.

Contact Lenses and their Evaluation in Athletes

Six tests are available where the fitter can see the performance of the athlete after fitting contact lenses. This will evaluate athlete's ability when he is confronted with environment similar to his game. *These tests basically are:*

No. 1.   Visual contraction—where candidate has to put a soft ball.

No. 2.   Information processing where the candidate has to respond to a projected slide.

No. 3.   *Anticipated timing:* This is judged by seeing the performance by throwing the object in space.

No. 4.   *Eye hand reaction:* Patient points to a projected light.

No. 5.   *Eye foot quickness:* Seeing on a check board pattern made on the floor, for a soccer player.

No. 6.   *Peripheral awareness:* This is tested with peripheral stimuli. It is applicable to athletes who play games along with partners as in doubles.

RGP for sports is usually bigger, i.e. 9.6–9.8.

Soft lens for sport should be of 38% hydration and bigger in OD, i.e. 13.5–14.00 mm.

Under water lenses: There are two types of lenses for seeing under water (a) a lens with an air cell on front surface (b) a lens with +150.00 D power in air and + 50.00 D under water.

Fenestrated lenses: Lenses with a hole for better circulation has been documented to be of limited value for corneal oxygenation by the author. Lens with multiple holes have been found to be useful in low vision.

Aspheric lenses: The back curves are aspheric. The lenses have different rate of flattening.

Fitting is done by a trial lens method and a lens just flatter than the corneal conoid is the final choice. It fits the cornea better as cornea is aspheric.

Offset lenses: The lenses have peripheral curves ground in a way that their center does not coincide with the physical center of the lens.

Disposable lenses: This is being tried and seems to be the lens of the future. It may be changed every 15–30 days. Daily disposable is the ideal soft lens as it does not require contact lens care solutions containing preservatives. It will be most useful for sensitive eyes as it is stored in saline without any preservative.

Indications for Daily Disposables

- Patients with allergic background
- Patient allergic to care products
- Intermittent wearers
- Unhygienic wearers
- Patients with lot of money and lot of travel.

The available disposable lenses are—Acuvue, Sequence, Mewvues, Surivue, SofLens, Freshlook, Optima, Purevision, AirOptix.

Ultrathin Polymethylmethacrylate Lens

Lenses are having diameter of 8–9 mm, most common being 8.2 and thickness of 0.08–0.09 mm. It is indicated in low riding lens, in cornea showing distortion, edema and discomfort with other lenses. It has advantage of better vision, comfort centering, minimal edema and distortion, and less or residual astigmatism. It is fitted with trial set varying in base curves form 41 to 46 D in 0.5 steps having a diameter of 8.2 mm.

Bifocal Lenses

The consensus among contact lens practitioners is that bifocals are a futile idea. However, bifocals are basically of two types. Soft bifocals are also available.

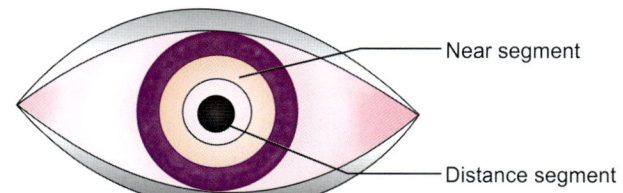

Fig. 16.1 Simultaneous vision type bifocal lens

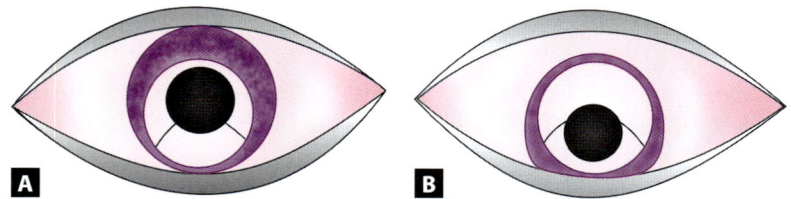

Figs 16.2A and B Kryptok bifocal-shaped like a cut bifocal (a camp type)

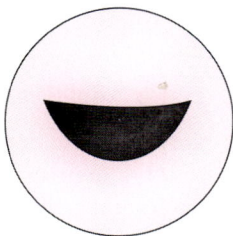

Fig. 16.3 Kryptok bifocal-shaped like inverted D shape

- *Simultaneous vision type:* This uses a central dot for distance and an annular ring for near vision. The images of near and distant objects keep disturbing during distant and near work (Fig. 16.1).
- *Bivision type:* This is like a kryptok bifocal. It may be shaped like a cut bifocal (a camp type) or inverted D shape or Black type. This is more popular than the simultaneous type (Figs 16.2 and 16.3).
- *Aspheric type:* These lenses have aspheric periphery which gives aid for the near.
- *Diffractive type:* These lenses have concentric steps and each step splits the bundle of rays into bundles, one for distance and the other for near.
- *Mono vision:* Dominant eye is used for distance and other eye is used for near.
- *Modified monovision:* One eye is used distance and the other eye has bifocal lens.

Fitting

The patient is fitted with the conventional lens. He/she is given a bifocal lens of the same dimensions. It is seen that the upper part of the bifocal just enters the pupil during distant viewing. Orientation is achieved by lower truncation or prisms ballast.

PIGGYBACK CONTACT LENS

Sometimes, GP lenses will provide excellent vision for a person with irregular cornea, but the wearer finds the rigid lenses uncomfortable and cannot wear them for a long period. In these cases, a fitting technique called piggybacking may be used. In piggybacking, a soft contact lens is worn under the gas permeable lens, acting as a cushion to reduce or eliminate any discomfort caused by the GP lens.

Hybrid Contact Lenses

Hybrid contact lenses are large-diameter lenses that have a rigid gas permeable central zone, surrounded by a peripheral zone made of soft or silicone hydrogel material. The purpose of this design is to provide the visual clarity of GP lenses, combined with wearing comfort that is comparable to soft lenses.

Soft Contact Lenses for Keratoconus

Custom soft contact lenses are available today that can correct mild to moderate keratoconus. These special, made-to-order soft lenses sometimes are more comfortable than gas permeable or hybrid contact lenses for people with keratoconus or irregular corneas.

Custom soft contacts for keratoconus typically have a larger diameter than regular soft lenses and have either a medium or high water content. Examples include KeraSoft IC lenses (Bausch + Lomb) and NovaKone contact lenses (Alden Optical). Custom soft lenses are usually recommended for people with keratoconus who enjoy excellent vision with GP or scleral lenses but cannot wear rigid lenses comfortably all day.

CHAPTER 17

Soft Lenses

In 1950 Professor Otto Wicherle, a polymer chemist from Czechoslovakia conceived the idea of soft lenses while working on hydrogels for possible biological application. Chemically it is hydroxyethylmethacrylate (HEMA) which is cross linked with EDMA, ethyl dimethyl acrylate or polyvinylpyrrolidone (PVP) and ethylene glycol dimethacrylate.

The author has documented similar biological tolerance with four polymers manufactured from HEMA in combination with methylacrylate, methyl methacrylate, ethyl acrylate and butyl acrylate. The water content of commercially used soft lens varies between 25% and 85%. Refractive index and dimensions vary with hydration, tonicity of hydrating fluid and a little with pH.

There is a considerable variation in the oxygen permeability of the lenses. The higher the hydration the greater the oxygen permeability. In general, the thinnest lens with highest water content transmits maximum oxygen which rarely meets corneal demand. Besides this transmission by diffusion gel lens. The size of lens is usually larger than cornea. Softness of lens is variable. It is hard and brittle when dry and it becomes soft and flexible when fully hydrated. Drugs, chemicals and vapors easily penetrate the lens while bacteria being larger than the pore size of the lens cannot pass through the lens.

Comparison with a hard lens: A gel is advantageous due to more comfort, minimum spectacle blur, least displacement, lack of entry of dust and particles behind the lens, quick adaptation with rare causation of flare, less photophobia, easy fitting and infrequent corneal staining.

Unfortunately, gel lens has a few limitations due to comparatively poor visual acuity especially in loose and tight lenses. Limitations of correction (astigmatism), especially higher cylinders along or in combination with low spheres, possibility of tearing and splitting, difficulty in verifications of fit, difficult to sterilize, or clean the deposits like protein and lipids and finally difficulty to manufacturers to duplicate and modify make them a bit challenging. However, with the improvement in manufacturing technology and materials like silicone hydrogel, soft lenses have become the contact lens of choice except in cases where the correction is only possible with rigid gas permeable lens.

Manufacturing involves methodologies, like spun cast, lathe cut and mould. In spun cast a small amount of monomer is polymerized in a revolving mould. In spun cast lens, duplication and thin edge are advantageous. Outer surface of lens is spherical. Inner surface is aspheric and curvature depends upon speed of mould, amount of the monomer, shape of mould, and characteristics of the monomer. The lens is solid after polymerization. In lathe cut lens there is greater flexibility in power, base curve, and diameter for individual fitting that can be assessed by trial lens methodology, as in hard lenses. Lathe cut lenses are thicker and are difficult to duplicate (Table 17.1).

Physical characteristics of Bausch and Lomb soft lens: Water content is 38%. It has a refractive index of 1.43 in water; water content by weight in water and saline are 41.7% and 38.6% respectively. The linear swelling by normal saline is 18%.

SILICONE HYDROGEL LENS

Silicone hydrogels are the latest in a line of developments aimed at increasing the oxygen permeability (increased comfort, longer wear and better eye health), wettability (better comfort) and clinical performance of contact lenses. They are healthier than conventional soft lenses because they allow up to 6 times more oxygen to pass through them and increased oxygen transmission results in better overall eye health. Silicone has higher oxygen permeability, allowing more oxygen to pass, than water, so oxygen permeability is no longer tied to how much water is present in each lens.

Types of Silicone Hydrogels

There are many types, even generations, of silicone hydrogels used to manufacture contact lenses today. These come with technical names such as galyfilcon, senofilcon, comfilcon and enfilcon.

The primary benefit of silicone hydrogel lenses is that they reduce the trade-off between oxygen permeability and wettability. *This opens up many possibilities for silicone hydrogel contacts, including:*

• Extended wear (sometimes for up to six straight nights and days)
• Continuous wear (sometimes for up to thirty days before replacement)
• Increased comfort and performance.

Table 17.1 Comparison of spin casting and lathe-cutting process of soft contact lenses		
	Spin casting	*Lathe*
Manufacturer	Liquid plastic is injected into spinning molds polymerized and hydrated	Unhydated polymeric material is cut into buttons lathe cut, polished and hydrated
Lens power governed	Posterior lens curvature	Anterior lens curvature
By peripheral construction	Bevel is present on anterior surface	Bevel is present on posterior surface
Anterior optical zone (AOZ)	Corresponds to front surface of the lens minus the anterior peripheral curve	Corresponds to the optical portion of the lens (i.e. front surface minus carrier portion of the lens)
Posterior optical zone (POZ)	Includes the entire diameter of the back surface of the lens	Is the back surface of the lens minus the posterior peripheral curve

The current brands of spherical silicone hydrogel lenses available, in order of highest oxygen transmissibility to lowest, are:

- Ciba Focus night and day which is approved for 30 day continuous wear
- Vistakon's Acuvue Oasys which is approved for 2 weeks daily wear use or 6 night extended wear and is designed to be more wettable than the others and is therefore beneficial for people who have dry eyes
- Ciba's O2 Optix which is approved for 6 days continuous wear or 2 weeks daily wear
- Bausch and Lomb's PureVision which is approved for 30 days continuous wear
- Vistakon Acuvue Advance which is a 2 weeks disposable lens and has not yet been approved for extended wear.

There are also currently two toric silicone hydrogel lenses available in the market.
- Bausch and Lomb PureVision Toric is a silicone hydrogel toric lens approved for 30 days extended wear use
- Acuvue Advance For Astigmatism—currently approved as a 2 weeks daily wear lens.

VERIFICATION OF SOFT LENSES

Overall diameter, edges and surface qualities are assessed by hand held magnifier. Base curve is measured by placing the lens over plastic templates of known radii. A central bubble and edge stand off indicate a steep and flat lens respectively.

For more accurate information the following instruments are used to verify base curve.
- The Carl Zeiss (Oberkochen) ophthalmometer uses keratometry to measure the base curve of a soft lens mounted convex-side-up in a liquid cell. The mire images are reflected by a mounted prism cell into the telescope and the resultant reading is multiplied by the refractive index of the saline. A compensation factor of about 0.03 mm is added to compensate for the convex calibration of the instrument.
- The Nissel ultra radiuscope is basically a Drysdale microscope with a sealed objective lens directly immersed into a liquid cell in which the lens is centered concave-side-up. As the light only travels through a single medium, a direct reading is possible, although a high luminosity bulb is necessary to compensate for the light lost by reflection.
- The wet cell gauge (Contact Lens Manufacturing Ltd.) is a magnified vertex depth gauge that permits the approximate determination of the base curve of an immersed lens.
- The Wohlk microspherometer also uses sagometry to measure the primary sag of the lens mounted in air on a holding ring. The reading is taken from a clock dial calibrated to read the base curve at a point where the probe just touches the back surface of the lens.

- The Soehnges control and protection system projects the profile of a lens immersed in fluid at a previously calibrated distance onto a screen containing graduated annuli that may be adjusted vertically until alignment is achieved.

Power is measured by the lensometer after blotting the lens over a lint free tissue. Surface and edges can be assessed with loupe also. Radioscopy over a well fitted lens is a guide to the optical qualities of the lens.

Indications

Soft lenses have the same indications as detailed in hard lenses: Optical, therapeutic, cosmetic, occupational, diagnostic and research. Soft lenses have proved better as a therapeutic device. The author has reported excellent results in bullous keratopathy, neuroparalytic keratitis, recurrent corneal erosion, desiccating diseases of the cornea, preventing symplepharon in glaucoma and as bandage lenses after cataract extraction. The author has also found them of immense value in cases of unilateral traumatic aphakia ametropia with or without corneal tears in cases of unilateral or bilateral aphakia ametropic anisometropia in infants. Contraindications to soft lenses are acute and sub-acute inflammations of the anterior segment, affections of cornea and conjunctiva, lacrimal insufficiency, corneal hypoesthesia, early pregnancy and systemic diseases affecting the eyes.

Fitting of Soft Lenses

General principles: Soft lenses regardless of power, size, or manufacture should be fitted to obtain three point touch. They should be parallel to the superior and inferior sclera and the apex of the cornea. Hard lenses are fitted on a steeper than 'K' but soft lenses of 12 or 13 mm diameter are fitted 2–3 diopters flatter than 'K' and soft lenses of 13–15 mm diameters are fitted 3–5 diopters flatter than 'K.'

Differences in lens design and properties of various polymers affect the fit and need considerations (1) type of posterior curve; lathe cut lens have spherical and spun cast lenses have aspheric posterior curve which will behave flatter than the former (2) peripheral curve: A lens with same base curve but with a wider peripheral curve will be different on single cut, and lenticular lenses (4) Water content lenses with a higher water content demand a bigger diameter for better stability (5) thickness of lenses: thicker lenses are fitted large and steeper than thinner lenses; (6) lens weight: heavier lenses are usually fitted larger (7) lens rigidity (resiliency); less rigid lenses are fitted steeper.

Basic Guidelines

The following basic guidelines common to all types of soft lenses may be adhered, to get good scientific start:
- There should be a 3 point touch fitting, i.e. one at corneal apex and two at periphery.
- Diameter of lens is usually (12–15 mm) which is at least 0.75 mm bigger than the corneal diameter.

- Smaller eyes require smaller diameter lenses and steeper base curves.
- Soft lenses are fitted flatter than 'K' by 2.00–5.00 diopters (0.4–1.00 mm) depending on the diameter of the lens.
- In lathe cut lenses 0.50 mm increase in overall diameter demands 1.50 D flattening of the base curve to achieve similar fit.
- Bausch and Lomb lenses are spun cast in 13.5 and 14.5 mm diameters and lathe cut in 14 mm diameter.

Guidelines for Evaluating Fit

- Soft lenses must fulfil the following criteria to give an ideal fit—CMC.
  - C—*Centering:* Lenses must be centered well. There should not be more than 0.5 mm decentration on any side.
  - M—*Movement:* On blinking or looking up, movements should not exceed 0.5–1 mm.
  - C—*Coverage:* Total coverage of cornea.
- *Relationship reflex:* The reflex should be uniform in all the meridians.
- *Over-refraction:* There should not be any demand if the power is proper. Higher or lower minus than desired will indicate a steep or a flat lens.
- *Visual acuity:* It should be uniformly clear before during and after the blink. Flattest lens which fulfils all the above criteria is the ideal lens.

Additional Criteria for Best-Fit Assessment

- Position of air bubble
- Movement with blink
- Movement with up gaze
- *Edge examination of slit lamp:* Edge of a flat lens will stand away form conjunctiva and may show a bubble underneath. Edge of tight lens will impinge into the conjunctiva to create a "Circular seat". A tight edge will push the conjunctiva ahead as it moves. Edge of optimum fit will smoothly slide over the conjunctiva.
- *Corneal return test:* If a lens is displaced temporally with finger of suction cup so that it is only one third on cornea and two thirds on sclera and its return is watched, an idea of fit can be had. Easy displacement and easy return to cornea indicates an ideal fit. Resistance to displacement and momentary stay in decentered position indicate a steep fit. Easy displacement and slow return is characteristic of a flat lens.
- *Edge lift:* Displace the lens by pushing the lower edge upward with the help of the lower lid and observe the edge lift at 6 O'clock. This is a guide about the fit.
- Retinoscopic and keratometric observations are detailed earlier.

Lathe-cut lenses and their fitting: They are made in diameters of 13.00–15 mm in 0.50 mm steps and each diameter series has a base curve between 36 and 43 in 0.50 diopter steps. Trial lens is 0.5–1 mm bigger than spun cast.

Fitting Lenses for Myopia with B and L Series

Various Bausch and Lomb series are given in Table 17.2. All lenses have same front curves in the same series but variable posterior spheric curves which determine the power. Exception to this rule is that B_3 and F_3 series each having two different anterior curves. The diameters are 13.5 mm for B3, U3 and O3 and 14.5 mm for B4, U4, H4 and O4 series, 14 mm for sofspin and optima 38. Thickness of standard lenses like B series is 0.12 mm, and that of 'U' series is 0.06 mm, and for 'O' series is 0.035 mm.

FITTING METHODOLOGY

An ideally fitted lens should be well centered, comfortable and must provide crisp vision, proper corneal coverage and adequate oxygen supply to the cornea.

Choice of the Trial Lens

- Measure the horizontal diameter, i.e. horizontal visible iris diameter (HVID).
- B3, U3, or O3 lenses with diameter of 13.5 is the choice if HVID is <11.5 mm.
  - B4, U4, or O3 lenses with diameter of 14.5 mm is choice of HVID is more than 11.5 mm.
- U series is always the first choice. It should be tried in all cases of refitting, and in lenses with power more than –15.0 D.
  A change from B series to U series is advised if patient complains of excessive awareness or unstable vision with blink, or vertical endothelial stria after 4 hours wear with B series.
  - B3, B4 (standard thickness lenses) should remain the first choice in-patient with poor dexterity and in cry environments.
  - Once handling is learnt well with standard thickness lens, 'U' series should be tried again.
  - 'O' series are advised for patients who exhibit edema even with 'U' series.
- Inadequate corneal coverage demands lens of bigger diameter in the same series, i.e. U4 and B4 will replace U3 and B3 respectively. There is one exception that is U4 replaces B4 when latter gives inadequate coverage (Proper coverage means that the edge should extend about 0.75 mm beyond visible iris).
- Power is finalized by over-refraction.
- Lens finalization is complete when no untoward reaction is noted, after four hours of continuous wear (position, fit, movement, comfort and vision are evaluated).
- Final order will read (1) series and (2) power.

List of Daily-Wear Contact Lenses for Myopia

See Table 17.3.

Table 17.2 Design dimensions of Bausch and Lomb soft lens contact lenses

	Lens	Description	Powers (D)
Myopia	U3/U4	Thin daily wear	−0.25 to −900
	−B3	Standard daily wear	−0.25 to −20.00
	−B4	Standard daily wear	0.25 to −9.00
	Sofspin	Affordable daily wear	−0.25 to −6.00
	OPTIMA 38	Premium quality daily wear	−0.25 to 12.00
	Natural Tint:		
	(B3, U3, U4)	Cosmetic tinted daily wear	Plano to −6.00
	HO3/HO4	Thin high minus daily wear	−8.00 to −20.00
	03/04	Thin daily wear	−1.00 to −6.00
	03/04	Thin daily wear	−6.50 to −9.00
	B and L 70	High-water flexible wear	−0.25 to −9.00
Hyperopia	+U3/U4	Thin daily wear	+0.25 to +6.00
	+B3/B4	Mid-range daily wear	+0.25 to +6.00
	M3/M4	Mid-range daily wear	+3.00 to +6.00
	B and L 70	High water flexible wear	+0.25 to +6.00
	OPTIMA 38 (Low plus)	Premium quality daily wear	+0.25 to +6.00
Aphakia	H3/H4		+12.00 to +20.00
	B3 (High plus)	8.0 Optic zone daily	+11.00 to +20.00
	Wear (Flatter cornea)		+6.50 to +18.50
			+ 6.50 to +14.00
	High water extended wear		+10.00 to 20.00
Therapeutic	U/U3	Daily wear	Plano
	B4	Daily wear	Plano
	O4	Flexible wear	Plano
	T	Daily wear	Plano
	B and L 70	Flexible wear	Plano
Presbyopia	Crescent	Segmented daily wear	+6.00 to −6.00
	Near add		+ 1.50, 2.00, 2.50
	PA1	Simultaneous vision daily	+6.00 to −6.00
	Wear near add		+1.50 (nominal)
Astigmatism	B and L Toric		
	Standard daily wear	*Sphere:*	+4.00 to −6.00
		Cylinders:	−0.75, −1.25 and
			−17.5 (for minus):
			−1.25 and −1.75 (for plus) axes: 90° and 180° ± 20° in
			10° increments base curves
			8.3 and 8.6 mm

Table 17.3 Daily wear contact lenses for Myopia			
Lens/Manufacturer	*Polymer*	*Water contact*	*Power (%) Range (D)*
Softcon: American Optical Corporation	Wificon A	55	–0.25 to –8
Hydrocurve II: Barnes Hind/Hydrocurve	Bufilcon A	45	Plano to –20
CSI; Syntex Ophthalmics	Crofilcon A	38.5	Plano to –20
Soft lens: Bausch and Lomp	Polymacon	38.6	–0.25 to –20
Aquaflex; Cooper vision	Tetrafilcon A	42.5	Plano to –20
Dura soft; Wesley Jessen	Phemfilcon A	30, 38, 55	Plano to –20
Hydron: American Hydron	Polymacon	38	Plano to –20
Cibasoft Minus: Ciba Vision Care	Teflon	37.5	Plano to –10

FITTING OF LOW HYPEROPIA

Low plus lenses with power up to +7.00 can be fitted with N, B3 and B4. Fitting criteria is the same as for other Bausch and Lomb series.

Lathe Cut Soft Lenses

Lathe cut lenses are machined from dry hydrogel buttons. Process is the same as for polymethylmethacrylate (PMMA) lenses with the exception that the polishing compounds are oil based.

Fitting Methodology of Lathe Cut Lenses

Fitting is done by a trial lens set. The base curve of the trial lens varies from 36 to 42 in 0.5 dioptric steps, each base curve having a diameter of 13.5 and 14.00 mm. Power of all lenses is –3.00 D. There is a similar aphakic set with +12.00 power.

Fitting Procedure

- Verify spectacle refraction in minus cylinder.
- Do Keratometry.
- Put a trial lens and wait for 15–20 minutes. (Base curve chosen is 1.00 mm or 5.00 D flatter than the K in 44–60% hydration, base curve chosen is 0.5 or 2.5 D flatter than the 'K').
  (Power preferably should not deviate more that ± 4.00 from patients demand at corneal level).
- Correct base curve and diameter will show
  – Movement about 1 mm
  – Stable vision
  – Normal retinoscopic reflex on over refraction and
  – Undistorted mires on keratometry.

- In order to have a bigger or a smaller lens, a well fitted lens shall have to be changed in its base curve proportionately to avoid a change in fit, 0.5 mm increases in diameter demands 0.3 mm or 1.5 D flattening of the base curve.
- Final order is constituted by (1) Base curve (2) Power (3) Diameter.

Specifications of Available Lenses

- Base curve   7.5–9.5 mm in 0.1, 0.2, 0.3 steps
- Power   0 to ± 20.00 D
- Diameter   12–16 mm in 0.5 mm steps
- Thickness   0.03–0.07 mm depending on power
- Peripheral curve   11–13 mm depending on power
- Lens design   Higher plus and minus lens are made in lenticular design

Authors also use lathe-cut trial lens set which has been detailed in Table 17.4.

In India, lathe cut sauflon 70% and 55% and sauflex 44% are popularly used in diameters 13–15 mm in 0.5 steps. Fitting is done by trial lens method detailed earlier. Base curve is finalized on the basis of centering, movements, sharp retinoscopic reflex and stable visual acuity before, during and after the blink.

Fitting Recommendations

General guidelines for selection of lathe cut trial lens:
- *Diameter*: Choice of lens diameter depend on the visible iris diameter, generally 13.50 mm diameter lenses would satisfy majority of the cases, however lenses up to 15 mm are used in practice.

Table 17.4	RAPCOS trial set		
D	mm	Power	Diameter
36.00	(9.37)	–3.00	14.40 mm
36.50	(9.25)	–3.00	14.20 mm
37.00	(9.12)	–3.00	14.2 mm
37.50	(9.00)	–3.00	14.0 mm
38.00	(8.87)	–3.00	14.0 mm
38.50	(8.16)	–3.00	13.8 mm
39.00	(8.65)	–3.00	13.8 mm
39.50	(8.54)	–3.00	13.6 mm
40.00	(8.44)	–3.00	13.6 mm
40.50	(8.33)	–3.00	13.4 mm
41.00	(8.23)	–3.00	13.2 mm
41.50	(8.13)	–3.00	13.2 mm
42.00	(8.04)	–3.00	13.2 mm
42.50	(7.94)	–3.00	13.0 mm
43.00	(7.85)	–3.00	13.0 mm

- *Choice of base curve of trial lens:*
  - Soflex 44 and Soflex 66—A trial lens of 13.00 diameter should be 0.8 mm flatter than flattest "K"—A trial lens of 13.50 mm diameter should be 1.00 mm flatter than flattest "K" example—7.5 at 90°: 7.8 at 180°, so BC would be 8.8 mm—A trial lens of 14.00 mm diameter should be 1.10 mm flatter than flattest "K".
  - Soflex 88—A trial lens of 13.00 mm diameter should be 0.30 mm flatter than flattest "K"—A trial lens of 13.50 mm diameter should be 0.40 mm flatter than flattest "K"—A trial lens of 14.00 mm diameter should be 0.50 mm flatter than flattest "K".

Lathe-cut Lenses for Aphakia

The base curve of initial trial aphakic lens is 4.00 D flatter than the flattest, 'K' trial set 36.00–43.00 mm in 0.50 steps. Finalization is on the basis of centering movements, retinoscopic reflex and visual acuity. Trial power will be algebraic sum of trial soft lens power plus additional power of trial lenses in trial frame. Astigmatism of 2.00 or over may surface cylinder which are, oriented either with prism ballast or single truncation or double truncation of soft lenses. A double slab off lens with thinner upper and lower half is also good for cylinder orientation.

Bausch and Lomb Spun Cast Lenses for Aphakia

There are two series H3 and H4 for aphakia.

Fitting of aphakia with Bausch and Lomb series lenses:
- Note the flattest 'K'
- Find the effectivity of back vertex power at the cornea (adding half of minus cylinder to the sphere).
- Try H3 (13.5 mm) and see the fit. If the fit eccentric, or movements are more than 1 mm replace it by H4. Their powers are in range for aphakes suitability.

EXTENDED WEAR LENSES

There are lenses which are worn day and night for a definite period in contrast to permanent or continuous wear lenses which are worn day and night indefinitely. The extended wear lenses have the advantage of (a) normal vision at odd waking hours, (b) lack of difficulties due to handling disinfecting solutions and lens loss and damage while handling, and (c) excellent proposition during travel. There are physiological disadvantages with the extended wear which may build up especially during night wear. These are caused due to lesser oxygen supply, lid inaction, raised temperature of cornea, change in pH and lower osmolarity of tears.

There is an agreement after extensive experimental and clinical trial that extended wear lenses does not permit adequate corneal oxygenation during sleep.

Indications

- Patient with handling problems, e.g. children, old arthritic patients
- Patient with poor vision in the fellow eye
- Aphakes who fail to tolerate daily wear lens
- All candidates of intraocular implants
- All candidates where spectacles stand as obstacle in the job selection.

Contraindications

- Un-cooperative and unhygienic patients
- Patients who cannot come for a follow-up
- Patient who develop more than 6–8% edema with daily wear lenses
- Astigmatism more than 2.00 D.

Extended Wear Lenses

See Table 17.5.

For time to time removal sauflon lens is preferred because it is tougher than Permalens.

Fitting Methodology

- Do spectacle refraction in minus cylinder and transpose the value at corneal level
- Do keratometry
- Put a trial lens (0.5 mm or 2.50 D flatter than the 'K', i.e. if keratometry is 7.3 and 7.5, the trial lens is 8.00 mm in base curve)
- Evaluation is same as in daily wear.

Post Fitting Care

Patient should be called after 1st week, 1st month and then every three months. Disinfection and cleaning is same as for soft lens. A 5th day heat disinfection and 5th day overnight enzyme cleaning is a simple and effective regime.

Table 17.5 Extended wear lenses				
Lens	Hydration	Power (%)	Diameter	Base curve
Hydro curve II	55	0 to ± 20	14 and 14.5	8.5 and 8.8
Saulfon	70 to 85 (in 0.3 steps)	0 to ± 20	13.7 to 14.4	8.1 to 9.00
Permalens (lathe-cut)	71	0 to ± 20	11.5 to 13.5	6.5 to 8.8
Soflens (O series)	38 (in 0.3 steps)	−1.00 to −9.00	13.5 and 14.5	Aspheric

Complications

Following complications can occur but can be minimized if careful fitting, follow-up and instructions are adhered to.

- *Conjunctival:* Conjunctivitis, papillary hypertrophy
- *Corneal:* Epithelial edema, necrosis, endothelial stria, allergic and infective inflammations. Infection can be due to indolent bacteria and fungus that may lead to endophthalmitis
- *Lens:* Fracture, deposits, discoloration.

Astigmatism and Soft Lenses

Ultimate positioning and physiological outcome of the soft toric lens on the cornea is an outcome of certain anatomical ocular factors and physical lens factors. These may be individual corneal, limbal, conjunctival and palpebral anatomy and blinking characteristics.

Cylinder up to 1.00 D can be easily fitted with spheric lens. Higher cylinder presents a problem of residual cylinder. It is more with low sphere rather than a higher sphere, i.e. –1.00 sphere –0.75 cylinder is more significant than –7.00 sphere –0.75 cylinder. Significant residual cylinder with spherical trial lenses is fitted with toric lens. Toric lenses may be front or back toric. Cylinders higher than 2.50 D are fitted by front toric lenses and they are marketed as Durasoft, Miracon and Hydron and Optima torics. Cylinders below 2.5 are fitted with back toric lenses and are marketed as Hydrocurve and hydro Marc.

Positional stabilization is achieved by (a) Truncation-single or double (b) Prism ballast (c) Superior and inferior marginal thinning (d) Superior slab-off lenticular (This behaves like a prism ballast).

SOFT LENS PROBLEMS

Signs and symptoms of a fitted soft lens may be classified as follows:

- Procedural
- Extraneous
- Fitting
- Faulty lens
- Psychological problems.

Procedural

- *Faulty insertion and removal:* Rarely, in soft lenses, patients find difficulty in insertion or removal. The latter, however is more common than former more so in older persons lacking manual dexterity. Proper instructions and asking the patient to demonstrate overcomes this problem.
- *Eversion of lenses:* This is very common and the patient should be taught to recognize and rectify it (details in instructions).

- *Storage problems*: It is wrong to store soft lenses in water or solutions other than saline, which is the only vehicle in which soft lenses must be equilibrated before use.
- *Switched lenses*: This is quite common. Patients will complain of blurred vision or discomfort due to faulty fit. A check of specifications will rectify this problems.
- *Overwear syndrome*: This is exactly like that found in hard lenses. History, symptoms, signs and treatment are also the same. This is a problem with low water content lenses. It happens when patients sleep with these lenses. The author has seen it often, when a patient slept with 55% aphakic lenses. Proper instructions should be religiously adhered to avoid this.

Faulty Lens

A lens on inspection may be found to have different specifications in diameter, power, thickness and base curve. It may also have a bad or chipped edge, unblended or badly blended peripheral curves. Lenses can have bad optical quality. A lathe cut lens may show unpolished lathe marks.

All these may be verified in inspection of the lens.

Wrongly powered lens may be due to one of the following factors (a) wrong spectacles (b) wrong accounting for affectivity (c) incorrect methodology of power calculation (d) wrongly ordered or fabricated lens (e) increase in myopia (f) wrong keratometry.

If ordering is done by refracting through a trial lens of known and verified specifications errors are minimized. Weekly calibration of the keratometer and verification of the final lens parameters before ordering and verification after fabrication will also avoid residual error in power. Six monthly patient's check-up will exclude power error due to increase in error of refraction.

Fitting Problems

A fitted lens may start creating problems due to a variety of reasons. Problems basically arise due to metabolic or physical factors or both.

Soft Lens Post Fitting Care

Essentially soft lens after care is same as that of hard lenses. Some additional features for soft lenses and general comments will be highlighted here. The symptoms and signs may be mild, moderate and severe. Milder reaction includes mild spectacle blur, mild corneal edema, few corneal stains and one to four endothelial stria. The milder symptom may be adaptive and if so they should not continue beyond 2–3 weeks. If they continue, a thorough check and rectification needed, lens change is demanded if they persist.

Moderate symptoms and signs include a significant spectacle blur which does not correct itself fully within the same day, moderate corneal edema and corneal staining, four or more corneal stria, obvious papillary hypertrophy, mild neovascularization up to 1 mm and slight conjunctivitis or keratitis. These symptoms are treated symptomatically and lens is changed when required.

Severe problems constitute abrasion, ulcer and infection which require immediate ophthalmic attention.

Physical Problems in Soft Lenses

This is an important subject which should be known not only to the contact lens fitter but to every optometrist and ophthalmologist.

The main problem is that of a dirty lens. The debris on the lens is dependent on the composition of the patient's tears and on the methodology of handling, disinfection, hygienic habits, environment and other variables. Age of the lens, surface finish, porosity difference and hydration play a role. Soft lenses carry a net negative charge and readily combine with cations. Typical cations known are calcium, chlorhexidine gluconate, ethylmercuric chloride derived from thimerosal guide about the nature of debris likely to deposit. A lens that has been worn may show complex debris that may have constituents of tears, preservatives and substances deposited after chemical interactions amongst them. Debris has many ill-effects, it may cause hazy vision, irritation watering and reduced wear. Debris may not allow proper wetting and proper disinfection. It may cause discoloration and infection.

Protein build up: This develops with passage of time. It is present in most of the cases within 6 months. This deposit is dull white in color. It makes the lens rigid and impermeable to oxygen. Treatment is to clean the lens daily, or to instill acetyl cysteine 5% drops over the lens during wear, or to do enzyme treatment every week.

LENS DEPOSITS

Deposits may be inorganic and organic. Inorganic are more with chemical and organic more with thermal method of disinfection. The inorganic may be calcium phosphate, calcium carbonate, rust spots and mercurial. These can be prevented by thermal sterilization and cured by chelating agents like 5% EDTA. Organic deposits may be proteins, microorganisms, lipid, melanin, chlorhexidine, fluorescein and Rose Bengal. Best treatment is enzyme cleaning weekly and daily care by mechanical cleaning and boiling.

Deposits can be prevented by incorporation of sulfur, phosphorous and sulfonate (SO) to the plastic material. These impart a negative charge which repels the debris which is usually negatively charged.

Another method is to give an anticoating coat. This method makes the HEMA pores denser by a chemical treatment named HT90 by Diamond Shamrock. This treatment not only prevents deposits, but also increases the wettability and oxygen permeability.

Fungus growth: Fungi grow over and into the plastic. Fungal growth is usually due to lack of disinfection of a duplicate pair. Disinfection by boiling or by chemicals should be done every day.

Discoloration: Lenses with 55% hydration turned yellow in some cases with passage of time. Fluorescein discolors the lens immediately and requires 2–3 saline changes for rendering it possible for reuse. Epinephrine like compounds used as decongestant or mydriatic may discolor the lenses. Lenses have been found to turn yellow after continued washing with germicidal solution. Treatment with hydrogen peroxide 3% for 96 hours or more will bleach the tinted lens in most of the cases. Overnight soakage in saline containing "softab" (an effervescent tablet of dichloroisocyanurate) sterilizes the lens and deals with discoloration.

Infection: Serious conjunctival and corneal infection with contaminated lenses has been documented by the author. It can be viral, fungal and bacterial. Usual sources are lens case, lens solution saline, tweezer, and patient's hands. Treatment is to observe hygienic handling and to carry out instructions properly.

Lens spoliation: Soft lens spoliation can be initiated and perpetuated by the following factors, operating singly or in combination. They are trauma with boiling, chemical cleaning, preservatives, fungal and bacterial enzymes, self oxidation (OH), lid action and deposits.

Besides deposit and debris problems, these lenses may get split or displaced.

Loose Lens

Symptoms and Signs

A loose lens fit is indicated by: (1) Poor centering (2) Excessive movements, i.e. more than 1 mm on blinking or lateral gaze, (3) Variable vision which blurs on blinking (4) More awareness of the lens, (5) Edge stand off (6) Lens falling out of the eye (7) Bubble under the edge of the lens, (8) Keratometric mires on blinking blurred (9) Retinoscopic reflex blurs on blinking.

Treatment

- *Replace the loose lens by a steeper or larger lens*: In lathe cut lenses 0.5 mm increase in diameter or 0.20–0.30 mm decrease in base curve will tighten the lens. In spun cast change to steeper or larger series is desired to tighten the loose fit.
- *Splitting of lenses*: Being softer they are likely to get chipped. Soft lenses are approximately one fifteenth in hardness compared to PMMA hard lenses. The higher the water content, the greater is their fragility. Splitting starts as a small nick in the edge which extends into a split. A piece of soft lens may lie in the upper fornix for days together, without any symptom.
- *Lens displacement*: This can occur in flat lenses, in patients with wide palpebral apertures, in conditions where lens gets dried up as in dry eye syndromes, or in dry and hot atmosphere where prolonged exposure will dry the lenses. Treatment is symptomatic.

Metabolic Problems in Tight Lens

Symptoms and Signs

- Fluctuating vision that clears for a moment on blinking.
- Initially comfortable but becomes progressively uncomfortable as the day passes.
- Lack of movements after blink.
- Circumcorneal injection.
- Edge indentation of limbus or sclera to create a depression and obstruction in the flow of blood.
- Keratometric mires clear on blinking.
- Retinoscopic reflex is fuzzy and clears on blinking. An extremely tight lens will show excessive movements.

Treatment

- Replace the tight lens by flatter or a smaller lens.
- Blurred or unstable vision. This may be due to a combination of metabolic and physical factors.
  Most common cause is the protein build-up over the lens. *Other causes of reduced vision may be:*
  - A steep or a loose lens
  - Switched lenses (check specification to know this)
  - Inverted lens
  - Other deposits over the lens
  - Change in corneal curvature.
  Slit lamp examination helps to solve the above problems. Vision may become dim when the lens gets dried up during prolonged driving exposure to hot atmosphere, reduced blinking during the evening due to mental and physical fatigue. If change with similar lens gives clarity, it is a pointer towards bad optics of the lens. Blurred vision during reading is caused either by partial blinking and consequent lens dryness or by lens flexure by looking down. This is treated by holding the book at higher level.
- *Burning and irritation*
- This may be immediate or delayed. Immediate burning is caused by a contaminated lens due to chemical cleaner, toxic fumes, nicotine and hypo-or hypertonic saline. Protein build up can also cause irritation. Chemical contamination of lenses is treated by boiling the lenses.
- *Staining*
  - Continuous arcuate staining in the periphery of the cornea is indicative of dryness of the cornea or epithelial damage caused by the decentered lens. This is treated by a larger lens.
  - A patchy arcuate staining is indicative of a bad edge or bad blending. This is treated by a new lens with better blending of peripheral posterior curves.
  - Chaffing at the edge of the cornea is due to decentered lens. It is treated by using a lens with a bigger diameter.

- Scattered stippling of the cornea is due to dirty lens or anoxia caused by protein build-up. It is treated by cleaning the lens or by lens replacement.
- Diffuse generalized toxicity as in chemical, oil or grease. It can be due to hypersensitivity to chemical cleaner, or it can also be due to a viral infection.
- Stains due to foreign bodies are usually zigzag in configuration.
- A linear scratchy superficial staining at lower cornea is indicative or nail trauma during lens removal.

- *Corneal edema:* It is seen by slit lamp by retroillumination under high power. It is indicative of anoxia, commonly caused by a tight lens. Lower oxygen supply to the cornea can result from sleeping with lenses having water content below 60%. In environments with lower oxygen content as in congested places or at altitudes above 8000 feet, cornea will show edema due to anoxia.

  Edema of the cornea may be mild epithelial, or moderate epitheliostromal or severe, affecting the whole thickness of the cornea. It extends from limbus to limbus. Moderate and severe grades of edema are generally associated with swelling of lids, chemosis and circumcorneal injection. Edema, if left untreated leads to vascularization, and decline in comfort, clarity of vision and tolerance.

  Acute epithelial anoxic necrosis: It is due to severe and serious corneal anoxia, caused by over wear of low water content soft lenses (below 60%). The author has noted in two aphakic patients, acute pain, redness, chemosis, watering and photophobia. Cornea shows epithelial bullae. It shows central superficial feathery desquamation. The whole epithelium may be shed off like corn flakes. Stroma is grossly edematous and endothelium shows stria. Mild aqueous flare is noted in the anterior chamber. It is treated by antibiotic drops pad and bandage. Pain and apprehension are dealt by analgesics and sedatives. Serious trouble may be prevented by proper instructions to the patient.

- *Vertical stria in the cornea:* These are wrinkles in Descemet's membrane, indicative of corneal edema and treated by a flatter lens.
- *Fixed folds in Descemet's membrane:* Due to acute anoxia of the cornea, it is usually caused by prolonged wear, such as after overnight sleep with the lenses.
- *Indentation:* It is a circular groove created by the burrowing effect of the edge of a steep lens.
- *Vascularization:* It is indicative of a prolonged anoxia of the cornea, treated by a flatter or a smaller lens or by reducing the wearing time or may be by total discontinuation of lenses.
- *Photophobia:* This is induced by corneal irritation due to flat or steep lens, dirty lens, chemical contamination of lens or by hypo or hypertonic saline.
- *Excessive tearing:* This may be induced by improper lens fitting (flat or steep), damaged lens, contaminated lens or foreign body under the lens.

- *Giant papillary hypertrophy of tarsal conjunctiva*: This is an adverse reaction to lens wear material or lens deposits. It is treated symptomatically by lens refinement, lens replacement or lens discontinuation.
- *Patient dropouts:* This may be at the fitter's discretion. Lens is commonly withdrawn for vascularization, repeated infections and inability of the patient to come for a follow-up. Patients may stop using lenses due to persistence of complaints like discomfort, photophobia, reduced acuity or infection or replacements.
- *Psychological:* If a patient has a lot of symptoms and the fitter fails to find any sign, the problem is labeled as psychological.
- *Extraneous:* These problems are detailed under physical problems.

SOFT LENSES AS A THERAPEUTIC DEVICE

By now the therapeutic role of soft lenses is well established in the following medical and surgical conditions.
- Medical
    - *Corneal:* Chronic corneal edema (bullous-keratopathy).
      Abrasion, erosion, ulcerations.
      Filamentary keratitis.
      Chemical keratitis.
      Neurotropic and neuroparalytic keratitis.
      Herpetic keratitis.
      Dry eye syndromes
      Keratoconus.
      Anterior corneal dystrophies
    - *Lid:* Entropion, trichiasis, colobomas
- *Surgical:* To avoid postoperative discomforts.
  Corneal lacerations
  Corneal perforations
  Keratoplasties and keratectomies.
  Thermokeratoplasties.

The mode of action of soft lenses may be summarized as follows:
- It protects the eye from wind, dust, foreign bodies, cilia, lid concretions.
- Soft contact lens preserves secretions by reducing evaporation.
- It insulates corneal surface and promotes healing of epithelium by rising temperature.
- *Round the clock release of medication in medicated lenses*: As pilocarpine soaked lenses.
- It prevents symplepharon before and after surgery.
- Corneal pathology or wound healing can be observed without disturbing tissue.
- Epithelialization forms on smooth optical surface beneath contact lens, wound edges remain compressed.
- Wounds are packed (hard).

- Blinking allows better tear circulation than with patching.
- Lid action on damaged epithelium avoided by soft lenses.
- It reduces pain from exposed or damaged nerve endings.
- Vision is not obstructed as in patching, conjunctional flap or tarsorrhaphy as it is a transparent bandage.

The author has documented the successful use of the soft lenses as a therapeutic device in the following diseases and adjunctive therapy is also mentioned (Table 17.6).

Handling of soft lenses: Insertion, removal cleaning disinfection

General instructions: Keep the nails short, wash your hands thoroughly before handling lenses.

Table 17.6 Indications of therapeutic soft contact lens and adjunctive therapy in these conditions	
Diseases	*Adjunctive therapy*
Bullous keratopathy	• Five per cent saline 5 times a day
	• Tablet diamox (raised IOP) thrice daily
	• S/conj. Decadron (iritis) daily
	• Soda Bicarb washes (meibomitis) (Mechanically with lid massage)
	• 20% glycerin 5 times a day
Dry eyes	• 0.9% salien 4–8 times a day
(Keratoconjunctivities sicca	• Moisol 4–8 times a day
Pemphigus	• Change of pH
Xerosis	• Adapt drops—one drop hourly
Steven-Johnson Syndrome	• Adapt drops 2 hourly
Trachoma IV-S)	• Soda bicarb washes (3%) for blepharitis
Indolent ulcer	• Depending on cause
Graft ulcer	• IDU one hourly
Indolent keratitis	• Fungizone four hourly
Recurrent erosions	• Gentamycin four hourly
Corneal fistula	• Mucomyst thrice daily
Filamentary keratitis	• 1:10 Decadron drops
Chemical keratitis (Alkali and Acid)	
Lagophthalmos with external	Mechanical movement of lens and saline
Ophthalmoplegia	Washes 4 times a day
	Postoperative bandage lens Remove the discharge that collects under the lens every 24 hourly
Glaucoma	Use pilocarpine soaked lenses
Neuroparalytic keratitis	Saline drops thrice daily
	Bausch and Lomb O4 and B4 are used as therapeutic lenses also

Insertion: Insertion of soft lenses is exactly the same as in hard lenses.

A trapped bubble behind the lens may be massaged out. This is done by gentle rubbing of the upper lid over the soft lens.

Removal: It is different from hard lenses. Hard lenses are popped out by lid action but soft lenses are pinched out. Eye ball is moved up. The lens slips toward the lower fornix and is pinched out by holding between index finger and the thumb. Right and left hands are used for respective lenses.

In older patients, insertion and removal difficulties are common. Some inmate of the house may learn this handling to help the patient.

Taco test: Before insertion of lenses, one should be sure that the lens is not inside out. This can be verified by gently folding the lens between the thumb and forefinger. In normal lens edges should point inward and look like a Mexican taco with the edges touching. When the edges roll outwards rather than inwards the lens is inside out and must be reversed.

It is important that the lens be grasped and folded near the apex of the lens rather than at its edges.

Soft Lens Care and Solutions

Various solutions are used for cleaning, rinsing, storage and disinfection.
- *Saline:* It is best to use small packages of unpreserved saline (0.9% Sodium Chloride). Injectable saline is used alternatively.
- *Lens cleaners:* Essentially have non ionic detergents which remove surface deposits. Besides it contains sodium chloride, buffer hydroxyethylcellulose and polyvinyl alcohol. Usual preservatives are 0.004% thiomersal and 0.2% disodium edetate. Pliagel has 0.1% sorbic acid and 0.5% disodium edetate.
- *Lens storage and rinsing solution:* This is essentially normal saline and buffer which is preserved with 0.001% thiomersal, 0.1% disodium edetate and 0.005% chlorhexidine. The solution with chlorhexidine cannot be used for boiling as it makes lens milky white. Pliagel is a thiomersal free lens cleaner.
- *Disinfecting solution:* This is constituted of saline, buffer, wetting agents and 0.001% thiomersal and 0.005% chlorhexidine.
- *Enzyme tablet:* This is dissolved in distilled water and lens is put in this solution for at least 6 hours. It acts best at a temperature of 37°C. Low water content for 3 hours and high water content for 15 minutes.
- *5% hydrogen peroxide:* Five minutes soakage in this solution disinfects and cleans the lens. It should be followed by two washings with saline as hydrogen peroxide cannot be put in the eye.

New Care Systems

- Hydrogen peroxide with enzyme
- Hydrogen peroxide with neutralizing tablet for neutralization, one can also use saline, platinum, catalase thiosulfate, sodium bicarbonate.

Daily Care

- Store it overnight in saline with 0.1% disodium edetate
- Keep the bottle in steam for 15 minutes for disinfection
- Do enzyme cleaning every week.

Caution

- Do not instil any medicine in the eye over the lens.
- Do not wear lenses if the eye has
  – Constant irritation
  – Constant blurring
  – Constant watering
  – Constant pain
  – Constant redness
  – Constant discharge
  – Broken lens
- Do not prescribe lenses to patient who do not follow instructions.
- Never use hard lens solutions for soft lenses, as preservative especially benzalkonium chloride binds itself with soft lens and causes serious corneal damage.

Soft Lens Inspection and Verification

The tabulated scheme highlights the soft lens specification and the instruments for their verification (Table 17.7).

Table 17.7 Evaluation of soft contact lens	
Specifications	*Methodology*
Diameter	• Measuring magnifier
	• Wet cell
Base curve	• Soft lens analyzer (template mounted projector viewing)
	• Keratometer (lens in liquid cell)
	• Radioscope (lens in liquid cell)
	• Spherometer
	• Spherical templates
Thickness	• Radiuscope
	• Electronic thickness gauge
Power	• Lensometer
	• Water cell method
Surface quality	• Biomicroscope
	• Stereoscope
	• Loupe

CIBA VISION SOFT CONTACT LENSES (TEFILCON)

CIBA vision (tefilcon) soft (hydrophilic) contact lenses are made from hydroxyethylmethacrylate (HEMA) with a water content of 37.5% by weight.

For a complete listing of available lens parameters, please refer lens parameters available.

Fitting soft contact lenses is easy and predictable. Custom fitting of each eye is recommended. This can be accomplished by using a small trial set or by fitting from inventory.

CIBA vision (tefilcon) soft contact lenses are suitable for daily wear. Choosing CIBA vision (tefilcon) soft contact lenses requires a professional judgment by the fitter.

Clinical evaluation of fitting performance is described below:
Lenses which satisfy the criteria of a well-fitted lens listed in this fitting guide may be dispensed. A gradual increase in lens wearing time is recommended. Satisfactory physiological response after full adaptation to daily wear is a requirement for acceptable lens performance. This should be determined with a thorough biomicroscopy examination after at least four hours of lens wear at all follow-up visits.

PARAMETERS AVAILABLE

Diameter	13.8 mm	14.5 mm		
Base curve	8.3 mm	9.6 mm	8.9 mm	9.2 mm
Power range	–10.00 D to –6.00 D (in steps of 0.50 D)			
	–6.00 D to + 4.00 D (insteps of 0.25 D)			

(Special parameter also available see annexure)
Center thickness 0.1 mm at –3.00 D.

FITTING PROCEDURE OUTLINE

- Prefitting examination
- Initial lens power selection
- Initial lens diameter selection
- Initial lens base curve selection
- Initial lens evaluation
- Follow-up care.

FITTING PROCEDURE

- *Prefitting examination is necessary to:*
  - Determine whether a patient is a suitable candidate for contact lenses
  - Assess whether a patient is suitable for daily wear.
  - Make ocular measurements for initial contact lens parameter selection

- Collect baseline clinical information to which postfitting examination results can be compared.

A prefitting examination should include a thorough case history, spherocylindrical refraction, measurement of horizontal visible iris diameter (HVID), keratometry, tear assessment and biomicroscopy.

- *Initial lens power selection*
  - To determine initial lens power, convert the spherocylindrical spectacle Rx to its spherical equivalent as follow:
    Spherical equivalent = sphere power + 1/2 cylinder power
  - If the spherical equivalent is greater than ± 4 D a vertex distance correction is necessary (see vertex distance conversion chart) to determine the lens power required at the corneal plane.
- *Initial lens base curve selection*
  - In general, most patients accept 8.6 mm base curve. Begin with this base curve.

Note: If keratometry readings indicate that the central cornea is unusually steep or flat, the fitter may wish to exercise professional judgment and start with a steeper or flatter base curve, respectively.

- *Initial lens evaluation*
  - Select an initial lens from inventory or a diagnostic fitting set for each eye of the power and base curve as determined in steps 2 and 3.
  - Allow the lenses to settle on the eye for approximately 15 minutes.
  - Evaluate the lenses (see criteria of a well-fitted lens)
  - If an acceptable fit is observed for both eyes, the lenses can be dispensed after instructing the patient on proper lens handling and cleaning/disinfecting. If trial lenses are used, a spherical over-refraction should be conducted to determine the proper lens power to be ordered. When the lenses are received they should be examined on the eye to assure that the criteria of well fitted lens are still satisfied. Wearing time should be gradually increased over a period of days.

CLINICAL ASSESSMENT

Criteria of a Well-fitted Lens

- Full corneal coverage
- Good centration (concentric about the visible iris)
- Satisfactory movements in up gaze, CIBA vision soft lenses should exhibit 0.2–0.5 mm of movement in up gaze.
- Satisfactory lens lag response by the patient.

In Office Care Regimen for Trial Lenses

- Clean front and back surface of lens with recommended surfactant cleaner
- Disinfect lens using a recommended hydrogen peroxide or chemical disinfection system

- Store lens in sterile saline or other recommended storage solution
- If a trail lens is not dispensed, you must clean and disinfect the lens prior to another trial fitting.

Characteristics of a Tight (Steep) Lens

A tight CIBA vision soft contact lens would display some or all of the following characteristics:

- Good centration
- Little or no up gaze movement with the blink
- Little or no up gaze lag
- Good comfort
- Blurred vision which clears immediately following blink
- Bubble(s) under the lens
- Conjunctival indentation and/or blanching of limbal vessels at the lens edge
- Limbal-conjunctival hyperemia.

Characteristics of a Loose (Flat) Lens

A loose CIBA vision SOFT (Tefilcon) contact lens would display some or all of the following characteristics:

- Decentration (usually temporally and/or superiorly)
- Excessive up gaze movement with the blink
- Excessive up gaze lag
- Reduced comfort response-usually lower lid sensation.
- Lens edge standoff
- Unstable vision.

Basic Instruction for Patient Cleaning and Disinfecting

The eye care practitioner's instructions to the patient concerning cleaning and disinfecting contact lenses should include the following:

- CIBA vision soft contact lenses are only recommended for use with chemical (not heat) disinfection system.
- CIBA vision recommended the use of one system of lens care. Unless specially indicated in the labeling, do not alternate, change, or mix lens care systems for any one pair of lenses.
- Do not reuse solution. Use fresh solutions for each step.
- Do not use saliva, tap water, distilled water, or anything, other than a recommended sterile solution labeled for the care of soft lenses.
- Lenses must be both cleaned and disinfected each time they are removed, for any reason. If removed while the patient is away from the lens care products, the lenses may not be re-inserted but should be stored until they can be cleaned and disinfected. Cleaning is necessary to remove mucus and film from the lens surface. Disinfecting is necessary to destroy harmful microorganisms.

- Clean one lens first (always the same lens first to avoid mix-ups) rinse the lens thoroughly with sterile saline or disinfecting solution to remove the cleaning solution, mucus, and film from the lens surface, and put the lens into the correct chamber of the lens storage case. Then repeat the procedure for the second lens.
- Stored lenses must be disinfected and left in the closed case until ready to wear.
- If the lenses have been stored for more than 24 hours, disinfect immediately before wearing and at least once a week. Put fresh solution inside the lens chambers completely covering the lenses, before each disinfecting.
- After removal of lenses from the lens case, the case should be emptied rinsed with sterile saline for disinfecting solution, and allowed to air dry. At the next use of the case, fill it with fresh solution.

Lens Deposits and Use of the Enzymatic Cleaning Procedure

In order to remove protein which may form on the lenses wearers should use enzymatic contact lens cleaning tablets according to the directions for use which accompany the tablets. The practitioner's instructions should emphasizes that the lenses must be disinfected after completing all cleaning procedures, including enzymatic cleaning.

Key Product Information

See Table 17.8.

Table 17.8 CIBA vision soft lenses	
Lens type	Soft lens
Design concept	Standard thickness
	Bicurve posterior surface
	Conventional edge
Wearing indication	Daily wear
Posterior design	Bicurve
Manufacture	Front surface lathe cut
Type	Back surface cast mould
Material	HEMA38 (Tefilcon)
Water content	37.5%
Oxygen permeability	8.9×10^{-11}
Central thickness	0.12 mm at −3.00 D
Edge thickness	50 microns
Oxygen transmission	$8.9 \text{ mm} \times 10^{-9}$
Lens diameters	13.8 mm
Base curves	8.3 mm/8.6 mm
Lot numbers	8.9 mm/9.2 mm

Contd...

Contd...

Power range	Category I (in steps of 0.50 D)					
	–60.50 D to + 4.00 D					
	–60.50 D to –20.00 D					
	+ 04.50 D to +20.00 D					
Optical zone size	8.35 mm					
Trial set parameter	13.8 mm	8.3 mm	8.6 mm	8.9 mm	9.2 mm	8.9/14–5
	–03.00 D	1	2	1	1	1
	–10.00 D	1	1			
	+03.00 D	1	1			
Fitting philosophy	Trial lens fitting start with BC nearest to the value 0.9 mm flatter than flattest K reading (Make flatter by 0.8–1.00 mm)					
Care system compatibility	Recommended for use with thermal, chemical hydrogen peroxide					

18 Contact Lens: Optics

INTRODUCTION

To understand the correction of ametropia by contact lens it is essential to understand the behavior of rays passing through the plastic contact lens and the tear lens before they hit the cornea.

EFFECTIVITY

A convergent or a divergent bundle has a power that is reciprocal of the length of the bundle in meters (Fig. 18.1A).

- Power of a bundle having a focal length fi is $1/f = f$
- The bundle after traveling a distance 'd' has a power $1/f - d$.

POWER OF A LENS IN AIR

A lens with a front and back surface power of F_1 and F_2 and radii of r_1 and r_2 having a thickness 't' and refractive index n, can have various powers such as front vertex power, back vertex power and equivalent power (Fig. 18.1B).

If the thickness is ignored the back vertex power (PVP) = $F_1 + F_2$. Considering the effect of thickness (t) and refractive index (n) apply the formula of effectivity to get the BVP.

$$BVP = F2 + F1/1 - F1 \times t/n$$

TWO LENSES IN AIR

If two lenses have the same radius but are of opposite sign, it does not matter whether they are placed in touch with each other or with a thin air film in between them. So a contact lens, whose back surface radius is the same as the front surface of the cornea, will correct the refractive error whether you place it over the cornea or at a little distance from the cornea provided the back vertex power is equal to the refractive error of the eye.

Example: Two lenses, one with surface power of + 10.00 D and –5.00 D (refractive index = 1.5) and the second of surface powers + 6.00 D and + 10.00 D (refractive index = 1.6) are placed together with –5.00 D of the first touching the + 6.00 D of the second.

Considering the separate powers of the total power = + 10.00 – 5.00 + 6.00 + 10.00 = 21.00 D

Radius (r2) of the second concave surface of the first lens
$$r2 = 1 - n/f2 = 1.15/5.0 = 0.1 \text{ m}$$
Radius (r2) of the +6.00 D surface of the second lens
$$n - 1/F3 = 1.6 - 1/ + 6 = 0.1 \text{ m}$$
Total power of the interface when lenses are placed in closed apposition
$$n - n/r = 1.6 - 1.5/0.1 = 1.00 \text{ D}$$
Considering the total system the power
$$+10.00 + 10.00 = 21.00 \text{ D}$$

FLUID LENS

When a contact lens is placed over the cornea it always traps a tear film behind it. To consider the power of the trapped fluid (fluid lens) one has to consider the radii or curvature of the bordering surfaces, i.e. back surface of the lens and front surface of the cornea. There are three separate systems (Fig. 18.1C). One is contact lens in air, second is fluid lens in air and third is corneal lens.

$$\text{The fluid lens power} = n - 1/f2 + 1 - n/rc$$

whereas, n = 1.3375 and r2 is the curvature of the back surface of contact lens and rc is radius of front surface of cornea.

CHANGE IN BASE CURVE

When the base curve is fitted parallel to the cornea, the fluid does not have any power. If the base curve is steepened by 0.5 D then there is a corresponding steepening of the anterior surface of the fluid lens which becomes more convex or more (+) by 0.50 D. This direct relationship is due to fact that all the calculations are made on the basis of refractive index 1.3375 which is used for cornea, fluid lens and the base curve of the plastic lens.

Examples

1. K	42.00 × 180		2. K	48.00 × 90	
	42.50 × 90			46.00 × 180	
Px	−4.00−0.25 × 180		Px	−1.00 − 2.00 × 90	
BC	41.00		BC	48.00	
P	−3.00		P	−3.00	

CALCULATION OF THE OUTER OPTIC RADIUS AND POWER OF THE CONTACT LENS

After finalizing the base curve, power, thickness and refractive index one needs to calculate the required outer optic radius and power. The problem may be solved by tracing a pencil in the reverse direction through the lens starting from the back focus, and finding the front surface power required to render the rays parallel on emergence (Fig. 18.1D).

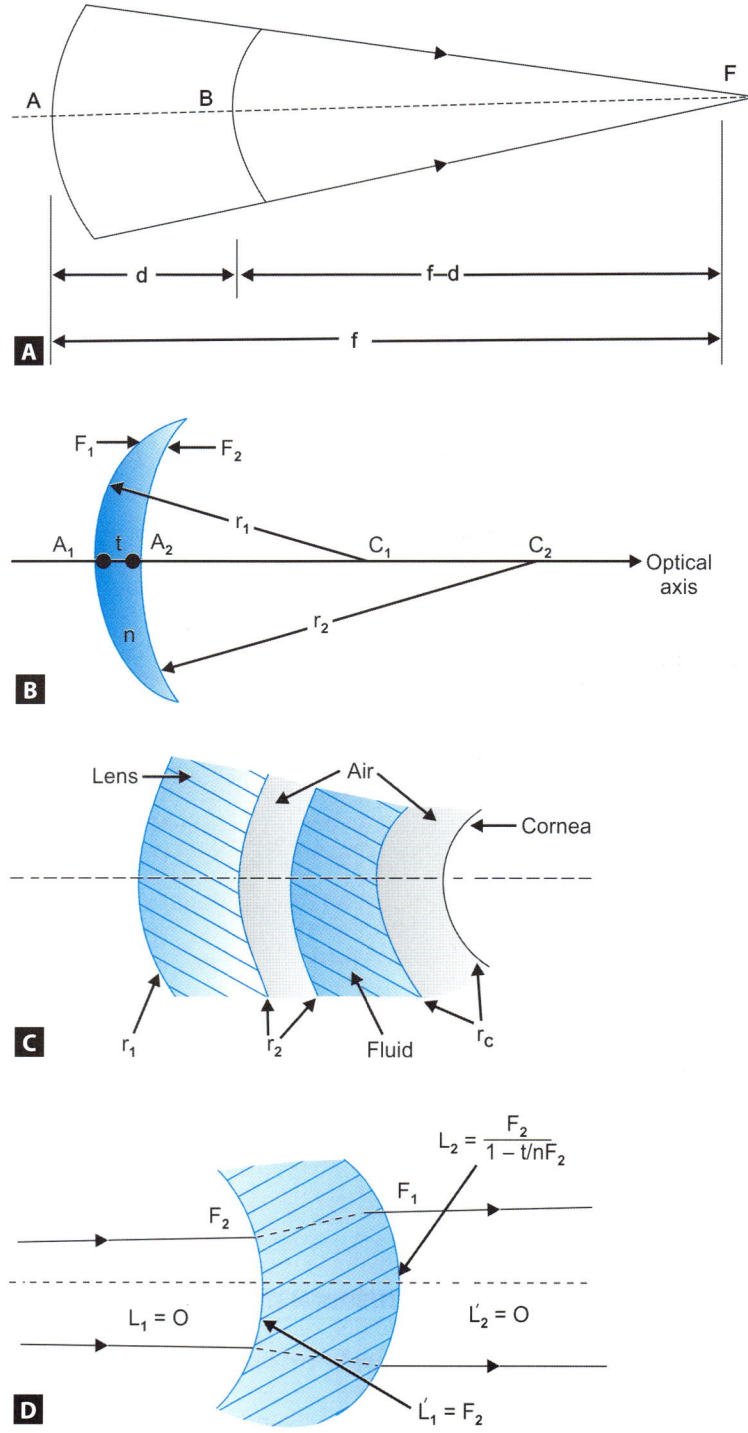

Figs 18.1A to D Refraction of rays through various lenses

Example: If the base curve is 8.5 mm, power –5.00 D, thickness 0.6 mm, refractive index 1.49 the outer optic radius is calculated as follows: Back surface power is

$$n - 1/r2 = 1.49 - 1/.0085 = .490/.0085 = 57.65 \text{ D}$$

Tracing the divergent bundle of –5.0 D backward, it becomes a convergent bundle of +5.0 D hitting –57.65 D. So net power at the back surface is –57.65 + 5.00 = –52.65 D. Effectivity of –52.65 D after passing through the above thickness and medium –51.57. This is the strength of bundle, which is just to emerge out of the front surface of the contact lens. This must be neutralized by a front surface outer optic power of +51.57 to render the emergent rays parallel and the radius of the outer surface will be

$$n - 1/F1 = 490/51.57 = +9.5 \text{ mm}$$

PRISM EFFECT

Prism effect in the two eyes may be variable if the contact lenses do not center well on the cornea. It is calculated according to Prentice's rule, i.e. power in diopters multiplied by displacement from the optical center in centimeters.

ACCOMMODATION

With spectacles there is less accommodation in myopes and more in hypermetropes compared to an emmetrope (Figs 18.2A to C). If spectacle power of 9 ± 7.00 D are compared at cornea (vertex distance of 15 mm), it will be +8.47 and –6.33, which will be the contact lens power. Now if print at 33.33 cm form spectacles is considered then net vergence reaching the cornea through the spectacles ± 7.00 will be +4.26 and –8.70. So the net accommodation at corneal level is +4.26 – (8.47) = –4.21 for hyperope and –8.70 – (3.33) = –2.37 for myope and emmetrope will accommodate –2.87 (the effectivity of –3.00 D at 15 mm). With contact lenses there will be equal accommodation for hyperope, myope and emmetropes as the lenses are now over the cornea.

CONVERGENCE

To relieve convergence weakness base in prism is usually prescribed. With spectacles a myope converges more compared to an emmetrope (Fig. 18.3). This is due to base in and the base out prism effect of minus and plus spectacle lenses. Due to the contact lens, the convergence is exerted equally in hyperope, myope and emmetrope. This is because optical axis passes through the optical center of the contact lens in all positions of gaze.

MAGNIFICATION

Magnification needs a special mention in contact lenses because here the size of retinal image differs considerably from image formed with glasses (Fig. 18.4). Comparison of image formed by glasses (or contact lens) with the image without

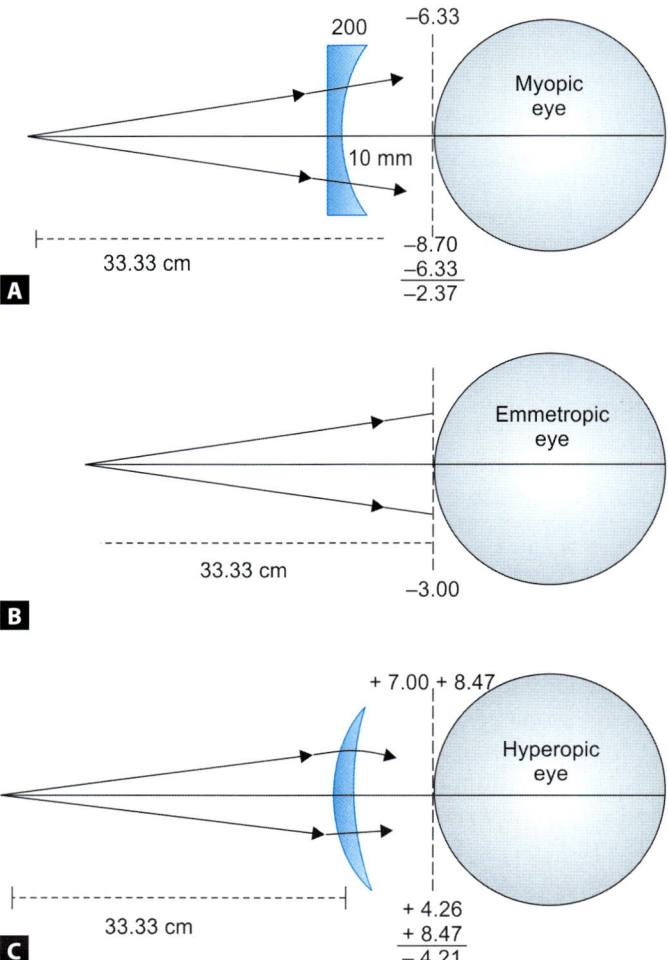

Figs 18.2A to C Accommodation in myopia, emmetropia and hyperopia

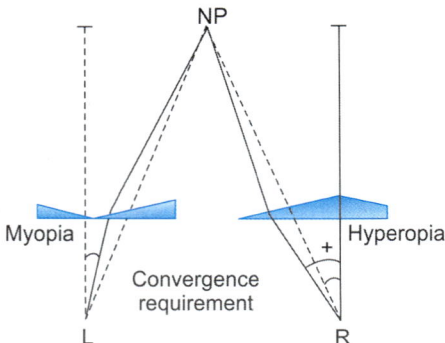

Fig. 18.3 Convergence in different refractive errors

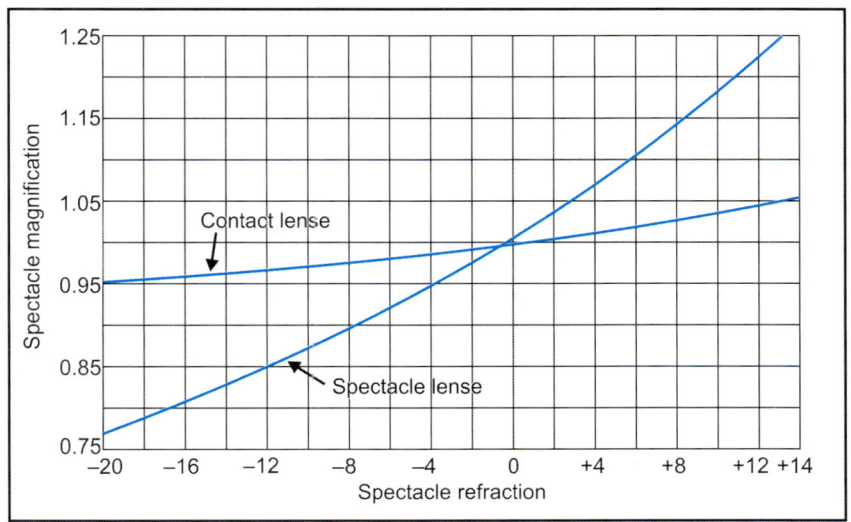

Fig. 18.4 Spectacle magnification in different powers

glasses and with image in a schematic eye is called spectacle and relative spectacle magnification can be calculated by the following formula:

$$1/1-aF$$

where 'F' is the power of the lens and "a" is the distance between entrance pupil and the lens in meters. Example F = 10.00 D and a = 15 mm hence spectacle magnification = 1/1 – (0.015 × 10) = 1/0.85 = 1/0.85 = 1.176. This is equivalent to increase of 17.6% similarly for minus lenses, example F = 10.50 D "a" in contact lenses is 3 mm. So spectacle magnification is 1/1 – (0.003 × 10.5) = 1/1.0315 = 0.97. This is equivalent to a decrease by 3%.

Relative spectacle magnification (RSM). This is a ratio of retinal image in corrected ametropic eye to that in the schematic eye having a reference to a distant object (Figs 18.5A and B). This is given by the formula:

$$Fo+Fs -d Fs Fe$$

where Fo is the power of the schematic eye, Fs is the spectacle refraction, Fe is the power of given ametropic eye and 'd' is the distance from spectacle point to the eye's first principle point. Power of the ametropic eye is difficult to measure, a rough estimate can be attained from axial length, RSM is considered, separately for axial and refractive errors, for example + 10.00 at 15 m in eye of 43.00 diopters will have RSM 27% as given below. RSM is

$$9/10 + 43 -0.015 × 10 × 43 = 59/46.5 = 1.27$$

where, 59 is the value of schematic eye. Contact lens image can be compared to orthodox spectacle by the formula 1/dFs for example –20.00 at 12 mm form eye, will yield 1.24 indicating that contact lens image will be 24% larger than equivalent spectacles.

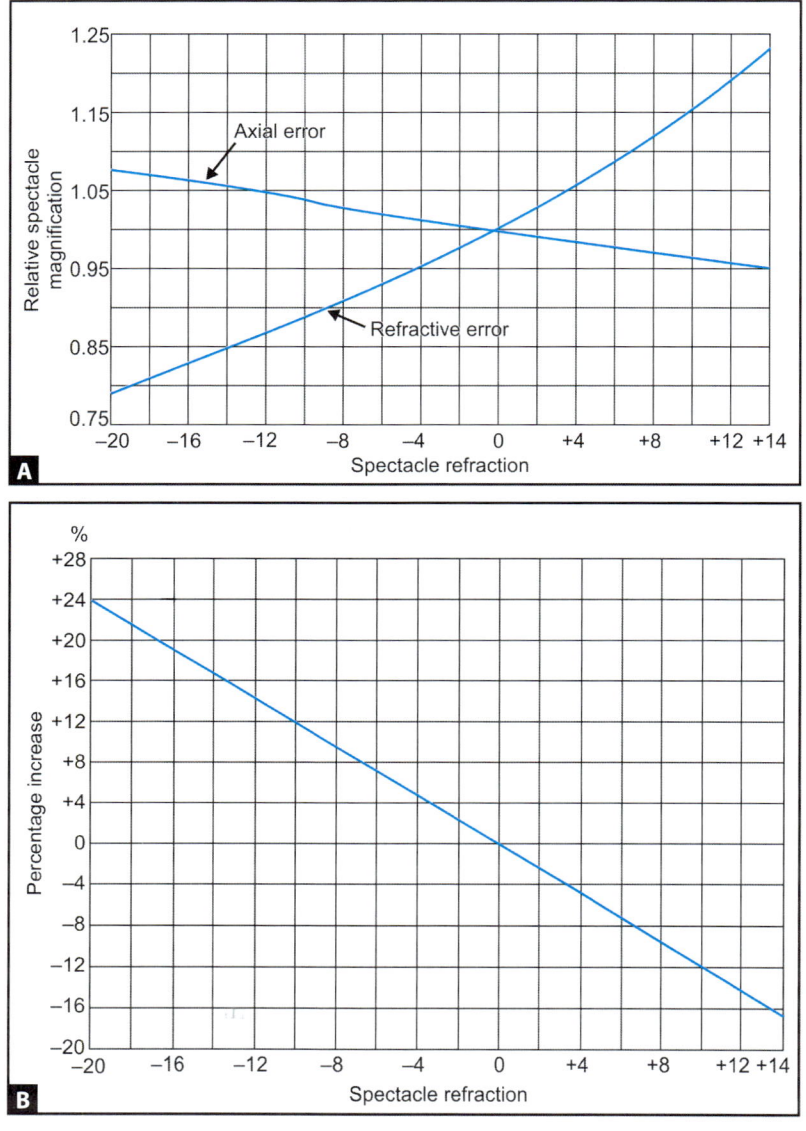

Figs 18.5A and B Relative spectacle magnification

Magnification in aphakia with spectacles and contact lenses: Considering schematic eye 59.60 D, power of aphakic is equivalent to 43.08 D and spectacle of 11.12 D at 12 mm from cornea. RSM I this case would be 59.60/43.08 + 11.12 – 0.012 × 43.08 × 11.12 = 1.23.

This would amount to an increase of 23% with spectacle. The contact lens gives an image 12% smaller compared to spectacle refraction of +11.12 or 0.88 compared to unity. Hence, contact lens image compared to unity in schematic eye would be 0.88 × 1.23 = 1.08 so the disparity is reduced from 1.23 to 1.08 or 23% to 8% magnification.

CHAPTER 19

Ocular Response to Contact Lens Wear

INTRODUCTION

Successful contact lens wear depends on adequate oxygen supply to the cornea; proper tear exchange and unchanging biocompatibility of the lens material. Any hindrance in these particularly a lack of good oxygen supply leads to corneal intolerance and subsequent discontinuation of the lens wear.

Any lens material that transmits inadequate oxygen if worn for a long duration leads to a syndrome known as corneal exhaustion syndrome or corneal fatigue syndrome. This is characterized by episodes of corneal edema after 6–8 hours, intolerance to lens wear, changes in posterior corneal translucency and endothelial irregularity (Holden et al.).

Despite the well-established fact that polymethyl methacrylate (PMMA) has undesirable, long lasting effects on the cornea, they are still being widely used. Daily wear of these lenses can also lead to corneal exhaustion syndrome. Low water content hydrogel with thickness of 0.2–0.3 mm also produces this syndrome.

Given a choice between daily wear and extended or continuous wear most patients opt for extended wear lenses because of their convenience Extended wear lenses are used by 20–30% of contact lens wearers in USA.

RELEVANT HISTORY

When De-Carle launched extended wear lenses he reported no side effects. This prompted contact lens practitioners to prescribe these lenses with little reason for added concern. Later studies by Ruben, Cooper, and Constable, etc. brought to light the serious ocular problems caused by these lenses. Having confirmed these, Holden et al. advised the practitioners to be more cautious than before while prescribing extended wear lenses.

CONTRIBUTING FACTORS

Factors contributing to ocular problems with contact lens wear are hypoxia, increased tear osmolality, increased temperature, reduced pH, increased carbon dioxide accumulation and lens effect.

The biochemical and physiochemical changes in the epithelium in response to EW/continuous wear were found to be decreased oxygen uptake, lactate accumulation, acid shift, enzyme shifts and probably changes in DNA and RNA synthesis, decrease in hemidesmosome numbers, reduced nerve density and altered cell shape has been noted.

Flow chart 19.1 Ocular effects of extended wear (EW) lens

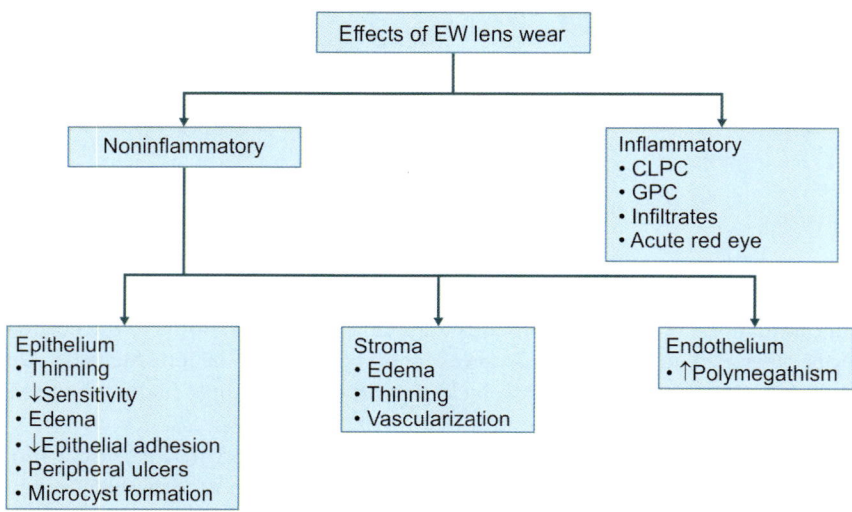

Abbreviations: CLPC, contact lens papillary conjunctivitis; GPC, giant papillary conjunctivitis.

Flow chart 19.2 Effect of extended wear lens on corneal epithelium

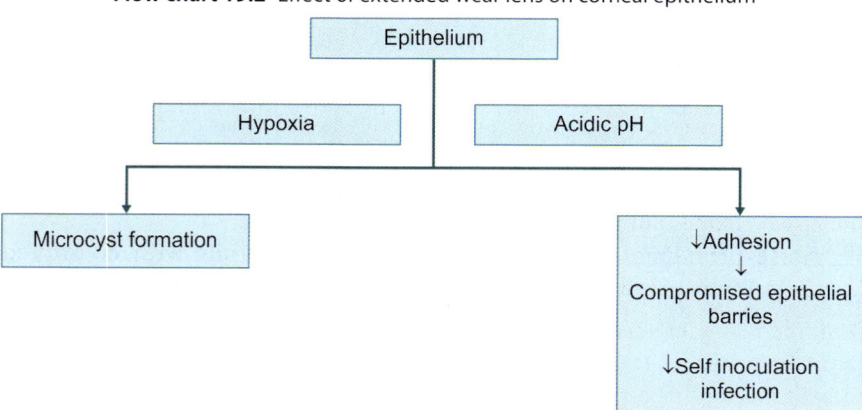

EFFECTS

Effects of extended wear lenses on the cornea may manifest as changes in the epithelium, stroma and endothelium, if undetected early they may become irreversible. The changes have been summarized by Holden et al. as under (Flow charts 19.1 to 19.3).

Polymethyl methacrylate (PMMA) and rigid gas-permeable (RGP) lenses show little macroscopic changes in lid, hyperemia/follicles probably because of lower deposit levels, better lens movement, tear exchange and reduced area of contact.

Flow chart 19.3 Effect of extended wear lens on corneal stroma

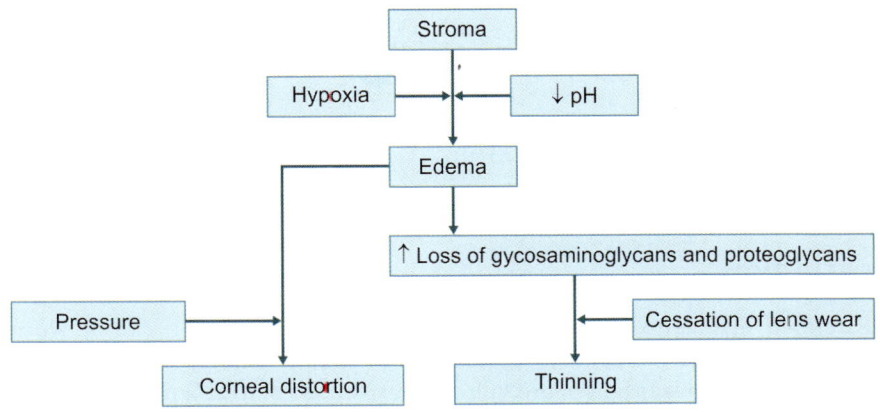

Acute red eye (ARE) usually occurs when flexible contact lenses become bound overnight. The cause is probably related to a build-up of debris under the lens and to tightening of the lens fit which results in clamping of the limbal conjunctiva.

Microcyst formation was first reported by Ruben et al. It is a delayed response to chronic epithelial hypoxia and clinically becomes evident as small, rounded, well-circumscribed transparent inclusions. They appear after 8–12 weeks of lens wear and clear in about 12 weeks following cessation of lens wear. They are probably degenerate, apoptotic cells. Prolonged daily wear of thick low water content lens for months and years by professional actor have shown irreversible corneal edema and fine surface irregularities causing disturbed catadioptric image which does not permit keratometry.

These problems can be avoided by using materials with continued biocompatibility, high DK values and careful examination followed by regular supervision.

CHAPTER 20

Extended Wear Lenses

DEFINITION

Extended wear lenses (EWL) can be defined as lenses which can be worn continuously day and night for several days, weeks, or months without removal. Since extended wear lenses are lathe-cut except for silicon lenses, there is a great future both for hydrophilic and nonhydrophilic extended wear lenses with improvement in manufacturing technology and polymers. The day is not far when all the small manufacturing laboratories will fabricate all types of lenses and cater to custom design as we do today with utmost ease for polymethylmethacrylate (PMMA) lenses. Extended wear lenses give additional benefit of comfort, better centration, convenience and above all improved corneal function. Being more fragile, these lenses are more difficult to handle, clean and get easily damaged. They are more costly due to high basic cost and need for early replacement due to deposit and damage.

CLASSIFICATION

On the basis of hydration they can be classified into low, medium and high water content lenses. Another way to classify is on the basis of relative hardness and least water content, and this group includes silicon, CAB and mixed lenses like polycon. By mistake patients have also used PMMA lenses as well for years. The former classification on the basis of hydration includes soft lenses, i.e.

- *Low water content (below 40%)*: Such lenses have to be very thin for successful extended wear as CSI lens is 39% water (thickness 0.03 and 0.08 mm), if other lenses are not available rarely Bausch and Lomb Polycon with 39% water (thickness 0.35 mm) have been used.
- *Medium water content (40–60% water)*: Hydrocurve I is 45% water (thickness 0.06–0.07 mm). Hydrocurve II is 55% water (thickness 0.08–0.29 mm), softcon is 55% water (thickness 0.25–0.60).
- *High water content lenses (more than 60% water)*: This group includes Permalens with 69–72% water (thickness 0.24–0.43 mm), and Sauflon with 70–85% water (thickness 0.05 mm).

CHEMICAL COMPOSITION

It is important to know the chemical constituents of each of the gas permeable lenses because physical properties are dependent on chemical structure. *Briefly the lenses are constituted of:*

Permalens	—	HEMA + VP + MA
Sauflon	—	HEMA + NVP
Hydrocurve	—	HEMA + Copolymer
Softcon	—	HEMA + POVIDONE
TC 75	—	HEMA + MA
CSI	—	Glyceryl + MA + MMA
SILSOFT	—	SILICON + O_2 + CH_3
POLYCON		
BOSTON	—	SILICON + PMMA
ALBERTA		

Abbreviations: HEMA, hydroxyethylmethylacrylate; VP, vinyl pyrrolidone; MA, methylacrylate; MMA, methylmethacrylate.

Any co-polymer must possess the following properties before it is adopted for biological use over the eye; chemical inertness, optical transparency, wettability, mechanical and dimensional stability, adequate oxygen permeation and biological tolerance.

Hydration

Hydration is an important consideration because this determines the physical properties and oxygen permeability. Percentage hydration of commonly used lenses is as follow.

Perma 71	Softcon 55
Sauflon 79	CSI 39
Hydrocurve 55	Silicon 0

Oxygen Permeability

Comparative oxygen permeability of PMMA, PHEMA and silicon are 1,15 and 2000 respectively. If DK value is considered, comparative value for commonly used lenses is as follows.

Perma 33
Sauflon 47
Hydrocurve 14
TC 75 32
Sisoft 340

Table 20.1 Parameters of extended wear lenses	
Lens	Permalens, Sauflon, Hydrocurve, Softcon, CSI, TC 75, Silsoft
Base curve	8–8.9 (0.3 steps) A, 8.1–8.7 (0.3) A, 8.5–9.8 A, 7.8–8.7 (0.3), 8.6–8.9, 7.8–9 (0.3), 7.3–8.3 7.7–8.9 (0.3 step) C, 7.8–8.4 (0.3) C, 8–8.5 C (80% S fit with 8.9) (0.2)
Diameter	13.5–14.5 (0.5) A, 14.4 A–14.5, 13.5–14, 14.5–14.8 A and T 13 14.5 11.3 and 13.5 C 12 C–15.5 A 15.5, 16 A (0.5)A 12.5 15.5 T 14.14.5 C 13.5, 14.0 C A and C 13.7 C
Power	+ 10 to + 20 (0.5)A, + 10 to 20A, +7.25 to + 2A, – 8 to +18.0 to + 20 Plan to A and C + 1 to 10C, –0.5 to –8, +0.25 to + 7.0 and Plan A and C + 20 0 to –12.5 C, C and A –1.5 to –6 (0.5)

Abbreviations: A, Aphakic; C, Cosmetic; T, Therapeutic.

Hydration percentage is a function of number of cross linkages between polymer chains, number of hydroxyl groups, tear pH, osmotic and hydrostatic pressure and environment, i.e. high temperature and high altitude, both require more oxygen for proper corneal function. Oxygen demand of the cornea fitted with a lens of 40% hydration in the day and night can be met by using a lens thickness up to 0.15–0.5 and 0.05 respectively. Similarly for a lens of 70% hydration adequate oxygen can be furnished in the day and night by using a thickness up to 0.45 and 0.20. These values are inadequate for aphakic cornea, which may still remain normal during extended wear. In aphakia this may be due to decreased oxygen demand and relatively increased oxygen availability (lens is absent), or due to involuntary ocular movements during sleep which furnish addition oxygen by tear pump mechanism. The parameters of extended wear lenses is described in Table 20.1.

Night Wear

Night wear is the critical period that determines whether a contact lens can be worn continuously or not. *At night the following physiological changes occur when contact lenses are in place:*
- The contacts become tighter because of increased acidity of tears
- Increased corneal thickness also increases lens tightness
- Tear osmolarity increases and contact adheres to cornea more
- Decreased lacrimation during sleep causes lens to dry up, resulting occasionally in a loss of lens
- The temperature of the cornea increases 3–4°C with the eye closed, consequently increasing oxygen demand
- Oxygen pressure falls 150–155 mm Hg on lid closure
- There is subacute inflammatory response on lid closure at night as shown by increased tear proteins, polymorphs and complement.

RELEVANT HISTORY

- Besides ocular history, which has been detailed in the contact lens book, history of certain medical, systemic and surgical ocular affections must be elicited as they can affect ocular tissues by causing ocular inflammation (noninfective or allergic type), delayed healing, tear dysfunction, corneal hydration, neurotrophic disturbances, exposure, infection, surgical trauma.
  - *Ocular inflammation:* This can be initiated by systemic infection. Besides systemic infection, certain noninfective affections like collagen disorders such as rheumatoid arthritis, systemic lupus erythematous, polyarteritis nodosa, polymyositis, Sjögren's syndrome, cranial, psoriatic and others can also involve the ocular tissues.
  - *Delayed healing:* Healing in the ocular tissues may be delayed by diabetes 5th cranial nerve paralysis, exposure, chronic ill health, chronic debilitating disease, malnutrition, anemia, jaundice, scurvy, malignancy and immunosuppressive drugs.
  - *Tear dysfunction:* Besides collagen disorders, tear layer is disturbed in its water, lipid protein constituents by a lacrimal gland inflammation by xerosis, trachoma, vitamin 'A' deficiency or conjunctival inflammations as in pemphigoid, acid/alkali burns and drug allergies (Stevens Johnson) and blepharitis. Drugs like diuretics, tranquillizers, parasympatholytic, β-blockers and antihistaminics tend to reduce tear secretions.
  - *Corneal hydration/edema:* Body hydration due to any cause or drug intake contraceptive pills, estrogen, pregnancy and allergic and other nephropathies is shared by the cornea. A well-fitted lens may start bothering after the initiation of above drugs or diseases.
  - *Neurotropic disturbances:* Corneal nutrition is disturbed in fifth nerve paralysis, and it becomes more vulnerable due to lowered vitality for insult, initiated by the microtrauma of the contact lenses. Similar nerve disturbance occurs after keratoplasty and partly after cataract operation. Nerve disturbances can also happen after herpes and zoster infection.
  - *Exposure:* Cornea and conjunctiva may show severe inflammation just due to desiccation by exposure. This may happen in seventh nerve paralysis, lid colobomas, malignant exophthalmos, proptosis, and surgical trauma as after operations on lid or around the eye as on face and sac, unconsciousness and during anesthesia if eye is not lubricated by ointment.
  - *Infection:* Infection anywhere in the body can settle in the eye. Patients with bed sore, urinary or fecal incontinence can easily pass on infection to the eye.
- *Personal:* It is important to know visual needs of the patient, motivation, and aptitude for compliance of instruction. Allergy and addiction must also be noted. Former are more sensitive and latter can contaminate the lens with nicotine or show exposure due to disturbed blinking.

Contraindications

Contraindications include inflammations of lids, conjunctiva, cornea uvea, raised intraocular pressure lagophthalmos (detailed earlier) and corneal nerve disturbances. The fitter must treat the above conditions and the eye must be quiet for at least 3 months before fitting contact lens. It is better to know the endothelial status also.

Endothelium Assessment

Besides indirect assessment of endothelial status through pachymetry, direct visualization can be done by specular microscopy. Heterogeneity in size, shape and number below 1000/sq mm is a bad sign and forms a relative contraindication.

Vitreous touch with adherence over 50% area of endothelium forms an absolute contraindication.

Selection of Cases for Cosmetic Wear Extended Wear Lenses

The following are the indications for cosmetic wear of extended wear lenses:
- Irregular working hours like air hostesses, doctors, emergency staff, police and firemen
- Working in irregular shifts
- Problems in daily wear
- Lifestyle does not permit them to be without lenses.

Aphakic Correction

An aphake can be corrected with a variety of optical aids as:
- Spectacles (optically inferior)
- DWL (50% failure due to handling difficulty)
- Intraocular implant (ideal but at present not practical for the masses)
- Keratophakia (technical problems)
- EWL 70–90% success.

Peculiarities of Aphakic Cornea

Cornea in aphakic differs from cornea in phakic person because:
- Sensations are reduced so warning symptoms are delayed
- Decreased threshold for trauma to produce corneal edema
- Decreased number of endothelial cells
- Disturbed corneal topography due to scar
- Vitreous touch may further decompensate the cornea depending on its location, area of touch density, duration and state of endothelium (LADDE)
- Oxygen requirement of aphakic cornea is lesser than cornea in phakes.

Selection of Aphakic Patient

An aphake with normal corneal and tear function forms a good candidate for extended wear lens in:

- Lack of manual dexterity resulting in difficulty in handling
- Infants and children who cannot handle the lens
- Inability to tolerate aphakic glasses which result in giddiness
- In aborted intraocular implant operation, this lens is the nearest substitute
- An attendant should be available at home in a situation which demands lens removal
- Nearness to ophthalmologist for looking after the lens-induced problems.

Fitting Basics

- Mechanism of lens movement on the cornea is the main concern
- Movement though absolutely critical for tear exchange and debris removal, must be permitted within reasonable limits
- All the available methods to determine the shape of the cornea are limited in about 11 mm diameter of the cornea. This area is not very significant for lens mechanics
- Central lens thickness makes little sense. It should be taken as average thickness, ultrathin lens is not ultrathin in the periphery
- Diameter is determined by corneal curvature, pupillary and corneal diameter, lens chemistry and extend of cosmetic coverage
- We fit purely by empirical methods. Our current approach to fitting represents the weakest point in the soft lens development
- A well-fitted lens starts behaving as tight lens on dehydration
- As a general rule permalens, Sauflon, TC 75, scan lens are fitted 2.5–3.5 D flatter than 'K' Silicon, CAB and polycon are fitted on K.

General Guidelines for Lens Finalization

Following methodology should be adopted for finalizing the lens specifications:
- Verify refraction, transpose spectacles power in minus cylinder
- Drop cylinder and find effectivity at corneal level
- Do keratometry and find the 'K'
- Measure the corneal diameter
- Select appropriate lens base curve by fitting on 'K' or flatter than 'K' as given in the general rule above
- Power is finalized by refracting over the trial lens.

Best Fit Criteria

After equilibration with tears ideally fitting trial lens must be:
- Well centered
- Should not move more than 1 mm on blinking elevation and versions

- Should exhibit a stable visual acuity that remains so before, during and after blinking
- Should show crisp retinoscopic reflex and
- Undistorted mires over the contact lens
- The lens, conjunctiva and sclera should look normal by slit-lamp biomicroscopy
- There should be little or no awareness of lens
- Over refraction of residual astigmatism should yield adequate vision.

Follow-up

Having given a trial lens, follow-up examination is done after a wear of 30 minutes, 4 hours, 24 hours, 7 days, 15 days, 1 month and then 3–6 monthly depending upon individuals reaction. At each follow-up visit, examination of visual acuity refraction over the contact lens fit of the lens, corneal behavior and lens quality is seen.

Steep Fit

A lens with a steep or tight fit shows:
- Longer to settle
- Excessive movements initially
- No movements later on
- Indentation under the edge
- Blanching of vessels at lens periphery
- No motion when moved
- Vaulting over the central cornea
- Bubble within the edge
- Visual acuity and mires on blinking
- Circumcorneal injection
- Corneal edema
- Striae on endothelium
- Blurring due to apical dehydration of lens.

Marginally Tight Lens

Marginally tight lens is typically slightly decentered, evokes mild awareness, has satisfactory but fluctuating vision, and induces corneal staining and mild limbal or conjunctival hyperemia. Final decision is made after few days wear.

Tight Lens Syndrome

This usually occurs in aphakic eye. A well-fitted lens after a week or a month initiate symptoms like over wear syndrome. There may be even hypopyon. The reaction usually occurs in Perma and Hydrocurve lenses containing methacrylic acid which is pH sensitive. A shift to acidic pH makes the lens shrink and give a tight fit. The episode can be prevented by instillation of alkaline saline drops at night.

Loose Lens

A loose lens can be judged by the following behavior:
- Excessive movements and awareness
- Eccentric placement and displacement
- Visual acuity and keratometric mires blur on blinking
- Retinoscopic reflexes darkens.

UNIQUE FEATURES OF EXTENDED WEAR LENSES

- Permalens
  - Small optic zone 6.5 mm (unsuitable for big pupil)
  - Thin
  - Fragile (Handling difficulty)
  - Limited parameters (cannot be a choice for all patients)
  - Inspection difficult, reproducibility judged only on patients eye
  - Only nonthermal disinfection.
- Hydrocurve 55%
  - Thinnest aphakic lens
  - Lower deposit rate
  - Durable
  - More oxygen permeable than Perma per unit thickness.
- Sauflon
  - Bigger optic zone 8 mm (suitable for big and distorted pupil)
  - More oxygen permeable
  - Less fragile and tougher than perma
  - Larger range in base curves and diameters
  - Higher affinity for fluorescein
  - Edges are thicker and blunter than perma
  - Limited parameters, so cannot fit all.
- CSI
  - Non-Hema (Glyceryl + MA + MMA)
  - Membrane concept
  - 40% hydration
  - Durable and elastic
  - Equilibrates in 5 minutes
  - Over refraction possible after 5 minutes
  - Resistant to deposits, discoloration and effect of environment.
- Silsoft
  - Highest oxygen permeability
  - Less wettable
  - Tougher
  - Thicker and elastic.

When to Remove Extended Wear Lens?

This is dependent on individual constitution and behavior. An EWL should be removed when it shows significant deposits or lens damage. Lens should be removed as an emergency by the patient, his attendant or doctor if there is a persistent complaint of watering, redness, discharge, pain and blurred vision.

DISINFECTION

Lens Cleaning/Disinfection

Disinfection of the lenses can be done by thermal and chemical methods, proportion being 65:35 respectively. Use of thermal technique degrades the plastic and induces discoloration and chemical methodology produces more allergic reaction and plastic degradation.

Besides the usual heat sterilization as described in soft lens chapter (15 minutes steam exposure of lens case containing lens in saline solution), certain solutions need special mention due to their unique properties to eliminate specific problems.

- *Allergen preserved saline*: Disinfected by heat in this solution can do away with the calcium deposits.
- *LC 65*: It is disinfecting and rinsing solution and is specific for lipoid deposits.
- *Opticlean*: The solution has a wide range of cleaning property for protein, calcium and lipoid and can be used safely for all types of hard and soft lenses.

AO Septicon

This is a unique disinfection and cleaning kit, where the lid of container has platinum. The lens is immersed for ten minutes in the container having hydrogen peroxide. The container is now turned into saline and the lens can now be placed directly over the eye.

Pligel is disinfecting solution which does not contain thiomersol or chlorhexidine. The former is notorious for allergy and latter for accumulation in the lens.

Heat Disinfection

Heat disinfection is used for hydrophilic soft lenses, mainly lower water content gel lenses (below 40%). High water content contact lenses show premature ageing with repetitive heat disinfection. At 80°C, the minimal effective time of 20 minutes is required.

- *Electrical (dry heat case but lenses in saline case):* This method ensures a rapid rise in temperature to almost 100°C and then a slow decline which exposes the lenses to over 80°C over a period of 40 minutes. This is effective against most bacterial contaminants but not fungal spores.

- *Thermos flask:* The cleaned lens is placed into its case with fresh saline and then into a thermos containing boiling water will show a slow decay of heat, from a peak of 90°C, for several hours. This is a safe and inexpensive method of disinfection.

Chemical Disinfection

Several chemicals are commonly used to disinfect contact lenses chlorhexidine, thimerosal (mercury salts), hypochlorite, quaternary ammonia compounds, hydrogen peroxide, benzalkonium chloride (nonhydrophilic only) and ascorbic acid for example. The concentration has to be such that a rapid kill time of microorganisms can be proven, especially the viruses—adenovirus and HIVs for example. The final solution must not be toxic to eye tissues. In most instances a neutralizing process of saline rinsing is required. Processes avoiding chemicals that selectively bind with the plastic of the case or lens are preferable. For example, chlorine is an effective disinfectant at 4–8 parts per million. With the lens wet, microwave techniques do not damage the lens but if the lens is dry, this method will seriously damage the lens surface. Soft lens solution should not contain chlorhexidine and thimerosal.

Lubricants

Lens wear in dry environments and by the borderline dry eye patients can be made more comfortable by the use of lubricant drops like Clerz, comfort drops and Bausch and Lomb Lubricant.

Detergents

Surface of the lens can be cleaned by the use of surfactants. Commonly used detergents are Mirasol, Clerz and Pligel. Their basic ingredient is poloaxamer 407 which is an excellent surfactant cleaner.

VARIOUS CATEGORIES OF EXTENDED WEAR LENSES

Permalens

The lens is being marketed by Global vision of England and Cooper lab of USA. It is a high water content (71%) lathe cut lens which is chemically constituted of 2HEMA vinyl pyrrolidone and methacrylates. It is available for aphakes in base curves of 8.3, 8.6 and 8.9 mm in power of + 10 to 20 D and diameters of 13 and 13.5 D. Plano or low powers in 14 mm diameter can also be used as therapeutic lenses.

It may take a month or two for final refraction to settle and due to dehydration, lens may show a lot of power variation even up to 2.00 especially in the morning. Final visual acuity may be line or two lower than visual acuity with spectacles or hard lenses.

It is fitted approximately 2.5 D flatter than 'K'. Lens chemistry, parameters unique features, fitting philosophy, follow-up, disinfection and problems have been described in general information on extended wear in the preceding pages.

The author has experienced excellent visual results with aphakic contact lens. Being softer, the lenses get easily torn. Deposits and lens loss constitute other problems. Cosmetic permalenses gave excellent visual results but early deposits fracture and acute loss and cumulative corneal insult, were noted after few hours (same day) and 7 days respectively. Author did a clinical comparison on the same aphakic patients between permalens and scanlens. Scanlens was found to be tougher and crisper in optics showing less breakage and less visual fluctuations.

Sauflon

The Sauflon lens was made by Phiip Cordery of England and was popularized by Heyer Schulte Medical Optic USA.

Chemically it is made up of HEMA and N-Vinyl 12 pyrrolidone. It has 79% water content. It is used for aphakia in base curves of 8.1, 8.4 and 8.7 and in diameter of 14.4 and power 0 to +20; for myopia in base curves of 7.8, 8.1 and diameter of 13.7 and power 0 to 8.00 for therapeutic purposes in base curves of 8.4 and diameter of 15.5 in plano power it is fitted 2.5 flatter than 'K' nearly 75% get visual acuity of 6/12 and above. General information on parameters, unique features fitting methodology follow-up, after care and problem is highlighted in preceding pages.

The author has documented therapeutic use of Sauflon lenses in a wide variety of pathological conditions (Table 20.2).

Other lenses for therapeutic purposes include plano 'T' U_4, O_4, Permalens, sauflon, softcon.

Table 20.2 Therapeautic use of soft contact lens			
Diseases	No. of eyes	Success	Failure
• Bullous keratopathy	37	30 (81%)	7 (19%)
• Indolent keratitis	20	18 (90%)	2 (10%)
• Desiccating diseases including SJ syndrome	40	35 (87.5%)	5 (12.5%)
• Postoperative bandage	20	20 (100%)	0 (0%)
• Recurrent corneal erosions	6	4 (66.66%)	2 (33.33%)
• Neuroparalytic keratitis	8	8 (100%)	0 (0%)
• Corneal perforations	21	21 (100%)	0 (0%)
• Chemical burns	6	2 (33.33%)	4 (66.66%)
• Postoperative exposure keratitis	22	22 (100%)	0 (0%)
• Herpetic keratitis	8	7 (87.5%)	1 (12%)
• Filamentary keratitis	6	6 (100%)	0 (0%)
Total	194	173 (89.2%)	21 (10.8%)

Table 20.3 Hydrocurve 55 parameters			
	Base curve	*Diameter*	*Power*
Aphakia	8.5/8.1	14/14.50	+7.25 to 20
Cosmetic	8.5	14	0 to –12
	8.8	14.5	+ 0.25 to + 7

Hydrocurve

It is a HEMA copolymer. It is used in hydration of 55% and 45%. The hydrocurve 55 parameters are tabulated in Table 20.3.

Even though the lenses have 55% hydration oxygen permeability is kept up to optimum levels by marking them ultrathin. At a thickness of 0.3 mm which is usual for high plus lenses, oxygen transmission is 5.6% and permeability in DK = 15×10^{-11}.

Fitting

Lens with base curve of 8.8 and diameter of 14.5 is the first choice both for aphakic and cosmetic fitting. Bigger diameter, i.e. 15.5 and 16 are chosen if initial lens remains decentered.

CSI

This is lens with 40% hydration, minimal possible thickness, very small optic zone requiring minimal movement and large lenticular zone.

Chemically it is constituted of glycerine, methylmethacrylate and methylacrylate. It is available in diameter of 14.8 and base curve of 8.6, 8.9 and 9.35, 80% of the patients get fitted with a base curve of 8.9 mm for 'K' below 42 and above 46, base curve of 9.35 and 8.6 is the first choice. Power varies between plano + 20.00. Other details are given in the preceding pages.

Softon

It is a 55% hydration lens which is chemically constituted of HEMA and povidone, it is available in base curve of 7.8, 8.1, 8.4 and 8.7, diameters of 13.5, 14.0 and 14.5 and powers ranging between –8.00 and + 18.00 including plano. It is relatively a thicker proposition (0.17–0.64 mm depending on power).

Fitting

First choice is 8.1/14.0. If the initial lens is too flat or sleep try 7.8/13.5 and 8.1/14.5 respectively. Other relevant information is given in the preceding pages.

TC 75

TC 75, is manufactured by Transcanada Contact Lens Ltd. It is used on extended wear basis in contrast to TC 50, which is a daily wear lens.

Chemically the lens is constituted of HEMA and methacrylic acid. For aphake it is available in base curves of 7.8, 8.1, 8.4, 8.7 and 9.0 diameters of 13.0, 13.5, 14.0 and 14.5 and in power varying between plano and + 20.00 D. For myopia base curves vary between 7.8 mm and 9.00 mm (0.3 mm steps) power –1.5 D to 6–.00 D, and diameter 13.5 for base curves of 7.8 and all other base curve have diameters of 14.0 mm.

Fitting

The initial lens is fitted 3–4 diopters flatter than 'K' and change of base curve is done on the basis of lens behavior.

SILICON LENSES

Silicon is a synthetic rubber that is unique in its oxygen transmissibility, rigidity, elasticity, stability, inertness and hydrophobicity. These physical properties make silicon lenses more biologically tolerable on cornea, optically crisp, resistant to warpage flexible, dimensionally stable.

Other properties are impermeability to fluorescein and bacteria, good thermal conduction and modern silicon lenses are subjected to ionic bombardment to make them wettable (changes contact angle 10°–30°–50°). The process basically is passage of electric current of 10,000 volts when the lens is placed in water. This replaces 40–50% of CH_3 by OH. Another process is dipping in Titante solution. Silicon is impermeable to hydrogen, hydroxyl and products of metabolism and it will never be able to compete with hydrogels which readily permit their permeability. The lenses are manufactured by moulding and edges are polished mechanically.

Indications

Silicon lens is problem solver. Metabolic and allergic corneal and conjunctival insults like injection, edema, staining and neovascularization induced by other lenses are relieved by this lens.

Fitting

Most of the silicon lenses are fitted on 'K' or 0.5 steeper or flatter than 'K'. The final lens must have stable visual acuity, movements of 1–2 mm. centering, and comfort. Fluorescein can be used for evaluation of fit. Silsoft (corning) is available in diameters of 11.3 and 12.5 base curves of 7.5–8.3 (in 0.2 mm steps) and powers of –20.00 to + 20.00. They are fitted on 'K'. The lens with diameter of 12.5 is reserved for corneal diameter larger than 12.00 mm or corneal curvature flatter than 42.

Silicon (corning) is available in diameter of 8.9 mm and being less flexible it can be used to correct astigmatism of 3–4 diopters. It is fitted on 'K'.

Silfex is available in diameters of 11.7, 12.2, 12.7 and 13.2 with base cures of 7.3–9.00 (in 0.1 mm steps) and power varying between –20.00 + 20.00.

Silflex is fitted 0.1 m flatter than K.

Dunker lenses have diameter of 11.00 mm, powers 20.00–28.00 and are fitted 0.5–1.50 D steeper than 'K'.

After care of lenses: Lenses can be sterilized by standard lens solutions and by thermal disinfection. Hydrogen peroxide should not be used because the lens holds it up.

Summary of Silicon Lens Fitting

- Do refraction and transpose cylinder into minus and drop it.
- Do keratometry and fit the trial lens of 'K'.
- Do fluorescein assessment for verification of tight or loose fit and give a proper fitting lens if fit is not proper.
- Do refraction over the trial lens for exact power calculations.
- Final order will include base curve power and diameter.

MIXED LENSES

Besides silicon and CAB, there are other gas permeable lenses which are cross linked polymers, the usual combinations being Silicon + PMMA and silicon + PMMA + CAB. These mixed lenses have the advantage of causing less corneal edema, less photophobia, better wearing time, less spectacle blur and fewer lens changes.

The main disadvantages of these lenses are bigger diameter, hydrophobic surface, instability in parameters and warpage.

The mixed lenses are listed in descending order to their oxygen permeability as Silicon, Boston, Alberta, Polycon, CAB, HEMA, modified PMMA.

Polycon

Polycon lens is a combination of 35% silicon and 65% PMMA. Polycon lenses unlike lenses made from other rigid permeable material, are extremely stable. The added dimension of oxygen permeability helps to eliminate compromises, which are often necessary with PMMA to overcome the problems of edema, spectacle blur, corneal changes, photophobia and flare. This new material because of its permeability and stability permits the use of larger lenses, larger optic zones, thinner lenses and reduced lens movements. These factors can result in greater comfort, accelerated adaptation and normal corneal and visual response. It is available in 9.5 and 8.5 diameters for phakes and in 9.5 and 10 mm diameters for aphakes. Fitting is done by trial lenses.

9.5 lenses are fitted (by Korb philosophy of lid attachment, i.e. moving with lid during blinking) flatter than 'K' by 0.15–0.25 mm and 8.5 lenses are fitted on K. For aphakia 9.5 and 10.00 mm diameter lenses are used and they are fitted flatter than 'K' by 0.15–0.25 mm (base curve of all polycon lenses are steepened 0.5 mm for every 1.00 D of stigmatism).

CHAPTER 21

Gas Permeable Cellulose Acetate Butyrate (Hard Lenses)

INTRODUCTION

Cellulose acetate butyrate (CAB) lenses are fabricated by taking cellulose from wood and cotton, acetic acid from vinegar and butyric acid from natural gas. CAB lens is 40 times more oxygen permeable and 320 times more permeable to carbon dioxide compared to soft lens. It has 25% greater thermal conduction; hence there is a better heat dissipation. It has a wetting angle of 18.5 and is easily flexible.

The above properties make CAB lens a better choice for patients who exhibit problems due to lesser oxygen exchange, unstable visual acuity, discomfort, unsatisfactory wetting and residual astigmatism.

The disadvantages include more thickness, more awareness, lesser stability in base curve of thin lenses, more cost and different refractive index than conventional hard lenses. Silvo makes the CAB soft, more prone to scratch and petroleum products make it opaque and both should be avoided. Currently available lenses are CAB curve, meso and Rx56. In present day context this chapter is only of historic interest.

FITTING OF CELLULOSE ACETATE BUTYRATE LENSES

Fitting is done by trial lenses which vary in base curves from 39 to 50 in 0.5 steps and in diameter from 9.4 to 8.5 in 0.1 steps for phakic patients (Table 21.1). In aphakes base curves vary between 41 and 45 in 0.5 D steps, diameters vary between 9.7–9.4 and power +11 to +20 in 0.50 D steps (Table 21.2).

Choice for Trial Lens

Trial lens is fitted 0.5 D steeper than 'K' and for each diopter of astigmatism steeper by 0.25 D but never more than 1.00 D. It is better to err on steeper side as lenses tend to flatten with passage of time especially in minus series.

Evaluation of Fit

This is exactly like hard lenses. Author did a clinical comparison with the continuous use of CAB and XL 30 lenses. XL 30 was fitted on one eye and the fellow eye was fitted with CAB lens. It was observed that irritation was more with CAB lens. Further surface deposits occurred 3 times more on CAB lenses. Corneal edema however was 4% both in XL 30 and CAB after 6 hours and 7 days.

Table 21.1 CAB diameter selection in phakics

Base curve (Diopters)	Diameter (mm) (Diopters)	Base curve	Diameter (mm)
39.00	9.4	45.00	8.9
39.50	9.4	45.50	8.9
40.00	9.3	46.00	8.8
40.50	9.3	46.50	8.8
41.00	9.2	47.00	8.7
41.50	9.2	47.50	8.7
42.00	9.2	48.00	8.6
42.50	9.1	48.50	8.6
43.00	9.1	49.00	8.6
43.50	9.0	49.50	8.6
44.00	8.0	50.00	9.5
44.50	8.9		

Table 21.2 CAB diameter selection in aphakes (+11 to +16 in 0.50 D steps)

Base curve	Diameter
41.00	9.7
41.50	9.7
42.00	9.6
42.50	9.6
43.00	9.5
43.50	9.5
44.00	9.5
44.50	9.4
50.00	9.4

Further, author has established the superiority of XL 30 over CAB. Oxford and Boston lenses. Clinical use of these lenses of extended wear basis with a central thickness of 0.20 mm corneal edema was minimum with XL 30 and on closure of eyes for half an hour anoxic endothelial bullae were least with XL 30.

Problems of Extended Wear Lenses and their Treatment

Problem in extended wear lenses (EWL) can be initiated by lack of lens movements, bad edge, lack of timely cleaning and follow-up, delay in reporting to competent fitter, dry eyes lid dysfunction and infection. Following problems may be encountered:

Dry Eyes

Dry eyes while wearing the contact lenses may be due to nocturnal exposure, dry environment, drugs like diuretics, sedatives, antihistaminics, beta blockers, and parasympatholytics.

Treatment: Besides treatment of the basic cause of dry eyes, symptomatic treatment includes instillation of preservative free artificial tears over the lens 3–8 times/day. Lubricant can also be used before starting the job entailing visual attention.

Tight Lens

Signs of the tight fitting lens are detailed earlier. This is treated by smaller and flatter lens. Symptoms may be temporarily alleviated by instillation of balanced salt solution or 3% sodabicarb.

These drops will deal with the problem induced due to drying and shrinkage.

Torn or Lost Lens

This can be due to tight lens or in those who rub their eyes.

Allergic Reaction

Allergic reaction starts immediately after coming in touch with the solution or lens. This can start after few months and years of their usage. Patient complains of itching and watering. There is a pale edema of conjunctiva, and cornea may show epithelial swelling and punctate staining. Author noted allergy to thiomersal, polymethylmethacrylate (PMMA) and hydroxyethyl methacrylate (HEMA). It is confirmed by doing a patch test.

Treatment: Eliminate allergen and substitute by another solution or plastic.

Giant Papillary Conjunctivitis

Giant papillary conjunctivitis is another allergic manifestation or irritation which can be produced by the hard and soft lenses, artificial eyes and stitch irritation after keratoplasty and cataract. There is giant papillary reaction of conjunctiva like spring catarrh.

Treatment: Giant papillary conjunctivitis can be treated by substituting other type of plastic, i.e. from hard to soft of gas permeable. Symptomatic treatment can be given with local cortisone drops. If the irritation still persists lens should be discontinued.

Meibomianitis and Blepharitis

These may be present before or after the use of contact lenses. Eliminate the cause such as dandruff, wart, herpes, molluscum, staphylococcal infection and allergic manifestation to solution, plastic or cosmetics.

Treatment: Lenses are withdrawn till complete recovery. Symptomatic treatment includes local hygiene, lid massage, scrubs and antibiotic and use of broad spectrum antibiotics.

Conjunctivitis

This may be induced by unhygienic patient, solution, contaminated environment and incompetent fitter.

Treatment: Lenses are discontinued for a week. Conjunctivitis is treated by local lavage with saline and appropriate antibiotic drops (after culture and sensitivity).

Keratitis

Keratitis is induced by injury, foreign body, hypoxia and dry eyes.

Treatment: Withdraw lenses and treat the cause.

Symptomatic treatment includes topical antibiotic drops, cycloplegic and dark glasses.

Edema

Lens can induce edema if it is thick, dried, low water-content or made up of material which is less oxygen permeable. Edema can also occur in environment with a low oxygen content or by drugs which produce general body hydration like contraceptive pills. Acute edema can occur with aphakic lens over an eye which has not healed yet. Author has noted it as acute edema after few hours or as cumulative edema occurring after 7 days.

Treatment: Besides treatment of the above causes, a flat and a small lens helps to improve the edema.

Foreign Body

The foreign bodies can be deposited by automobile exhaust or dust. They may result in irritation and spots in the visual fields.

Treatment: Use of goggles especially driving goggles and replace the lens for embedded foreign body.

Superficial Punctate Keratitis

This may occur due to drug, preservatives, hypoxia, tight fit, lens dehydration and infection with virus or bacteria. If superficial punctate keratitis (SPK) is singularly present, it may be due to drug, preservative or bad fit. However, association of chemosis and discharge indicates bacterial infection. Hypoxic superficial punctate keratitis (SPK) is quite common, author warns not to treat this antiviral drugs and find the cause and treat it.

Treatment: Withdraw lenses, find the cause and treat. Patching clean (uninfected) eye is helpful.

Neovascularization

This can be initiated by any of the following factors, i.e. dry eyes, old age, bullous keratopathy, tight lens, deposits and exposure. New vessels may be superficial or deep.

Treatment: Treat the cause like tight, loose, decentered or torn lens and give a well fitted, high hydration, more oxygen permeable lens. Reduce wearing time and use daily wear lens. Avoid chemical irritation. If neovascularization is still progressive, discontinue the lens.

Faulty Lens

Lens may be defective in parameters, i.e. thickness, power, base, edge, flange and surface.

Treatment: Get lenses from standard firm and check in your own laboratory.

Lens Deposits

Lens deposits are usually mixed and are constituted of calcium, lipoid and proteins.

Treatment: Deposits can be treated by observing following line of action:
- Observe local hygiene, treat acne, rosacea and blepharitis.
- Do mechanical cleaning by placing it in the palm of left hand and cleaning it with index finger of right hand by radial motion for centre of the lens to its edge.
- Instill alkaline saline drops at night.
- Get diamond shamrock 90 treatment to prevent deposit.
- Clean the lens with surfactant like clerz or pliagel.
- Do enzyme treatment depending upon individual's reaction of lens.
- Do septicon treatment, i.e. hydrogen peroxide soakage for 10 minutes.
- Ultrasonic cleaning of dirty lens in hydrogen peroxide is very helpful.

Lens Coloring

Lens may be colored during wear. The causes are local instillation of epinephrine, fluorescein and systemic use of rifampicin.

Treatment: Avoid instillation of drugs over the lens and treat the colored lens with 3% hydrogen peroxide overnight. A new lens is ordered if color persists.

Discontinuation of Extended Wear Lenses

During clinical practice author has observed that lens wear was discontinued due to lack of motivation, discomfort, poor vision, handling difficulty, lens loss/damage, pathology and ill health.

Replacement

Common causes for replacement have been lens loss/damage, discomfort, and blurred vision due to improper lens power.

Tinted Lens

Lenses are tinted for easy identification to enhance the facial appearance, for occlusion, and to hide the cosmetic blemish in corneal opacities, complicated cataract, aniridia, and disfigured eyes. Lenses are available in green, blue, pink and red colors. Besides transparent tints for cosmetic enhancement, opaque tints of varying sizes and shapes are used to cover the pupil, to mimic iris and hide the corneal opacities and disfigured eyes.

CHAPTER 22

Toric Soft Lenses

INTRODUCTION

These are lenses for astigmatism higher than 1.5 D, where hard lenses are uncomfortable. Toric lenses are usually more stable and provide more vision than spherical lenses. Toric lens in general provides less comfort, less wearing time, less reproducibility, less success in oblique astigmatism, less stable, less oxygen permeable (thicker), and more thick, more difficult to fit, and more expensive than a spherical soft lens.

RESIDUAL ASTIGMATISM

This is the astigmatism left after a well-fitted and well-centered lens. This may be same or different compared to prefitting astigmatism. This is dependent on lens molding on the cornea as its back and initial curvature of the front surface, i.e. whether it is plano, plus, low or high minus.

Soft Lenses and Astigmatism

A variety of soft lens propositions can serve the astigmatism.
- *Standard spherical soft lens:* Residual astigmatism might be a problem. It may be dealt with by glasses over the contact lenses. Aphakia is a good example for this. Author has prescribed 4 D cylinder in spectacles over spherical aphakic lens with 6/5 vision.
- *Hard lens over soft lens (piggy back):* This is less comfortable than soft and has more metabolic problems.
- *Thick spheric soft lens:* It moulds less but arouses more lid sensation and drags in more metabolic problems.
- *Toric lens:* This is ideal, but disadvantages have been highlighted earlier.

Lens Stabilization

A toric lens must show meridional stability. This will keep the cylinder at proper axis to ensure proper visual results.
- Stability can be achieved by incorporation of prism of up to 0.75 D or more
- Truncation—single or double as in hard lenses
- Back toricity
- Orientation grooves

- Carrier flange
- Combination of above.

Prerequisites of Successful Fit

- Lens must center well over the cornea
- Movements should not be more than 1.5 mm
- Rotation of axis should not be more than 15°
- Visual acuity should be stable before, during and after the blink.

Fitting

Spherical lens is first tried, the patient may accept it with some visual compromise. Fitting of toric lens is done with trial lens which has the same criteria of successful fit as for soft lenses and the above said criteria for toric lens.

Following lenses are available in various powers in sphere and cylinder Table 22.1.

TORIC LENSES

Hydrocurve II (45%)

The lens is basically meant for corneal toricity below 2 diopters. It is available in base curves of 8.6 and 8.9, power varying between +4 and −6; diameters of 13.5

Table 22.1 Toric soft lenses				
Lens name	Laboratory	% Water (Diopters)	Spherical power range (Diopters)	Cylindrical power range
Hydrocurve	Soft lenses	45	+3.00 to 6.00	−1.25 and −2.00
Hydrocurve II	Soft lenses	55	Plano to −.25	−1.25
Hydro-Marc	Fronter	43	Plano to −4.50	−0.75 to 1.50
Dura Soft TT Wesley-Jessen				
Standard	30/38	+1.00 to 6.00	−1.25 and −2.00	
Custom	30/38	+20.00 to −20.00	−0.75 to 4.00	
Hydron	American	38.6	+20.00 to −20.00	−0.50 to −6.00
Hydron				
Miracon	Bausch and Lomb	45	Plano to −6.00	−1.25 and −1.75
B and L Toric	Bushcn and Lomb	45	Plano to −6.00	−1.25 and −1.75
B and L Toric	Bausch and Limb	45	+0.25 to +4.00	−1.25 and −1.75
Torisoft	Ciba Vis. Care	38	Plano to −6.00	−1.00 and−1.75
Bal-Flange	Salvatori	43 (BP)*−0.75 to 4.00	−1.25 and −2.00	
*(BP) Burton, Parsons deltafilcon a				

Courtesy: Contact lens forum.

and 14.5; cylinder –1.25 and –2.00 and rotation of 25° on either side of 90° and 180° axis.

Lens of base curve 8.6 and diameter of 13.5 fits most of the cases.

Hydromarc (43%)

The lens is suitable for corneal toricity around 1.5 diopters. It is available in base curves of 8.45, 8.70 and 9.05 power +1 to –4.5; diameter 14.5, cylinder –0.75 to –1.50; and axis rotation 15° on either side of horizontal and vertical axis.

Fitting: Hydromarc is fitted by trial lens methodology. Base curve and diameter are chosen by adding 1 and 2, one-third in this is added to finalize base curve.

Dura Soft (30%)

The lens is available in base curve ranging between 7 and 9, power varying between +20 and –20; diameter of 12.8 and 13.5; cylinder –0.75 and –4.00, and axis rotation 15° on either side of 90 and 180 axis in 5° steps. Fitting the lens is done by trial lens methodology.

Hydron (38%)

The lens is available in base curves between 7.7 and 8.7 in 0.2 mm steps; powers ranging between +20 and –20; diameters 13.5, 14 and 14.5 and cylinder power ranging between 0.5 and 6. The lens has prism ballast (1.00 D) and truncation (1.5 mm).

Fitting: The lens is fitted flatter than the mean 'K' and diameter is 2–2.5 mm larger than the corneal diameter. Hydron lens is fitted by using a standard as aspheric trial set which is without prism and truncation.

Miracon (45%)

The lens is available in base curves of 8.6 and 8.9; power –0.5 to –6.0 D diameter of 14 mm cylinder of –1.25 to –1.75 and cylinder rotation 20° on either side of 90° and 180° axis.

Fitting: Miracon lens is fitted by trial lens methodology. Lens of 8.6/14 is the first choice. Bausch and Lomb has also made B and L toric lenses which are in half the thickness compared to Miracon (43% less thick).

Torisoft (38%)

It has a slabbed off top bottom. The lens is available in base curves of 8.6, 8.9 and 9.2; power +4 to –6, diameter of 14.35, a cylinder of 1 and 1.75; and axis rotation 20° on either side of 90° and 180° axis in 10° steps.

Bal-Flange Toric (43%)

The lens starts out just like any other soft lens except that the lenticular portion is made in minus lenticular form. Differential but partial removal of carrier more from bottom and less from the top, leaves the carrier flange at the top, like visior of Napoleon cap. The lens is available in spherical powers of –0.75 to –4.00 and cylinder of 1.25 to –2.00.

COMPARISON

Stability of Toric Lenses

Stability in nearly all the toric lenses is achieved by prism ballast. Durasoft lenses have truncation in addition and Torisoft lenses have slabbed off top and bottom (thin thick zones) and Bal-flange has a carrier flange at the top.

Surface Positioning of Cylinder

All the toric lenses have front surface cylinder except for hydrocurve and Hydron which have cylinder on the back surface. Basically back toric lenses are good in patients where astigmatism is corneal, and front toric lenses are indicated when the astigmatism is extracorneal.

Fitting of Soft Toric Contact Lens

The physical fit for a soft toric lens essentially remains the same as for a spherical soft lens. The lens should cover the cornea in all the gaze positions, allow adequate tear flow to enable metabolic debris to be removed and remain well-centered with respect to corneal center and visual axis. The choice of back optic zone radius (BOZR), total diameter (TD) and center thickness for a soft toric lens should be made in the same way as a spherical soft design. The power of the lens should be chosen with the spherical and, more importantly, the cylindrical power and axis as close as possible to the predicted final lens parameters. The aim of the trial fitting is two-fold: to assess the physical and physiological fit and response to the lens and to measure orientation position along with orientation stability. After insertion of the lens, it should be allowed to settle, as for a spherical soft lens, before the fit is assessed. The axis rotation provides necessary information to the practitioner to order the lens. The rotation of the lens indicates how far the axis of the cylinder will be mislocated when the final lens is placed on the eye. This mislocation can be compensated for by ordering a lens with the axis at a modified position. If, for example, an ocular refraction is –3.50/–1.50 × 180 and a trial lens rotates clockwise by 10° when placed on the eye, the final lens should be ordered as –3.00/–1.75 × 10; the 10° clockwise rotation will bring the axis round to 180° and vision will be clear. We follow the LARS (left add right subtract) rule, i.e. if the lens

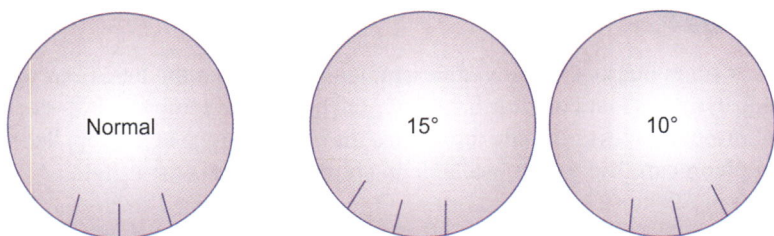

Fig. 22.1 Rotation of toric soft contact lens either in left or right side of 6 o'clock position requires modification of cylinder axis of final lens

rotates to the left the rotation should be added and if it is to the right it should be subtracted (Fig. 22.1). In current scenario of contact lens practice, fitting a soft toric lens is as simple as fitting a spherical lens for the majority of patients and with improving performance and patient satisfaction, it should continue to be an integral part of contact lens practice.

CHAPTER *23*

Special Lenses

In this chapter, lenses for specific purposes have been described. These include especially designed lenses for presbyopia, cosmetic, infants, amblyopia and lens spoliation.

BIFOCAL SOFT LENSES

These are lenses with bifocal proposition to attend presbyopia. Following lenses have been used for this purpose. Bi-Soft, Dura soft and crescent bifocal.

Fitting Bifocals

Bifocal lenses are fitted on the same general principals as soft lenses. Base curve diameter and segment height can be best judged with trial bifocal lens fitting. Lenses with different segment height are available. Segment top should be kept 1.5 mm below the visual axis.

Bi-Soft

This lens is in a concentric, two-zones 'thin lens' design. It is available in 3 base curves (8.3, 8.6 and 8.9 mm), distance power ±6.00 with add power of +1.25 + 1.75 and +2.25 D and diameter of 13.8 mm.

Dura Soft

This has a crescent segment. It has single truncation and prism ballast. It is available in base curves of 8.3, 8.45, 8.6, 8.8 and 9.0, distance powers of –2.5 to –4.50 and diameter of 13.5 mm. Near adds of 1.25, 1.75 and 2.50 D are available.

PAI

This aspheric bifocal lens is made by Bausch and Lomb. It is available in distant powers of –4 to +2 and the near add has a power of +1.25.

Crescent Bifocal

This lens is made by Neefe optical. It has 50% water. It is available in base curves of 8.5, 8.8, 9.10, 9.40 powers ranging between ±6.00 D; addition +2, +2.5 and +3, and segment height 3.5, 4 and 4.5 mm.

COSMETIC LENSES

Soft lenses are available in tinted and painted propositions to serve optical, cosmetic or both the purposes. Lens may have:

- *Painted iris:* These are available with iris details in blue, pink, yellow, red and green color. These are used in aniridia, ugly broad coloboma, in actors for changes of iris color and to cover peripheral or paracentral corneal scars.
- *Pupillary coverage lens:* These lenses are used for covering the odd pupillary reflex, as in complicated cataract, or young patients waiting for cataract operations central corneal scars, in amblyopic eyes and odd looking lenticular remnants.
- *Lenses with central painting:* These lenses are for providing a big central brown or black area for covering corneal scars or unsightly eyes. Such lens can also be used for occlusion.
- *Painted iris and black pupil:* These lenses are used purely for cosmetic reasons to cover corneal scars and unsightly eye with normal eyeball contour.

In all the painted lenses, color does fade away with passage of time (months), and a duplicate lens is required.

Soft Lens for Infants

It is an emergency to accomplish optical adequacy after operating a congenital cataract.

Fitting

Retinoscopy, fundus examination, contact lens trial and refraction through the contact lens can be done in a dark room with child in mothers lap. An idea of keratometry can be had by seeing the fluorescein pattern under a steeper trial rigid lens with base curve 7–7.5. The power needs to be modified every two months for the first year and then 6 monthly. Author has noted a wide variations the initial contact lens power between +10 and +44 dioters. Final power may be even 10 diopters less than the initial within 2 years. Starting diameter is usually 13.5 mm.

Author recommends that all infants be fitted with high gas permeable lenses of DK 90 or more on daily wear basis. Author has shown 70% loss of endothelial cells in infants with the use of even 85% hydration soft lenses within three months. Lens can be worn on alternate days to avoid endothelial insult.

TYPES OF LENS

Extended wear and gas permeable lenses should be used to avoid undue corneal insult while sleeping during the day or night.

Insertion and removal is taught to the mother. Follow-up must exclude watering, photophobia, lid edema, and corneal haze. This symptomatology indicates corneal edema and problems and calls for lens and fitting reassessment.

Critical period in infants is 4–6 months; add in infants over the refraction +3.00 <1 year of age; +1.0> 2 years of age and no additional add > 3 years of age. Silicon, RGP and soft contact lens can be used in infants. Silsoft is silicon lens used in infants, made by Bausch and Lomb. It is available in base curve 7.5, 7.7 and 7.9 in diameter 11.3 and 12.5 and power + 12–32.

Occlusion Lens

A high plus lens with a power around + 18.00 diopters serves a good occluder for treatment of amblyopia.

Disposable Lens

Patients with problem of heavy and early deposit formation should be given disposable lenses. This seems to be ideal lens proposition till a proper deposit resistant polymer is discovered. Such disposable lenses have already been marketed.

The disposable lenses have the same physical parameters as the daily wear or extended wear lenses. They are marketed by Bausch and Lomb and Johnson and Johnson. Acuvue is a popular trade name of disposable lens marketed by the latter.

Even if the lens is looking perfectly normal, it is replaced by a new lens every two to four weeks. This avoids inconvenience due to deposits, infection, discoloration and changes in physical parameters.

Advise to daily wear patient:
- The same scheme is followed, only the lenses should be removed at night, rinsed and stored in the disinfectant solution and in the morning rinsed with sterile saline, cleaned and inserted. The dirty or spoiled lens is replaced with a new lens.
- Lenses should be changed every two to four weeks.

Properties of a disposable lens:
- High DK/L
- Of sufficient tensile strength and surface to last two weeks wear
- Packed cases are water air tight and disposable after opening
- They must be an economical proposition to the patient.

Contact Lens for Athletes

In competition sports contact lenses offer special advantages as indicated below.

Contact lens gives you an edge because they:
- Increase peripheral vision by 15%
- Gives better depth perception
- Reduces visual distortion
- Object size is near normal size
- Increases visual stability

- Permits to use protective glasses over them
- Eliminates changes of ocular injury due to frame and glasses
- Offers more comfort.

Guidelines to Fit Contact Lens in Athletes

- Give maximum visual acuity
- Correct myopia even up to 0.25
- Correct anisometropia 0.50 or more
- Correct significant hyperopia
- Correct astigmatism over 1.0 with toric soft or RGP
- Permit least movement in dynamic sports
- Keep a duplicate pair with you
- Fit EWL as DWO to get maximum oxygen
- Avoid thick, low water, and EWL regimen
- Disposable are ideal for occasional or part time use
- Avoid flat or a steep lens.

Lenses for the sports may be fitted from the following lenses:
- Soft 55% water
- BC 8.9 and 9.2
- OD 15 mm
- Daily wear basis.

Overnight use of disposable lens is not advised because:
- Lens user more prone to risk
- His cornea may be compromised
- He may lack compliance
- And these were the reasons to switch on to disposable.

Daily disposable lenses have advantage which include:
- No inconvenience of care system
- No decrease in comfort with time
- No deposits
- No GPC, chemical conjunctivitis, acute red eye.

Lenses for infants include:
- Silicon
- RGP
- Soft.

Silicon lenses are available as silosoft in following specifications:

Base curve	7.5, 7.7, and 7.9
Diameter	11.3 and 12.50
Power	+12.00 to 32.00

Choice for Bifocals include:
- Monovision
- Simultaneous

- Alternating
- Aspehric
- Diffractive.

Monovision is a very simple philosophy because no extralenses are required. Dominant eye is fitted for distance and nondominant eye is fitted for near. This simple methodology costs binccularly of vision.

In astigmatism variety of methods are available for stabilization of axis. These include:

- Prism
- Truncation
- Dynamic stabilization
- Aspheric back
- Posterior toric
- Inferior negated
- Combination.

Author thinks that prism and truncation either alone or in combination is the best.

CHAPTER 24

Complications of Contact Lenses

INTRODUCTION

Complications have been discussed under many classifications by various authors. It is better to adopt a classification which has a wider coverage of the entire spectrum of complications and where each complications is discussed in a simplified manner. The description of each complication should include a brief introduction about disease, symptomatology, pathogenesis and treatment.

The following classification fulfils the above criteria (Fig. 24.1). *Contact lens complications can be classified broadly into:*

- Occlusive
- Microbial
- Allergic
- Toxic
- Traumatic
- Refractive
- Desiccation
- Lens spoliation
  (Physical deposits)

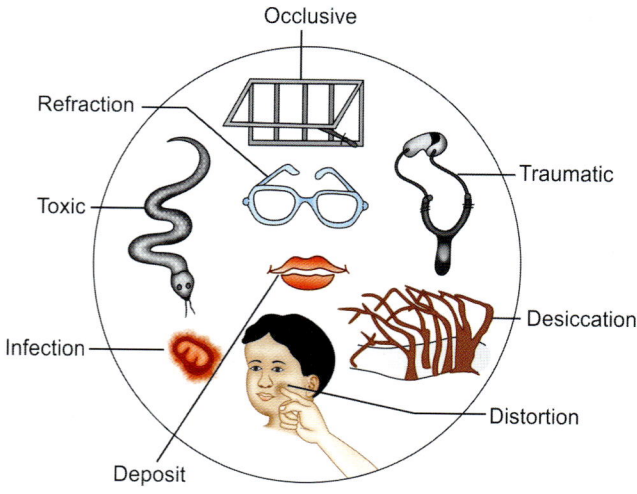

Fig. 24.1 Classification of types of contact lens complications

OCCLUSIVE

This is basically an oxygen deprivation problem. This is also used synonymously with hypoxic or anoxic problems.

Oxygen Requirement

Oxygen requirement of the cornea varies from 7.5% to 21%, the mean being 10%. This is supplied to the cornea by tear exchange during lens excursion while blinking and by diffusion through the substance of the material of the lens. Adequate exchange of tears means 10–20% exchange of tears with each blink. This is only true for hard and rigid lenses and not for soft hydrophilic lenses where tear exchange is only 1–2% with each blink.

Diffusion, which is main source of oxygen supply in hydrophilic lenses is determined by the physical and chemical property of the contact lens. Diffusion can be enhanced by
- Using a more hydrophilic material
- Using thin lenses
- Using high gas permeable materials like silicone and fluorocarbons

The oxygen permeability property is expressed by the DK/L value of the material where

D = Diffusion coefficient
K = Oxygen solubility
L = Lens thickness

For provision of adequate oxygenation, the DK value of the daily wear lens should be 20–25, and for extended wear lenses DK value should be 75.

The modern rigid gas permeable lenses have the dual property of efficient tear pump and diffusion property thereby maintaining good oxygen concentration under the lens.

Pathogenesis of Hypoxic Problems

Chronic lack of oxygen supply due to a gas impermeable lens. Lack of blinking, relatively hypoxic environment will alter the aerobic metabolism of the epithelium into anaerobic, with accumulation of lactate in the cornea and its diffusion into the anterior chamber, producing even sterile hypopyon.

Manifestation of Hypoxia (Fig. 24.2)

Cornea will become water logged in all the layers and may show the following clinical manifestations of hypoxia.
- Edema, of the epithelium, stroma and endothelium,
- Superficial punctuate keratitis (see in the end)
- Decreased sensations
- Decreased adhesion to basement membrane
- Corneal infiltrates
- Superficial and deep vascularization

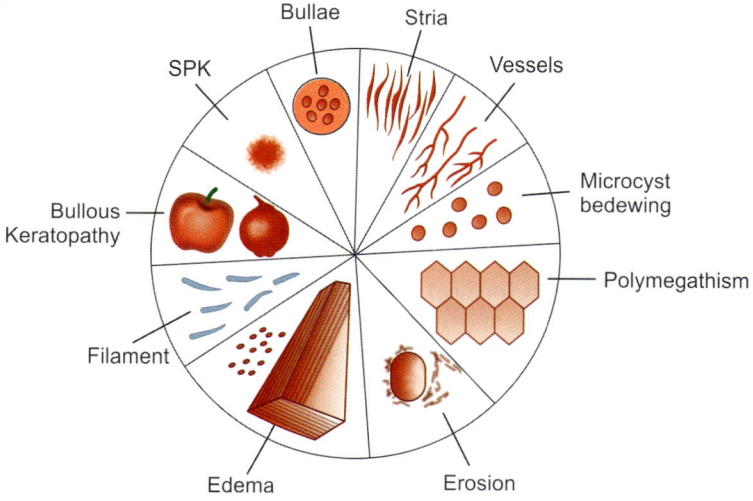

Fig. 24.2 Ocular manifestations of hypoxia

- Compromised corneas, more prone to infection.
- Superior limbal keratoconjunctivitis.

Epithelia microcysts: Epithelial microcysts are universally present in all the users of extended wear contact lenses. They are best seen by indirect diffuse illumination.

It seems to be a manifestation of chronic hypoxia. Such cases will also show swelling and polymegathism in the endothelium. Epithelial changes disappeared on lens withdrawal.

Subepithelial keratitis: These are present as subepithelial or anterior stromal opacities.

These may be central, paracentral or distributed over the entire cornea.

The lesion seems to be due to contact lens trauma toxic ingredient of accessory solutions and allergic phenomenon.

It is treated by eliminating the cause. Solutions should be preservative free. Use of corticoids minimized the symptoms. Contact lens withdrawal will eliminate the pathology.

Corneal edema: It used to be a common feature in contact lens wearers with PMMA use. The problem is less with rigid gas permeable lenses.

It is clinically seen by sclerotic scatter, optical section, direct and indirect focal.

It is seen as increase in corneal thickness, as confirmed quantitatively by pachymeter. There may be epithelial edema, increase in stromal thickness, corneal striae and Descemet's folds polymegathism and decrease in the number of endothelial cells.

It is caused by hypoxia, lack of adequate tear exchange, and pre-existing epithelial and endothelial pathology. It will create glare, drop in visual acuity, pain if the epithelial bullae rupture.

It is prevented by prefit assessment of the endothelial function giving a proper fit, choosing highly oxygen permeable lens material and using lens on daily wear basis rather than extended wear basis.

Treatment

Occlusive problems can be prevented by:
- Proper fit-ensuring tear exchange
- Choosing proper material with high DK value
- Using thinner and smaller lenses
- Proper blinking
- Avoiding hypoxic environment.

MICROBIAL

Microbes can have a hold on the cornea according to Rich's law. *The resistance of the cornea can be lowered due to a variety of:*
- Local and systemic factors
- Substandard contact lens solutions, physical, chemical buffer system
- Contact lens trauma
  (Imperfect finish)

The cornea may be infected by:
- A contaminated solution
- Lack of personal hygiene
- Contaminated water supply
- From the surrounding infected adnexa.

Common Pathogens (Fig. 24.3)

There has been a changing microbiological pattern in contact lens wearers showing severe infections. This has been documented to be due to:
- *Staph. aureus*
- *Pseudomonas pyocyaneus*
- *Serratia marcescens*
- Acanthamoeba
- Bacillus cereus

Causes of Serious Corneal Infection

This has been found to be due to:
- Lack of compliance to lens care instructions
- Delayed reporting
- Incompetent initial care
- Nonavailability of appropriate antibiotics and antifungals

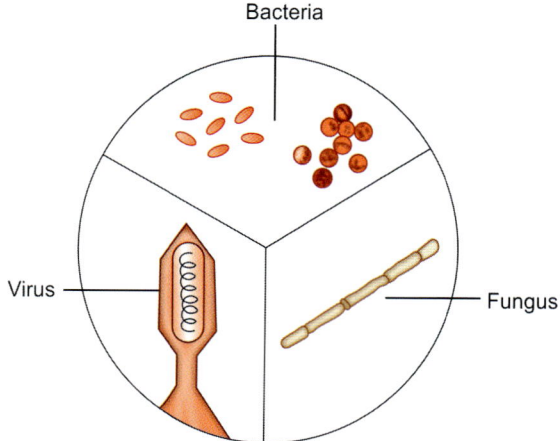

Fig. 24.3 Common pathogens causing corneal infections in contact lens wearers

Principles of Treatment

This includes a complete knowledge of:
- Antecedent history
- Knowledge of characteristic clinical picture of *Staph. aureus, Pseudomonas, Acanthamoeba* and fungus lesion on cornea.

  Infection has been noted more in PMMA than RGP, soft than RGP EWL than DWL, aphakia than myopia old than young, 7 day EW than 5d EW, < 45 day used solution than > 45d solution.

  Staph. aureus has dense localized infiltration with a clear surrounding cornea and purulent discharge; same is true for *Candida* and *Streptococcus pneumoniae.*

  Pseudomonas ulcer will show a dense infiltration within a hazy cornea and a mucinous discharge.

  Acanthamoeba ulcers have circular outlines, resistant to common medical treatment showing chronic ulceration unresponsive for weeks and months and are very painful.

  Fungal ulcers show dry cheesy slough, with satellite lesions, fixed hypopyon, clear surrounding cornea, though the signs are most severe but symptoms are almost absent except for the diminution of vision.

Laboratory diagnosis includes:
- Gram's staining
- Giemsa staining
- KOH preparation
- Slide for future use.

  Sensitivity pattern of the local pathogens to available antibiotics.

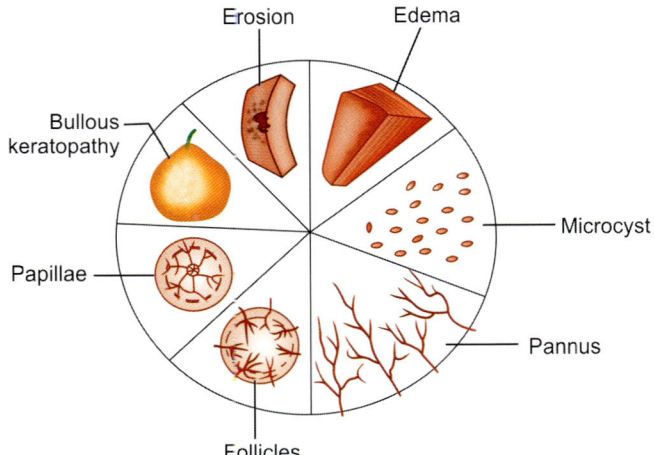

Fig. 24.4 Allergic manifestations due to contact lens use

ALLERGIC

Allergic manifestations in contact lenses (Fig. 24.4) are basically due to type-I hypersensitivity, where contact of immunogen with the target tissue disrupts the cell membrane of the mast cells and histamine and other mediators of inflammation are liberated to initiate inflammation.

The common immunogen includes:
- Thiomersal
- Chlorhexidine
- Chlorobutanol
- Papain
- PMMA
- HEMA

Symptomatology

Itching is the most important symptom which starts immediately with the contact of immunogen with the eye. The eye will show a pale swelling of the conjunctiva with watering.

Other modes of allergic presentations include:
- Hyperemia
- Follicular hypertrophy
- Sterile corneal infiltrates
- Superior limbal keratoconjunctivitis
- Pseudodendrites
- Microcyst
- Giant papillary conjunctivitis

Sterile corneal infiltrates are rare entity. They look quite alarming, but lack fiery ciliary congestion typical of microbial infiltrates. They can be situated anywhere in the cornea. They respond readily to corticosteroids.

Superficial Punctate Keratitis

This will show as pinhead white spots in the cornea which will readily take up fluorescein stain. This will be accompanied by chemosis of the entire conjunctiva.

Patient complains of itching, photophobia and watering.

Treatment

Withdrawal of contact lenses with treat the pathology within 24 hours. Immunogen responsible for the episode can be exactly known by performing a patch test and also by process of exclusion.

Patient can be made comfortable by the use of local sodium cromoglycate 3% drops and dexamethasone drops 0.1%.

The lens can be resumed by changing the:
- Schedule of wearing (reduced wearing time)
- Material of lens (PMMA to rigid GP to HEMA)
- Lens design
- Mechanical or enzyme cleaning
- Use of preservative free lubricating drugs

Superior Limbal Keratoconjunctivitis

This is characterized by:
- Superior limbal hyperemia
- Swelling
- Tongue shape superior corneal haze with vascularization at a later date
- Tarsal papillae

Patient's Complaints

Sudden irritation tearing redness and sensitivity to light after a prolonged uneventful contact lens wear for years he may present with history of change of contact lens solution, lens, or contact lens care regime.

Etiology

A combination of presence of contact lens and thiomersal exposure seem to be essential factor. Well established patients of SLKC may not show a universal response to conjunctival or skin challenge with thiomersal.

Prevention

Avoid thiomersal containing contact lens accessory solutions.

Treatment

- Discontinue lenses
- Re-fit when infiltration and vascularization have subsided.

Giant Papillary Conjunctivitis

Giant papillary conjunctivitis (GPC) is an extreme form of papillary hyperplasia in the upper tarsal conjunctiva which is seen in 10.15% of soft and 1–3% of hard lens wearer.

The onset comes after several weeks or years of contact lens use.

Symptomatology

- Increase of awareness of lens wear
- Increasing irritation
- Blurred vision
- Mucinous discharge
- Marked lens movement
- Intolerance of contact lens
- Drooping of lid or lids.

Signs

Hard lens GPC in contrast to soft lens GPC is characterized by:
- Fewer papillae
- More elevated apices
- Located near lid margins

Whereas soft lens GPC shows:
- Papillae more in number
- Apices are round and flat
- Located closer to tarsal fold
  Cellular profile for the smear shows mast cells in the epithelium.
- Eosinophils and basophils in epithelium and substantia propria
- Increase in lymphocytes and plasma cells.
  Author has failed to show presence of basophils and eosinophils in the typical cases of GPC. This alteration might be due treatment with corticoids.

Treatment

Wear can be made more comfortable in early cases by the use of:
- Lubricants
- Vasoconstrictors
- Cromoglycate drops
- Olopatadine drops
- Corticosteroids (for short intervals)
  It is best to withdraw the lenses and switch on the glasses for few months before restarting the lens wear.

The restarting of lenses should include changing the
- Schedule of wearing
- Material of lens

- Edge design
- Mechanical or enzyme cleaning
- Use of lubricating drugs

Microcysts

This is one of the allergic manifestations which will present as small microcysts on the surface of the cornea.

This can be seen by slit lamp on indirect diffuse illumination and by retro-illumination. Examination of the cornea by direct oblique illumination might show disturbance in catoptric image.

Treatment

Withdrawal of contact lens makes them disappear within a month or two.

TOXIC

Toxicity can manifest over the cornea and conjunctiva. It is usually due to contact lens solutions or drugs. Most commonly known toxic substance include benzalkonium chloride, thiomersal, and IDU.

Patient may show it as cumulative effect over a period of time as in benzalkonium chloride which can accumulate in the lens or it may be of sudden onset. In sudden onset symptomatology might give history of change of lens or lens solution or care regime.

Clinical Picture Symptoms

Patient complains of irritation, gritty sensation, photophobia, watering and pain.

Signs

There is hyperemia, chemosis, diffuse SPK, corneal infiltrates, pannus and SLKC, there are no follicles or papillae.

Treatment

Prevention include exclusion of known toxin.
Treatment includes:
- Lens withdrawal
- Pad and bandage
- Change of lens care system
- Avoid solutions containing benzalkonium chloride, thiomersal, and prolonged use of corticoid, IDU, timolol and local anesthetics.

Cetavlon, carbon tetrachloride, and chloroform has been wrongly used some time by the patient to clean hard lenses and if such a lens is inserted in the eye without adequate washing, this results in coagulation and desquamation of the epithelium. This is an extreme example of accidental toxicity.

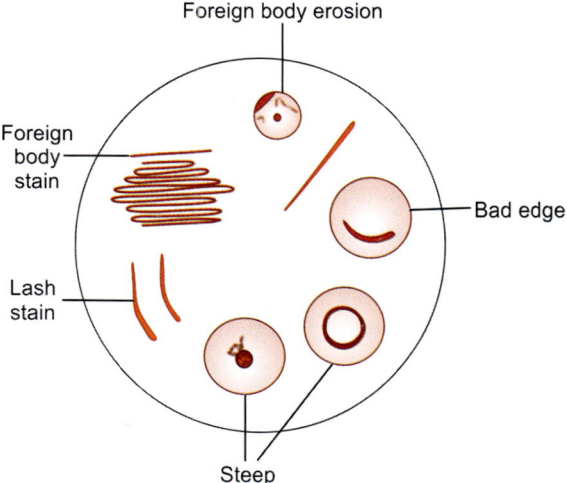

Fig. 24.5 Traumatic injury to the eye in a contact lens wearer

TRAUMATIC

Contact lens wearer can show traumatic injury to the eye (Fig. 24.5) which can be induced by:
- Contact lens (sharp edges, steep and flat fit)
- Nail
- Finger
- Lens remover
- Lash
- Foreign body
  Various traumatic lesions have been typically depicted in the figure.

Treatment

- Verify the lens specification, i.e. posterior curve, width and the blend of peripheral curves.
- Check the edges and redo the sharp edge if sharp.
- Do not go for a steep or a flat lens.
- Cut your nail before inserting lens.
- Do not use lens remover.
- If a foreign body goes under the lens. Remove the lens, wash the eyes, use antibiotic drop. Restart the lens next day especially if no irritation persists on removing the lens.

DESICCATION

These disturbances are due to tear film resurfacing disorders. These include:
- 3–9 O' clock staining

- 6 O' clock staining
- Dimple staining.

3–9 O'Clock Staining

This is dryness of conjunctiva and cornea at 3 and 9 O'clock or just below it at 4 and 8 O'clock or just below it at 4 and 8 O'clock. This is accompanied by conjunctival congestion in that area and corneal infiltration. This is basically due to thick corneal lens which produced tenting of the upper lid and consequent desiccation at 3 and 9 O'clock. This will result in infiltration, vascularization and if left unattended ulceration and even perforation can occur. Fenestrated scleral lenses with immobile bubble can produce similar lesion.

Symptoms

This will result in irritation, redness and photophobia and intolerance to contact lenses.

Treatment

It is treated by using:
- Lens of reduced thickness
- A large lens
- A soft lens

6 O' Clock Staining

This is a desiccation of conjunctiva and cornea at 6 O'clock, with hyperemia of conjunctiva and infiltration of the adjoining cornea.

This is caused by partial closure of the lid due to incomplete blinking. Lower part of the lens may be dry and dirty due to tear secretion desiccation. This result in lack of tear film resurfacing and desiccation. This area will take up fluorescein stain.

Symptoms

Symptoms will be similar to 3–9 O'clock staining.

Treatment

This is treated by stressing the role of complete blinking and demonstrating them methodology of complete blinking and its frequency during instruction. Complete blinking is done 20 times after every half an hour.

Dimple Staining

A tight fitting lens may trap air bubbles under its surface. Bubble will break up into small bubble which will stick on to corneal surface to create desiccation. This indicates a poor exchange symptom, patient may complain of slight visual haze.

Treatment

Give a new lens with good fit and see that the fluorescein exchange is adequate and quick.

LENS SPOLIATION

Lenses may get spoiled to create problems of various types. This spoliation may be physical due to alteration in the lens geometry and chemistry. Another common type of lens spoliation is by lens deposits.

Physical Change

The lens may get chipped, fractured while handling (insertion, removal, storage).

Lenses may get discolored due to local use of fluorescein and phenylephrine or due to systemic use of rifampicin. Lenses do show deterioration of plastic which tends to get easily fractured, or chipped. This is biochemically due to breakage of the old bonds, formation of new bonds and formation of new chains.

Lens Loss

This is much more common in hard than soft, and in extended wear than daily wear. It is much more often in children than adults. A loosely fitted lens is likely to be lost easily.

Symptoms

There might be more awareness of lens.

Sign

Lens may be more mobile (more than 2 mm on blinking).

Treatment

- Give proper fit
- Use soft lenses if losses are more.

Deposits

Deposits are seen in all type of lenses, i.e. extended wear, daily wear rigid gas permeable and hard lenses in order of the decreasing frequency.

The deposits may occur as diffuse milky coating over the entire surface of the lens, solitary pin head deposits, aggregated mulberry like and as patchy islands. They are constituted of inorganic, organic and mixed components. Calcium and proteins are the most common constituents. Tears and cleaning solutions are the ready sources.

Pathogenesis

Exact etiology is not clear but following factors constitute important contributory causes:
- Mode of handling and cleaning
- Material of lens
- Defects on the lens surface, aging and decay of plastic
- Accessory solution composition
- Care regime
- Use of local drug over the lens
- Intake of systemic drugs like rifampicin
- Local ocular environment as dry eyes, lagophthalmos, blepharitis and meibomianitis.
- Personal hygiene.

An interaction of lens factors and patient factors ultimately governs the deposit formation. Effect of deposits on the lens.

Deposit can affect the lens in the following ways:
- *Physically:* Cyst formation, bleb formation, discoloration
- *Physiologically:* To impair diffusion of gases
- *Optically:* To interfere with vision to cause retracted field haloes, distortion, polyopia, photophobia, aberration, astigmatism and ghost images.
- *Toxic:* Lens may accumulate toxic concentration of preservative to damage the cornea and both palpebral and bulbar conjunctiva.
- *Refractive:* Change in refractive index and fit of the lens.
- *Infective:* Deposits may harbour bacteria and fungi to infect the lens and cornea. Fungi can grow through the lens substance.
- *Allergic:* Altered protein in the deposits are well known immunogens. These may cause hyperemia, follicles, papillae, GPC and corneal infiltrates.

Management of Deposits

Best treatment for deposits is to replace the lens (Use of daily disposable lenses are the best).

Deposits may be prevented by:
- Proper patient selection seeing his lid, personal hygiene, tear functions and attitude towards compliance.
- Choose a proper lens material
- Choose a daily wear instead of extended wear lens
- Do proper monitoring (follow-up)
- Do proper cleaning (mechanical and chemical)
- Do weekly enzyme cleaning
- Do proper sterilization
  Note: A complete deposit resistant material is yet not known.

Superficial Punctate Keratitis

In contact lenses superficial punctate keratitis (SPK) can be seen for over the cornea in diffuse or localized form. In localized form it may be located at 3 and 9 O'clock, where it shows involvement of adjoining conjunctiva also. It may be seen over the center of cornea. It may be seen in paracentral region where it may be seen as arcuate stain, diffuse stain over the area under and outside the lens edge or localized within the edge only. SPK, in contact lens users may be due to the following causes. Contact lens induced SPK disappears within 24–48 hours with lens withdrawal but SPK due to associated conditions will remain unaffected with lens removal and requires specific treatment for the specific condition.

Mechanical

This SPK is due to imperfections on the edge or most common posterior imperfection is a bad blend or a rough edge which will produce SPK, in the paracentral area lying partly under the contact lens and partly outside the surface which will create a physical damage to the epithelium on the cornea. The contact lens over its excursion limits. Extremely flat lens will produce mechanical damage to corneal apex. It is treated by selecting a manufacturer with longest track record and inspecting each lens before fitting. Give optimum fit to avoid corneal apical damage by a flat fit

Occlusive

This is an altered physiological state due to corneal hypoxic state. Basically a bad fit or impermeable contact lens material does not permit adequate oxygenation of the cornea which shows edema. This edema is first intracellular and if hypoxic condition is allowed to continue the epithelial cells get damaged and they take up punctate stain. Such a situation of altered physiology is treated by giving an optimum fit and using a highly oxygen permeable material.

Toxic

Certain ingredients of accessory solutions are notorious for showing toxicity over cornea. The most common is the Benzalkonium chloride.

The SPK induced by such an ingredient is prevented and treated by eliminating the use of solutions having such a constituents.

Pathological

Pre-existing pathology like collagen diseases, dry eye, viral keratitis, and tyrosinemia can cause SPK. Such a lesion will persist even after contact lens withdrawal. Such pathologies are treated by specific therapies.

Infective

Infected SPK is usually a viral lesion. It might start or follow a systemic malaise and mild fever. Preauricular glands are enlarged. The lesion is very symptomatic. Viral lesion is usually unilateral. It will not heal with lens withdrawal and may progress to dendritic lesion and may show iridocyclitis. The cornea will remain hypoasthetic despite prolonged lens withdrawal.

Allergic

An asymptomatic contact lens user may become symptomatic contact lens user due to development of allergy. Common immunogens include thiomersal, papain, chlorhexidine, PMMA, HEMA and lens deposit. First symptoms is itching. There is a pale cold edema of the conjunctiva. Cornea may show SPK which will be diffuse over the entire surface of the cornea. SPK will persist till the cause is eliminated.

Accidental Drug-induced

Contact lens solutions for external use are sometimes put in the eye by mistake. Cetavlon is a common example. Entire cornea shows a diffuse SPK while epithelium looks like a ground glass. Abrasion might also develop. Such solutions should not be used, or kept beyond the reach of the patient with a bold red label "Not to be put in the eye".

Use of drugs which reduce the secretion of tears or which delay or alter healing might induce SPK on the cornea. Drugs like corticoids especially when used as suspension for days and weeks. Induces SPK timolol, IDU, local anesthetics, antihistaminic and central nervous system depressants also produce SPK. A contact lens wearer using these drugs might confuse the fitter who should elicit history of using such drugs locally or systemically.

Important Rigid Gas Permeable Patients: Symptoms and their Management

Blurred Vision

Symptom: Distant objects are blurred.

Sign
- Visual acuity is blurred
- Patient accepts minus sphere or minus cylinder or both
- Front surface shows deposits
- Lens may show toricity, i.e. warpage.

Time of onset: Gradually overtime, if it is deposit induced it comes later in the day.

Management
- Increase lens power
- Order a new lens with appropriate power
- Improve the lens cleaning regimen.

Fluctuating Vision

Symptom: Variable vision.

Sign
- Excessive lens motion
- Small optic zone
- Lens flexure
- Larger pupil
- Flat lens fitting
- Oily tears and lens surface film.

Time of onset
- Any time in the day
- Low illumination brings symptoms if pupil is larger or optic zone is small.

Management
- Refit to improve centration
- Increase the optic zone
- Change the central thickness
- Use rewetting drop
- Improve cleaning system.

Flare

Symptom: Distant things do not focus clearly.

Signs
- Decentered lens
- Smaller optic zone
- Larger pupil.

Time of onset
- Usually in the evening
- May be related to environment as overhead fluorescent lights.

Management
- Improve lens centration
- Use larger optic zone
- Use larger lens diameter.

Problems with Near Vision

Symptom: Asthenopia (fatigue and headache on prolonged near work).

Sign
- Reduced clarity at near
- Poor convergence amplitude
- Demands plus lens
- Cylindrical correction over 1 D.

Time of onset
- Builds more towards later part of the day
- After changing to contact lens from high minus spectacle prescription.

Management
- Give correct contact lens power
- Correct the cylinder
- Consider monovision in early presbyopia
- Inform high myopes or myopes in presbyopic age about near vision problem.
- Avoid excessive and prolonged use of computer over the contact lens and using lubricant drops while working on computer.

CHAPTER 25

Ocular Changes with Contact Lenses

OXYGENATION IN CONTACT LENSES

Oxygen is an essential requirement for corneal metabolism. The oxygen requirement of cornea is 5 mm^3/cm^3. Cornea utilizes atmospheric oxygen. Oxygen of 10% at cornea is the mean value and is taken to be usually adequate. In a contact lens user, oxygen requirement is furnished through the tear exchange which is pumped in and out of the space between lens and cornea. This pump has another very important function of draining out the debris. Only 10–20% of the tears trapped behind the contact lenses exchange with every blink which is sufficient to supply adequate oxygen to cornea. This is possible only with hard and rigid lenses whereas flexible soft lenses exchange only 1–3% of the trapped tears. This tear pump mechanism is not adequate for all the cases and the residual oxygen must be provided by diffusion through the body of the contact lens in such cases, as in gas permeable lenses. Lid closure results in fall of oxygen supply to 7% which is inadequate for maintaining normal corneal metabolism. The oxygen is required for cell integrity, cell division and repair. Relative oxygen requirement of epithelium, stroma and endothelium is in the ratio of 10:1:50.

GLUCOSE AND THE CORNEA

Glucose is the main substrate of the cornea and 90% of this comes from aqueous. Besides this, traces of amino acids, vitamins and mineral are also supplied through aqueous. The remaining 10% of glucose comes from the tears and limbus. 15% of glucose is utilized aerobically and 85% by anaerobic metabolism, hence lactate is the main byproduct of this pathway. Abundance of lactate in the cornea despite oxygen supply remains an unresolved problem. Further the glucose is metabolized through the following three pathways giving energy output (ATP) in the ratio of 2:36:1.

1. Embden Meyerhof (Generates 2 ATP's)
2. Kreb's cycle (36 ATP's)
3. Hexose MP shunt (1 ATP)

When a contact lens is placed over the cornea, it initiates physical, anoxic, metabolic occlusive problems to a varying degrees. These problems result in tremendous changes in all layers of cornea, uvea, conjunctiva and lids.

Physical Changes

Temperature rises from 32°C to 36°C; pH falls from 7.4 to 7.2.

Occlusive

There may be less of tear pump function causing trapping of the debris behind the lens, the dead cells undergo autolysis causing a chronically red eye.

Anoxia

Contact lens is a barrier to oxygenation of cornea by covering its surface and further if the fit is improper tear pump may not supply adequate oxygenation. This results in edema and a large variety of corneal insults detailed in contact lens problems.

Metabolic

Glycogen is decreased, lactic acid rises and LDH falls in epithelial cells.

With the use of contact lenses over the cornea, the epithelium, stroma, and the endothelium show a variety of morphological and functional changes which may be reversible or irreversible.

Epithelial Changes with Use of Contact Lens

Following changes had been seen in the epithelium of contact lens users.
- Loosening of cell junctions
- Decrease in surface microvilli
- Microvilli seen only towards the cell center
- Increase in cell permeability
- Cellular edema (intracellular)
- Decrease in trans-corneal potential
- Epithelial thinning (Removal of contact lens renders the epithelium normal within 30 days)
- Epithelial microcysts appear in 3 months much more with extended wear. They decrease with lens withdrawal after a temporary increase in size
- Epithelium becomes more fragile
- Decreased transparency
- Corneal sensations decreases due to decrease in acetylcholine.

Stromal Changes in Contact Lens Wearers

Stroma shows following changes:
- There is stromal edema, posterior stroma swells more than anterior Stria means 5–7% and folds mean 10–12% swelling of the cornea.
- Later on many cases may show thinning.

- Ultra microscopically degeneration and death of certain keratocytes due to metabolic toxins.
- Stromal infiltrates (infective, toxic, necrotic).
- Stromal vascularization. This is seen much more with aphakic and therapeutic lenses.

Endothelial Changes in Contact Lenses

Following changes were observed in endothelium.
- Decreased endothelial cells count.
- Pleomorphic (shape variation).
- More polymegathism (size variation).
- Endothelial bedewing.

Conjunctival Changes in Contact Lenses

Conjunctiva may show following changes:
- Hyperemia
- Papillae formation in lids giant papillary conjunctivitis (GPC)
- Superior limbal keratoconjunctivitis.
  (This is a tongue shaped haze in the upper third of cornea with swelling and hyperemia of conjunctiva over the superior limbus).
- Clumping of microvilli in the center of cells.

Lid Changes in Contact Lenses

Authors have observed many individuals with lack of blinking, infrequent blinking or more frequent blinking with or without head posture with the use of contact lenses. Lid margins become less sensitive.

Uveal Changes in Contact Lenses

Rarely hypopyon may be seen in contact lens wearer. This is due to occlusive effect which causes vasodilation (lactic acid induced). This happens more with aphakic lenses.

CHAPTER 26

Silicone Lenses

INTRODUCTION

It was in late 50's that Walter Wecker and Neil Bailey began experimenting with silicone for contact lenses. This process has been continued by Muller Welt Company and later by Dow Corning. Dow Corning has been marketing their silicone lenses under brand name "SILSOFT". SilSoft has been used with success and was approved as extended wear lens in 1981 in US. Bausch and Lomb has now taken the patent and is selling SilSoft, and research is continuing to improve the lens and to make it a viable extended wear lens.

ADVANTAGES

Silicone lenses were taken as lenses of future because of the following advantages:
- It is biologically inert.
- It has a thermal conductivity.
- It is flexible and gives comfort of the soft lens.
- It has no appreciable water content to absorb chemical and contaminants.
- It is not affected by temperature and pH changes.

DISADVANTAGES

As a contact lens material silicone has the following disadvantages:
- It is always in flexible state, so it is very difficult to fabricate it.
- It is basically hydrophobic unless surface is treated some way.
- It is prone to deposition of lipoid and proteins.
- It develops negative pressure or suction which makes the lens adhere to the cornea.
- The disadvantage of suction completely disrupts the tear pump and builds up resultant toxic metabolic waste. The autolytic enzyme of the trapped cellular debris will result in an irritable red eye and host of other metabolic problems.

The negative suction makes the hydrophobic lens surface to rub with the hydrophilic corneal surface causing contact adhesion phenomenon.

CLINICAL OBSERVATION

Japanese and German 100% silicon lenses have same parameters as soft. Their results were discouraging due to following clinical observations.

- Conjunctival injection
- Corneal edema
- Corneal erosions
- Breakdown of hydrophilic chemical coating within one hour
- Epithelial cells get stuck to the back of lens
- Sterile keratitis.

These observations by Japanese and German studies did bring out certain conclusion for silicone lenses and they were:

- Flatter and smaller lenses would be better
- Improvement on edges and in surface treatment is required.
- Tear exchange should be better.
- Per oxide should be used to sterilize and clean the lenses.

Dow Corning's silsoft lenses have already overcome these problems. This Dow's and now Bausch and Lomb's lens has number of advantages over the other extended wear lenses and they are:

- Tremendous ability to pass oxygen and carbon dioxide.
- It highly exceeds the criteria of oxygen permeability required for extended wear.
- The laser marking to indicate the lot number, base curve and power.
- Large range of available parameters to meet the requirement of aphakes at all the ages.

PARAMETERS OF BAUSCH AND LOMB SILICONE LENSES

Base Curve

- Base curves for adult age
  8.1, 8.3, 8.5 and 8.7
- Base curves for children
  7.5, 7.7 and 7.9

Power

- Power for adult aphakes
  +10.00 to 20.00 in 1.00D steps
- Power for pediatric age
  +23.00, +26.00, +29.00 and +32.00

Diameter

- 11.3 and 12.5 mm
- All pediatric lenses are available in 11.3 mm diameter only.

FITTING METHODOLOGY

Fitting of silicone lenses is done by trial lens methodology. The trial lenses have the above base curves and diameters.

Steps of Fitting

- Finalize spectacle prescription is minus cylinder and drop cylinder
- Transpose this power at corneal level (effectively).
- Do keratometry.
- Initial lens is 11.3 in diameter and of base curve akin to flat curvature of the cornea of the flattest lens near to the flat curvature.
- If the 11.3 lens is eccentric or unstable, try 12.50 mm lens.

Ideal lens fit criteria includes:
- Well centered.
- Movement not more than 1.5–2 mm.
- Uniform fluorescein scalloping film can be seen at the edges. This ensures a good exchange and avoid adhesion phenomenon.

Steep lens fit is indicated by:
- Big central fluorescein pooling.
- Gross peripheral ring touch within the edges.
- Immobile lens (on blinking).

Flat lens fit is indicated by:
- Fluorescein pool under edges, which are lifted.
- A touch over the cornea apex.
- A freely mobile lens.
- Eccentrically placed lens.

Note: In all the silicone and high DK value lenses the edges scallop due to spring like nature.

Awareness of lens in the eye is the only problem though it is less than the rigid permeable lenses and the previous silicone lenses and the patient gets used to the silicon lens in few days.

SilSoft super plus contact lenses have been used in children who have had cataract surgery where an intraocular lens has not been implanted (aphakia). The SilSoft material and customized design permit the eye to breathe and deliver outstanding vision, necessary elements for healthy development of pediatric eyes. Because the material allows oxygen to pass through it, SilSoft super plus lenses can even be worn overnight.

CHAPTER 27

Extended Wear Rigid Lenses

INTRODUCTION

The concept of extended wear was started in early 70's in England. It was a soft lens of high hydration and better oxygen permeability. In 80's, rigid polymers with very high oxygen permeability have been approved for extended wear.

METABOLIC CONSIDERATION

Aerobic metabolism of the cornea can be maintained only if partial pressure of oxygen is 10%. Though this is an average figure but the individual variations may range from 7.5 to 21%. Lenses with DK value of approximately 25 would supply sufficient oxygen during the day (open eyes). DK value of lenses used as extended wear must be higher, i.e. 85 and above to provide adequate oxygen to cornea during sleep (closed eyes). This metabolic oxygen requirement was possible with the hydrophilic extended wear lenses during the day only, because their DK value was between 30 and 40.

None of the previous generation hydrophilic soft extended wear lenses had this high DK value and consequently produced hypoxic embarrassment to the cornea resulting in:

- Corneal edema
- Superficial punctate keratopathy (SPK)
- Microcyst
- Bullous keratopathy
- Sterile infiltrates
- Epithelial erosion
- Epithelial ulcers
- Superior limbic keratoconjunctivitis.

The new generation of lenses which is essentially constituted of silicon and fluorocarbon has much higher DK values. The high DK value materials can supply oxygen to the cornea in quantity far excess than the basic metabolic need during the day and the night. These lenses are the modern rigid gas permeable extended wear lenses.

SOFT EXTENDED WEAR VS RIGID EXTENDED WEAR LENSES

A comparison between these two types of extended wear lens will clarify the exact status of each.

- Rigid lenses do not change their parameter on exposure to environment and pH change. They do not dehydrate. The soft lenses with high water content after few months of wear may create sudden redness and sore eyes. This is due to dehydration of lens. Lens may loose 8–10% water after taking it out of the bottle. The dehydrated lens fits steep, trapping tissue debris, metabolic wastes, lactic acid and pyruvate, resulting in a red eye. Dehydrated soft lens becomes tighter when the pH changes to acidic due to accumulation of lactic acid. The rigid lenses do not tighten even after years of use. The current generation silicone hydrogel lenses may be more suitable for extended wear purposes.
- Another major problem is soft lens spoilage by deposit formation on its surface. They may form a uniform sheet, or present as geographic island or appear as solitary jelly bump or as mulberry like deposits. They may appear within few hours over soft lenses. Some of them may remain permanently. Some of them resist all type of mechanical, enzymatic, chemical and ultrasonic treatment. In rigid lenses deposits do occur, but they can be removed completely by organic solvents or polishing.
- *Reproducibility of soft lenses:* This has been a problem to duplicate soft lenses in exact dimensions. This difficulty is more for low water ultrathin lenses. A change of thickness from 0.035 to 0.045 mm will reduce the oxygen transmission by 30%. Such a wrong replacement lens will initiate trouble, especially in complicated cases that are already or borderline oxygen supply. To avoid this problem with replacement lenses, follow-up should be the same as it is for the new lenses. Modern rigid gas permeable lens can be fabricated to an accuracy of one thousandth of 1 mm and this can be easily checked in the clinic on radiuscope and other gauges.
- Optical quality of rigid lenses is far superior to that of the soft lenses. In soft lenses hydration, dehydration and flexure decreases the vision. Patient may say that "I see everything but it is not clear".
- The number of potential extended wear patients is far greater in rigid extended wear lenses than it is for soft lens patients.
  - A fairly large number of astigmatic patients requiring toric soft lenses may fall outside the limited parameters of toric soft lenses.
  - Old PMMA and daily gas permeable lenses wearer having used to a crisp visual acuity will feel satisfied only with crisp optic of rigid extended wear lens.
  - Eventually we may have toric, bitoric and bifocals in rigid gas permeable to serve larger number of contact lens patients.
- Rigid extended wear lenses are much more durable than soft. Whereas a rigid lens can be worn for years without a change but the soft extended wear lens should be changed every 3–6 months.
- *Oxygen performance:* Adequate availability of oxygen to the cornea is dependent on
  - Tear pump
  - DK value of lens material
  - Corneal coverage (lens diameter)

- Hydration
- Thickness of the lens.

Oxygenation of cornea would be better if
- Tear pump works like that of the PMMA lens
- DK value of material is higher
- Lens diameter is smaller than corneal diameter
- Lens hydration is higher
- Lens thickness is reduced.

- Boston IV lens with 36 DK performs better than permalens of 34 DK because
  - Tear pump of rigid Boston IV lens exchanges 15–20% tear with each blink compared to 1–2% of tear exchange with permalens with each blink
  - Diameter of Boston IV lens is 9.2 and 9.5 which is smaller than the corneal diameter.
    The diameter of permalens is more than 13.5 mm which is bigger than that of cornea.
    Bigger diameter may also mean a poor exchange with collection of tissue debris and metabolic wastes resulting in a chronic red eye.
  - Rigid lenses have more thermal conductivity which keeps the temperature of cornea lower. Every one degree rise of corneal temperature raises the oxygen demand of cornea by 5% for its optimum functioning.
    Whereas fluoroperm has DK value of 61 DK/L and DK 92, Boston equalens has a DK of 71 and silicon has DK of 360. Many materials in the market have DK value of 90 and 100 and even more.

DISADVANTAGES OF RIGID EXTENDED WEAR LENSES

Comfort Factors

Soft lenses are the more popular lenses due to the initial comfortable insertion than the rigid lens. In US, 70% of lens wearers use soft lenses. A patient who wants comfort ahead of anything will always opt for a soft lens. By sleeping few nights with the rigid lens awareness may lessen considerably.

Fitting of Rigid Lens is more Exacting and Time-consuming

We will have to go to old technique of fitting the lenses on eyes rather than fitting the eyes to the lenses as we did in soft lenses.

There is a distinct advantage that the following parameters in the lens can be modified:
- Diameter
- Power
- Peripheral curves
- Blend of peripheral curves
- Edge.
  These demand more time.

Sleeping with Lenses on is an Initial Problem

A long time PMMA wearer who has been repeatedly told not to sleep with the lenses finds it difficult to sleep the first night. This may be more so if he has had abrasion when he slept with his PMMA lenses.

This is corrected by explaining the property of the lens material and reassuring the patient that corneal or ocular damage will not occur with this new material.

Adhesion Phenomenon

Rigid extended wear lenses do show adhesion phenomenon sometimes. This is basically due to the lens behaving as a suction cup causing first ring impression on the cornea and then adherence to the cornea. *This is likely to occur in*

- High DK value lenses
- Steep lenses
- Thin lenses.
  Patient is usually unaware of this adhesion.

On examination, a ring impression is seen over the cornea and lens may not move and remain adherent to the cornea. It was seen more with paraperm material (DK 56) than with Boston IV material (DK 26).

3–9 Staining

This is much more with extended wear than with daily wear.

It is seen more often with:

- Low riding lenses
- Thick edged lenses
- Partial blinkers.
  Furnishing a high riding, thin edged lens with good edge finish will correct the problem. Complete blinking should be stressed and demonstrated to the patient.

FITTING

Fitting is Done by Trial Lens

Fitting a low DK lens like Boston IV and paraperm demands fitting on flat K or slightly flatter than 'K', i.e. keratometry is 44 and 45, trial lens will be 44 or 43.75. The overall size of the lens is 9.2 and 9.5. Size of the lens and base curve is varied to achieve an upriding lens. This lens will be under the upper lid and hence comfortable.

Fluorescein pattern should indicate an alignment pattern and no bearing area. If the lens is low riding, it is made to ride up by flattening the base curve.

Even if the interpalpebral position is attained the lens will do well. Smaller lenses can easily achieve interpalpebral position. The diameter used here may be 9.00 mm.

Fitting of Higher DK Value Lenses (Like Equalens or Fluoroperm)

These lenses are basically more soft due to higher content of silicon and fluorine and hence springler. The edges turn is to create scalloping. The trial lens is fitted 0.5–1.00 diopter flatter than 'K', i.e. if keratometry is 44 and 45, the trial lens will be 43.50 or 43.00 of diameter 9 mm or more.

Fluorescein pattern should show a good corneal alignment. A steep lens with fluorescein pool in the center, showing no movement and creating a ring impression over the cornea will be loosened by giving a flatter base curve or reducing the diameter.

A flat lens with fluorescein pool at the edge, showing an edge lift, and excessive movement, is treated by using a steeper base curve or using a bigger diameter.

Prefit Examination

This is the same as for other lenses as highlighted in prefit assessment. *This includes examination of function and health of:*
- Facial muscle
- Lids
- Palpebral aperture
- Conjunctiva and cornea
- Tear status
- Visual functions.

Indications for Rigid Extended Wear Lenses

- Lack of dexterity as in old and infantile aphakes
- Metabolic problems with hydrophilic extended wear
- Visual problems with toric extended wear soft lenses
- Allergic problems with soft extended wear causing giant papillary conjunctivitis
- Superior limbic keratoconjunctivitis created due to soft extended wear
- All lenses where thickness is more as in high plus and minus, toric, bifocal, keratoconic, bigger diameter lenses.

Schedule: For the first week the lenses are given for a daily wear regime and then it is switched to an extended wear regime.

Written instruction are given for the care of lenses and schedule of wear. This also contains cautions which highlight when to report to the fitter on occurrence of certain specific problems like persistence of haze, discharge redness and pain.

MANAGEMENT OF RIGID GAS PERMEABLE EXTENDED WEAR

A successful rigid gas permeable (RGP) extended wear (EW) requires (1) a good lens, (2) a good patient, (3) a good contact lens fitter.

Patient selection for RGP EW: The patient for RGP EW should be a successful daily wearer, highly motivated and competent.

The patient should have adequate tear film and should not have allergies, lid abnormalities, regular medications.

Lens selection: The RGP EW lens should have DK value near 90. It should be wettable, durable and have stable parameters.

Lens design: It should give alignment fit with minimal bearing, slightly wide edge (maximum 0.5 mm) with a good clearance.

Edge should be rounded. The edge should be located either posteriorly or in the middle and never towards the front.

The lens design should avoid:
- Narrow tight edge
- Excessive mid peripheral bearing
- Poor tear exchange
- Excessive back surface debris
- Excessive flexure.

Patient should be given verbal and written information, instructions and consent taken. *Follow-up of RGP EW should be done on:*
- Day one in the morning at 9 AM
- Weeks—one and two
- Months—one, 2, 4, 8th, then every three months
- Check over night removal schedule which should be overnight removal every 5th night.

Follow-up day one: Look for
- Persistent haze after waking up
- Striae (edema)
- 3–9 stain
- Back surface debris
- Binding, arcuate stain, and indentation.

Subsequent visits follow-up: In addition to above look for epithelial microcysts and lens parameter changes.

Strategies for Success

- Persistent striae are dealt by
  - Increase of DK/L
  - Change from extended to daily wear
- 3–9 staining dealt by
  - Change diameter
  - Change edge design
  - Improve blinking
  - Use lubricant drops
  - Use daily wear regime.
- Lens binding is dealt by
  - Decrease in diameter
  - Increase in edge width (0.5 mm)

- Increase in edge clearance (75 mm)
- Use daily wear.
- Microcysts are dealt by
  - Increase of DK/L (above 90)
  - Use daily wear.

LENS CARE

- Dispense presoaked lenses
- Use manufacturers recommended solutions
- Give proper patient instructions and ask patient to repeat instructions
- Wash eyes with saline morning and evening
- Use eye drops
- Use cosmetics before inserting the lens in the eye
- Clean lenses with lens cleaner daily
- Avoid lenses with deposits.

Patient's education: Give the patient education about
- Lens care
- Wearing schedule
- Early warning signs and appropriate action.

Warning signs: Include persistence of the following complaints over an hour and if so run to the eye specialist and these warning signs are
- Persistent watering
- Persistent discharge
- Persistent pain
- Persistent foggy vision
- Persistent lens adhesion
- Persistent whiteness in the eye (localized or diffuse haziness of cornea).

Successful RGP EW can be achieved by proper patient, lens and fitter selection and they are:
- Patient should be
  - Suitable
  - Educated
  - Compliant
- Lens should
  - Fit well
  - High DK/L
  - Properly cared for
- Contact lens fitter
  - Educated
  - Motivated

CHAPTER 28

Contact Lens Fitting after Refractive Surgery

INTRODUCTION

Contact lens fitting after radial keratotomy or excimer laser refractive surgery poses problems psychologically to the patient and physically to the fitter. Patient's expectations to be free of lenses and contact lenses is not fulfilled and disturbed topography of cornea remains unclarified. Anatomically, epithelium may show dystrophic changes, punctuate lesions, and hypoesthesia. Topography shows central flattening and paracentral steepening. There may be gross surface irregularity in intersecting incisions after radial keratotomy or presence of surface haze after surface ablation. This might result in decentration, central pooling, intermediate touch and edge lift causing physical irritation. Pooled tears stagnate to initiate hypoxic damage.

FITTING METHODOLOGY

Large rigid highly gas permeable lenses are fitted by hit and trial method on the basis of the following physiological requisites.

- Tears must exchange
- Lens should not move excessively
- Lens weight should be uniformly distributed on a large part of the cornea.

Choice of trial lens: A large lens of 9.5 mm diameter is chosen on the basis of selecting a trial lens 2.5 D steeper than the postoperative keratometry.

Finalization is done on the basis of fluorescein pattern. It is better to choose a large diameter lens and achieve optimal fitting by changing the base curve; trapped air bubbles may be dealt with by fenestration.

Author had documented BC finalization by a regression formula which says;

Base curve of contact lens after RK = 6.5 + 0.9 postoperative 'K'; where 'K' stands for average postoperative keratometry.

Indications

- Under correction
- Over correction
- Regular astigmatism
- Irregular astigmatism
- Anisometropia
- Fluctuating vision
- Post-LASIK ectasia

Power Calculation

Power calculation is done by over-refraction. It may be as high as the preoperative refractive error due to additional minus which has been given to compensate the tear pool lens trapped behind the center of the contact lens.

Toric lenses may be given to attend to the residual astigmatism and are stabilized by prism or flange-edge.

Soft lenses are given for sensitive cases but with a great caution because of the risk of infection and vascularization.

Therapeutic lens have a role in high myopia showing postoperative under correction. The lenses will be used to mould the cornea (Orthokeratology).

Post-fitting Problems

Besides the usual problems of contact lenses, specific problem is that of a corneal vascularization which ascends into the incisions from the limbus. The reported incidence of neovascularization is 33 to 60%.

Contact Lens Failure

Author has found that contact lens failure is due to:
- Irritation
- Neovascularization
- Fluctuating vision
- Changes in refractive error.

One of the methodologies for Orthokeratology is as follows:
- Rigid gas permeable-extened wear (RGP-EW) lens
- Fit. Flat by 1.00 D
- Day and night wear 1 week
- Overnight rest
- Use for two weeks again
- So after 3 weeks again
- Go 1.00 more flat
- Replacement every 3 weeks
- Continue till 20/20 or + 0.5 SPH.
- Retainer one day
  - Rest 2 days
  - Retainer one day
  - Rest two days
  - Rest two days
- Aspheric lens flattens more than spheric
- Final reseat may be 05 to 2.5 rarely 5.00 flattening.

Post-LASIK Ectasia

Post-LASIK ectasia is rare but potentially serious complication after an uneventful LASIK. It is characterized by stromal thinning, progressive anterior and posterior corneal steepening with irregular astigmatism resulting in loss of corrected distance visual acuity. The accurate incidence of ectasia is still undetermined, but ranges from 0.04 to 0.6%. Although keratoconus and post-LASIK ectasia display similar corneal topographic picture, the histopathology, ultrastructure and biochemical features suggests that the pathophysiology is varied in either conditions. Post-LASIK ectasia is due to weakening of the biomechanical strength of cornea after LASIK. Dawson and Randleman showed that ectasia is probably due to interlamellar biomechanical slippage of corneal collagen fibrils (interlamellar fracture) followed by subseqent interfibrillar biomechanical slippage (interfibrillar fracture).

Although Barraquer initially described abnormal keratoconus like corneal curvature in patients after myopic keratomileusis, it was Seiler, who first reported the same corneal curvature changes in patients who had preoperative form fruste keratoconus. There are various risk factors associated with increased incidence of post-LASIK ectasia. These include younger patient age, abnormal corneal topography (i.e. forme fruste keratoconus), low residual stromal bed thickness, low preoperative CCT and high myopia. Klein et al. described idiopathic ectasia in a series of cases where there were no risk factors. In 2008, Randleman published Ectasia Risk Score system. This system correctly identified 91% of ectatic eyes (91% specificity).

Although there are several therapeutic options, the visual rehabilitation of patients with post-LASIK ectasia remains a therapeutic challenge for refractive surgeons. Various treatment modalities include corneal collgen crosslinking (CXL), rigid gas permeable contact lenses topography guided photorefractive keratectomy (PRK) with simultaneous CXL, intracorneal ring implantation and keratoplasty. In view of ectasia and corneal topographic irregularity, RGP contact

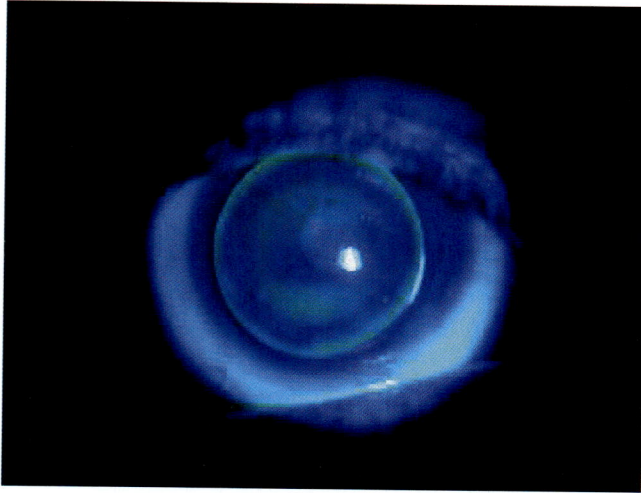

Fig. 28.1 Rose K contact lens in post-LASIK ectasia

lenses are most suitable ones for the visual rehabilitation in these cases. The introduction of Rose K2 aberration control lens heralded a new era for treating ectatic corneal disorders giving high quality of vision. Their complex geometry helps to fit any irregular corneal surface and bring all focal points on to the retina to a single point irrespective base curve radii or lens power. These are multicurve lenses and have the best comfort and acceptability in such patients. Most important advantage is their success of fitting reaching 80 to 90% in first fit in keratoconus.

Rose K2 lens may be a better therapeutic option in visual rehabilition of post-LASIK ectasia patients than conventional RGP lens (Fig. 28.1). Amongst the Rose K2 lenses, many can be fitted by keratoconic design, however some patients with grossly irregular corne, irregular cornea design may be needed. Although Rose K2 is expensive which makes it difficult to indicate in developing countries like India, the advantages (the quality of vision, ease of contact lens fitting and comfort in its usage) overweigh its cost.

Spectacle refraction or spectacle lens power (BVP) in dioptres	Ocular refraction in dioptres for distances in mm of:														
	6	7	8	9	10	11	12	13	14	15	16	17	18	19	20
+0.25	0.25	0.25	0.25	0.25	0.25	0.25	0.25	0.25	0.25	0.25	0.25	0.25	0.25	0.25	0.25
.50	0.50	0.50	0.50	0.50	0.50	0.50	0.50	0.50	0.50	0.50	0.50	0.50	0.50	0.50	0.51
.75	0.75	0.75	0.75	0.76	0.76	0.76	0.76	0.76	0.76	0.76	0.76	0.76	0.76	0.76	0.76
+1.00	1.01	1.01	1.01	1.01	1.01	1.01	1.01	1.01	1.01	1.02	1.02	1.02	1.01	1.02	1.02
.25	1.26	1.26	1.26	1.26	1.27	1.27	1.27	1.27	1.27	1.27	1.28	1.28	1.28	1.28	1.28
.50	1.51	1.52	1.52	1.52	1.52	1.52	1.53	1.53	1.53	1.53	1.54	1.54	1.54	1.54	1.55
.75	1.77	1.77	1.78	1.78	1.78	1.79	1.79	1.79	1.80	1.80	1.80	1.81	1.81	1.81	1.81
+2.00	2.02	2.03	2.03	2.04	2.04	2.04	2.05	2.05	2.06	2.06	2.07	2.07	2.07	2.08	2.08
.25	2.28	2.29	2.29	2.30	2.30	2.31	2.31	2.32	2.33	2.33	2.34	2.34	2.35	2.35	2.36
.50	2.54	2.54	2.55	2.56	2.56	2.57	2.58	2.58	2.59	2.60	2.60	2.61	2.62	2.62	2.63
.75	2.79	2.80	2.81	2.82	2.82	2.83	2.84	2.85	2.86	2.87	2.87	2.88	2.89	2.90	2.91
+3.00	3.06	3.06	3.07	3.08	3.09	3.10	3.11	3.12	3.13	3.14	3.15	3.16	3.17	3.18	3.19
.25	3.31	3.33	3.34	3.35	3.36	3.37	3.38	3.39	3.40	3.42	3.43	3.44	3.45	3.46	3.48
.50	3.58	3.59	3.60	3.61	3.63	3.64	3.65	3.67	3.68	3.69	3.71	3.72	3.74	3.75	3.76
.75	3.84	3.85	3.87	3.88	3.90	3.91	3.93	3.94	3.96	3.97	3.99	4.00	4.02	4.04	4.05
+4.00	4.10	4.12	4.13	4.15	4.17	4.18	4.20	4.22	4.24	4.26	4.27	4.29	4.31	4.33	4.35

(Contd...)

(Contd...)

	6	7	8	9	10	11	12	13	14	15	16	17	18	19	20
.25	4.36	4.38	4.40	4.42	4.44	4.46	4.48	4.50	4.52	4.54	4.56	4.58	4.60	4.62	4.64
.50	4.63	4.65	4.67	4.69	4.71	4.73	4.76	4.78	4.80	4.83	4.85	4.87	4.90	4.92	4.95
.75	4.89	4.91	4.94	4.96	4.99	5.01	5.04	5.06	5.09	5.12	5.14	5.17	5.19	5.22	5.25
+5.00	5.15	5.18	5.21	5.24	5.26	5.29	5.32	5.35	5.38	5.41	5.43	5.46	5.49	5.52	5.56
.25	5.42	5.45	5.48	5.51	5.54	5.57	5.60	5.63	5.67	5.70	5.73	5.76	5.80	5.83	5.87
.50	5.69	5.72	5.75	5.79	5.82	5.85	5.89	5.92	5.96	6.00	6.03	6.07	6.11	6.14	6.18
.75	5.96	5.99	6.03	6.06	6.10	6.14	6.18	6.22	6.25	6.29	6.33	6.37	6.41	6.46	6.50
+6.00	6.22	6.26	6.30	6.34	6.38	6.42	6.46	6.51	6.55	6.59	6.64	6.68	6.72	6.77	6.82
.25	6.49	6.54	6.58	6.62	6.67	6.71	6.76	6.80	6.85	6.90	6.94	6.99	7.04	7.09	7.14
.50	6.77	-6.81	6.86	6.91	6.95	7.00	7.05	7.10	7.15	7.20	7.26	7.31	7.36	7.42	7.47
.75	7.04	7.09	7.14	7.19	7.24	7.29	7.35	7.40	7.46	7.51	7.57	7.63	7.69	7.75	7.82
+7.00	7.30	7.36	7.41	7.47	7.52	7.58	7.64	7.70	7.76	7.82	7.88	7.94	8.01	8.07	8.14
.25	7.58	7.64	7.70	7.76	7.82	7.88	7.94	8.01	8.07	8.14	8.20	8.27	8.34	8.41	8.48
.50	7.86	7.92	7.98	8.05	8.11	8.18	8.24	8.31	8.38	8.45	8.53	8.60	8.67	8.75	8.83
.75	8.13	8.20	8.26	8.33	8.40	8.47	8.55	8.62	8.70	8.77	8.85	8.93	9.01	9.09	9.17
+8.00	8.40	8.47	8.55	8.62	8.70	8.77	8.85	8.93	9.01	9.09	9.17	9.26	9.35	9.43	9.52
.25	8.68	8.76	8.83	8.91	8.99	9.07	9.16	9.24	9.33	9.42	9.51	9.60	9.69	9.78	9.88
.50	8.96	9.04	9.12	9.21	9.29	9.38	9.47	9.56	9.65	9.75	9.84	9.94	10.04	10.14	10.25
.75	9.23	9.32	9.41	9.50	9.59	9.68	9.78	9.87	9.97	10.07	10.17	10.28	10.38	10.49	10.60
+9.00	9.51	9.61	9.70	9.79	9.89	9.98	10.09	10.19	10.30	10.41	10.52	10.63	10.74	10.86	10.98
.25	9.79	9.89	9.99	10.09	10.19	10.30	10.41	10.52	10.63	10.74	10.86	10.98	11.10	11.22	11.35

(Contd...)

(Contd...)

	6	7	8	9	10	11	12	13	14	15	16	17	18	19	20
.50	10.07	10.17	10.28	10.38	10.49	10.60	10.72	10.83	10.95	11.07	11.20	11.33	11.45	11.59	11.72
.75	10.35	10.46	10.57	10.68	10.80	10.92	11.04	11.16	11.29	11.42	11.55	11.68	11.82	11.96	12.11
+10.00	10.64	10.75	10.87	10.99	11.11	11.24	11.36	11.49	11.63	11.76	11.90	12.05	12.20	12.35	12.50
.25	10.92	11.04	11.17	11.29	11.42	11.55	11.69	11.83	11.97	12.11	12.26	12.41	12.57	12.73	12.89
.50	11.21	11.33	11.46	11.60	11.73	11.87	12.01	12.16	12.31	12.46	12.62	12.78	12.95	13.12	13.29
.75	11.49	11.63	11.76	11.90	12.05	12.19	12.34	12.50	12.66	12.82	12.98	13.15	13.33	13.51	13.69
+11.00	11.78	11.92	12.06	12.21	12.36	12.51	12.67	12.84	13.00	13.17	13.35	13.53	13.72	13.91	14.10
.25	12.06	12.21	12.36	12.52	12.68	12.84	13.01	13.18	13.35	13.53	13.72	13.91	14.11	14.31	14.57
.50	12.35	12.51	12.66	12.83	12.99	13.16	13.34	13.52	13.71	13.90	14.09	14.29	14.50	14.71	14.93
.75	12.64	12.80	12.97	13.14	13.31	13.49	13.68	13.87	14.06	14.26	14.47	14.68	14.90	15.13	15.36
+12.00	12.93	13.10	13.27	13.45	13.64	13.83	14.02	14.22	14.42	14.63	14.85	15.08	15.31	15.54	15.79
.25	13.22	13.40	13.58	13.77	13.96	14.16	14.36	14.57	14.79	15.01	15.24	15.47	15.72	15.97	16.23
.50	13.51	13.70	13.89	14.08	14.29	14.49	14.71	14.93	15.15	15.38	15.62	15.87	16.13	16.39	16.67
.75	13.81	14.00	14.20	14.40	14.61	14.83	15.05	15.28	15.52	15.77	16.02	16.28	16.55	16.83	17.11
+13.00	14.10	14.30	14.51	14.72	14.94	15.17	15.40	15.64	15.89	16.15	16.41	16.69	16.97	17.27	17.57
.25	14.39	14.60	14.82	15.04	15.27	15.51	15.76	16.01	16.27	16.54	16.82	17.10	17.40	17.71	18.03
.50	14.69	14.91	15.14	15.37	15.61	15.86	16.11	16.37	16.65	16.93	17.22	17.52	17.83	18.16	18.49
.75	14.99	15.21	15.45	15.69	15.94	16.20	16.47	16.74	17.03	17.32	17.63	17.94	18.27	18.61	18.96
+14.00	15.28	15.52	15.77	16.02	16.28	16.55	16.83	17.11	17.41	17.72	18.04	18.37	18.72	19.07	19.44
.25	15.58	15.83	16.08	16.35	16.62	16.90	17.19	17.49	17.80	18.12	18.46	18.80	19.16	19.54	19.93
.50	15.88	16.14	16.40	16.68	16.96	17.25	17.55	17.87	18.19	18.53	18.88	19.24	19.62	20.01	20.42

(Contd...)

(Contd...)

	6	7	8	9	10	11	12	13	14	15	16	17	18	19	20
.75	16.18	16.45	16.72	17.01	17.30	17.61	17.92	18.25	18.59	18.94	19.31	19.69	20.08	20.49	20.92
+15.00	16.48	16.76	17.04	17.34	17.65	17.96	18.29	18.63	18.99	19.35	19.74	20.13	20.55	20.98	21.43
.25	16.79	17.07	17.37	17.68	18.00	18.33	18.67	19.02	19.39	19.77	20.17	20.59	21.02	21.47	21.94
.50	17.09	17.39	17.69	18.01	18.34	18.68	19.04	19.41	19.79	20.19	20.61	21.04	21.50	21.97	22.46
.75	17.39	17.70	18.02	18.35	18.70	19.05	19.42	19.81	20.21	20.62	21.06	21.51	21.98	22.48	22.99
+16.00	17.70	18.02	18.35	18.69	19.05	19.42	19.80	20.20	20.62	21.05	21.51	21.98	22.47	22.99	23.53
.25	18.01	18.34	18.68	19.03	19.40	19.79	20.19	20.60	21.04	21.49	21.96	22.45	22.97	23.51	24.07
.50	18.31	18.65	19.01	19.38	19.76	20.16	20.57	21.01	21.46	21.93	22.42	22.93	23.47	24.03	24.63
.75	18.62	18.97	19.34	19.72	20.12	20.53	20.96	21.41	21.88	22.37	22.88	23.42	23.98	24.57	25.19
+17.00	18.93	19.30	19.68	20.07	20.48	20.91	21.36	21.82	22.31	22.82	23.35	23.91	24.50	25.11	25.76
.25	19.24	19.62	20.01	20.42	20.85	21.29	21.75	22.24	22.74	23.27	23.83	24.41	25.02	25.66	26.34
.50	19.55	19.94	20.35	20.77	21.21	21.67	22.15	22.65	23.18	23.73	24.31	24.91	25.55	26.22	26.92
.75	19.87	20.27	20.69	21.12	21.58	22.06	22.55	23.07	23.62	24.19	24.79	25.42	26.08	26.78	27.52
+18.00	20.18	20.59	21.03	21.48	21.95	22.44	22.96	23.50	24.06	24.66	25.28	25.94	26.63	27.36	28.12
.25	20.49	20.92	21.37	21.84	22.32	22.83	23.37	23.93	24.51	25.13	25.78	26.46	27.18	27.94	28.74
.50	20.81	21.25	21.71	22.20	22.70	23.23	23.78	24.36	24.97	25.61	26.28	26.99	27.74	28.53	29.37
.75	21.13	21.58	22.06	22.56	23.08	23.62	24.19	24.79	25.42	26.09	26.79	27.52	28.30	29.13	30.00
+19.00	21.44	21.91	22.41	22.92	23.46	24.02	24.61	25.23	25.89	26.57	27.30	28.06	28.88	29.73	30.65
.25	21.76	22.25	22.75	23.28	23.84	24.42	25.03	25.68	26.35	27.07	27.82	28.61	29.46	30.35	31.30
.50	22.08	22.58	23.10	23.65	24.22	24.82	25.46	26.12	26.82	27.56	28.34	29.17	30.05	30.98	31.97
.75	22.40	22.92	23.46	24.02	24.61	25.23	25.88	26.57	27.30	28.06	28.87	29.73	30.64	31.61	32.64
+20.00	22.73	23.26	23.81	24.39	25.00	25.64	26.32	27.03	27.78	28.57	29.41	30.30	31.25	32.26	33.33

Spectacle refraction or spectacle lens power (BVP) in dioptres	Ocular refraction in dioptres for vertex distances in mm of:														
	6	7	8	9	10	11	12	13	14	15	16	17	18	19	20
–0.25	0.25	0.25	0.25	0.25	0.25	0.25	0.25.	0.25	0.25	0.25	0.25	0.25	0.25	0.25	0.25
0.50	0.50	0.50	0.50	0.50	0.50	0.50	0.50	0.50	0.50	0.50	0.50	0.50	0.50	0.50	0.50
0.75	0.75	0.75	0.75	0.75	0.74	0.74	0.74	0.74	0.74	0.74	0.74	0.74	0.74	0.74	0.74
–1.00	0.99	0.99	0.99	0.99	0.99	0.99	0.99	0.99	0.99	0.99	0.98	0.98	0.98	0.98	0.98
.25	1.24	1.24	1.24	1.24	1.23	1.23	1.23	1.23	1.23	1.23	1.23	1.22	1.22	1.22	1.22
.50	1.49	1.48	1.48	1.48	1.48	1.48	1.47	1.47	1.47	1.47	1.46	1.46	1.46	1.46	1.46
.75	1.73	1.73	1.73	1.72	1.72	1.72	1.71	1.71	1.71	1.71	1.70	1.70	1.70	1.69	1.69
–2.00	1.98	1.97	1.97	1.96	1.96	1.96	1.95	1.95	1.95	1.94	1.94	1.93	1.93	1.93	1.92
.25	2.22	2.22	2.21	2.21	2.20	2.20	2.19	2.19	2.18	2.18	2.17	2.17	2.16	2.16	2.15
.50	2.46	2.46	2.45	2.44	2.44	2.43	2.43	2.42	2.42	2.41	2.40	2.40	2.39	2.39	2.38
.75	2.71	2.70	2.69	2.68	2.68	2.67	2.66	2.66	2.65	2.64	2.63	2.63	2.62	2.61	2.61
.3.00	2.95	2.94	2.93	2.92	2.91	2.90	2.90	2.89	2.88	2.87	2.86	2.85	2.85	2.84	2.83
.25	3.19	3.18	3.17	3.16	3.15	3.14	3.13	3.12	3.11	3.10	3.09	3.08	3.07	3.06	3.05
.50	3.43	3.42	3.40	3.39	3.38	3.37	3.36	3.35	3.34	3.33	3.31	3.30	3.29	3.28	3.27
.75	3.67	3.65	3.64	3.63	3.61	3.60	3.59	3.58	3.56	3.55	3.54	3.52	3.51	3.50	3.49
–4.00	3.91	3.89	3.88	3.86	3.85	3.83	3.82	3.80	3.79	3.77	3.76	3.75	3.73	3.72	3.70
.25	4.14	4.13	4.11	4.09	4.08	4.06	4.04	4.03	4.01	4.00	3.98	3.96	3.95	3.93	3.92

(Contd...)

(Contd...)

	6	7	8	9	10	11	12	13	14	15	16	17	18	19	20
.50	4.38	4.36	4.34	4.33	4.31	4.29	4.27	4.25	4.23	4.22	4.20	4.18	4.16	4.15	4.13
.75	4.62	4.60	4.58	4.56	4.54	4.51	4.49	4.47	4.45	4.43	4.42	4.40	4.38	4.36	4.34
−5.00	4.85	4.83	4.81	4.78	4.76	4.74	4.72	4.69	4.67	4.65	4.63	4.61	4.59	4.57	4.55
.25	5.09	5.06	5.04	5.01	4.99	4.96	4.94	4.91	4.89	4.87	4.84	4.82	4.80	4.77	4.75
.50	5.32	5.30	5.27	5.24	5.21	5.19	5.16	5.13	5.11	5.08	5.06	5.03	5.01	4.98	4.96
.75	5.56	5.53	5.50	5.47	5.44	5.41	5.38	5.35	5.32	5.29	5.27	5.24	5.21	5.18	5.16
−6.00	5.79	5.76	5.72	5.69	5.66	5.63	5.60	5.56	5.53	5.50	5.47	5.44	5.41	5.39	5.36
.25	6.02	5.99	5.95	5.92	5.88	5.85	5.81	5.78	5.75	5.71	5.68	5.65	5.62	5.59	5.56
.50	6.26	6.22	6.18	6.14	6.11	6.07	6.03	6.00	5.96	5.92	5.89	5.85	5.82	5.79	5.75
.75	6.49	6.45	6.41	6.37	6.33	6.29	6.25	6.21	6.17	6.13	6.09	6.06	6.02	5.98	5.95
−7.00	6.72	6.67	6.63	6.58	6.54	6.50	6.46	6.41	6.37	6.33	6.29	6.25	6.22	6.18	6.14
.25	6.94	6.90	6.85	6.81	6.76	6.72	6.67	6.63	6.58	6.54	6.50	6.46	6.41	6.37	6.33
.50	7.18	7.13	7.08	7.03	6.98	6.93	6.88	6.84	6.79	6.74	6.70	6.65	6.61	6.57	6.52
.75	7.41	7.35	7.30	7.25	7.19	7.14	7.09	7.04	6.99	6.94	6.90	6.85	6.80	6.76	6.71
−8.00	7.63	7.58	7.52	7.46	7.41	7.35	7.30	7.25	7.19	7.14	7.09	7.04	6.99	6.94	6.90
.25	7.86	7.80	7.74	7.68	7.62	7.56	7.51	7.45	7.40	7.34	7.29	7.24	7.18	7.13	7.08
.50	8.09	8.03	7.96	7.90	7.84	7.78	7.72	7.66	7.60	7.54	7.49	7.43	7.37	7.32	7.27
.75	8.31	8.24	8.18	8.11	8.05	7.98	7.92	7.86	7.79	7.73	7.67	7.62	7.56	7.50	7.45
−9.00	8.54	8.47	8.40	8.33	8.26	8.19	8.12	8.06	7.99	7.93	7.87	7.81	7.75	7.69	7.63
.25	8.76	8.69	8.61	8.54	8.47	8.40	8.33	8.26	8.19	8.12	8.06	7.99	7.93	7.87	7.81
.50	8.98	8.90	8.83	8.75	8.67	8.60	8.53	8.45	8.38	8.31	8.24	8.18	8.11	8.05	7.98
.75	9.21	9.12	9.04	8.96	8.88	8.80	8.73	8.65	8.58	8.50	8.43	8.36	8.29	8.22	8.16

(Contd...)

(Contd...)

	6	7	8	9	10	11	12	13	14	15	16	17	18	19	20
−10.00	9.43	9.35−	9.26	9.17	9.09	9.01	8.93	8.85	8.77	8.70	8.62	8.55−	8.47	8.40	8.33
.25	9.65+	9.56	9.47	9.38	9.29	9.21	9.12	9.04	8.96	8.88	8.80	8.73	8.65+	8.58	8.50
.50	9.88	9.78	9.69	9.59	9.50	9.41	9.32	9.24	9.15+	9.07	8.99	8.91	8.83	8.75+	8.68
.75	10.10	10.00	9.90	9.80	9.71	9.61	9.52	9.43	9.34	9.26	9.17	9.09	9.01	8.93	8.85
−11.00	10.32	10.21	10.11	10.01	9.91	9.81	9.72	9.62	9.53	9.44	9.35+	9.27	9.18	9.10	9.02
.25	10.54	10.43	10.32	10.22	10.11	10.01	9.91	9.81	9.72	9.63	9.53	9.44	9.36	9.27	9.18
.50	10.76	10.64	10.53	10.42	10.31	10.21	10.11	10.00	9.90	9.81	9.71	9.62	9.53	9.44	9.35
.75	10.98	10.86	10.74	10.63	10.51	10.40	10.30	10.19	10.09	9.99	9.89	9.79	9.70	9.61	9.51
−12.00	11.19	11.07	10.95−	10.83	10.71	10.60	10.49	10.38	10.27	10.17	10.07	9.97	9.87	9.77	9.68
.25	11.41	11.28	11.16	11.03	10.91	10.80	10.68	10.57	10.46	10.35	10.24	10.14	10.04	9.94	9.84
.50	11.63	11.49	11.36	11.24	11.11	10.99	10.87	10.75+	10.64	10.53	10.42	10.31	10.20	10.10	10.00
.75	11.84	11.71	11.57	11.44	11.31	11.18	11.06	10.94	10.82	10.70	10.59	10.48	10.37	10.26	10.16
−13.00	12.06	11.92	11.78	11.64	11.50	11.37	11.25	11.12	11.00	10.88	10.76	10.65−	10.54	10.43	10.32
.25	12.27	12.13	11.98	11.84	11.70	11.56	11.43	11.30	11.18	11.05+	10.93	10.81	10.70	10.59	10.47
.50	12.49	12.34	12.18	12.04	11.89	11.76	11.62	11.49	11.35+	11.23	11.10	10.98	10.86	10.74	10.63
.75	12.70	12.54	12.39	12.24	12.09	11.94	11.80	11.66	11.53	11.40	11.27	11.14	11.02	10.90	10.78
−14.00	12.91	12.75+	12.59	12.43	12.28	12.13	11.99	11.84	11.71	11.57	11.44	11.31	11.18	11.06	10.94
.25	13.13	12.96	12.79	12.63	12.47	12.32	12.17	12.02	11.88	11.74	11.60	11.47	11.34	11.21	11.09
.50	13.34	13.16	12.99	12.83	12.66	12.50	12.35+	12.20	12.05+	11.91	11.77	11.63	11.50	11.37	11.24
.75	13.55+	13.37	13.19	13.02	12.85+	12.69	12.53	12.38	12.22	12.08	11.93	11.79	11.66	11.52	11.39
−15.00	13.76	13.57	13.39	13.22	13.04	12.87	12.71	12.55+	12.40	12.24	12.10	11.95+	11.81	11.67	11.54
.25	13.97	13.78	13.59	13.41	13.23	13.06	12.89	12.73	12.57	12.41	12.26	12.11	11.97	11.82	11.69

(Contd...)

(Contd...)

	6	7	8	9	10	11	12	13	14	15	16	17	18	19	20
.50	14.18	13.98	13.79	13.60	13.42	13.24	13.07	12.90	12.74	12.58	12.42	12.27	12.12	11.97	11.83
.75	14.39	14.19	13.99	13.80	13.61	13.42	13.25−	13.07	12.90	12.74	12.58	12.42	12.27	12.12	11.98
−16.00	14.60	14.39	14.18	13.99	13.79	13.61	13.42	13.25	13.07	12.90	12.74	12.58	12.42	12.27	12.12
.25	14.81	14.59	14.38	14.18	13.98	13.79	13.60	13.42	13.24	13.07	12.90	12.73	12.57	12.42	12.26
.50	15.01	14.79	14.58	14.37	14.16	13.96	13.77	13.59	13.40	13.23	13.05+	12.88	12.72	12.56	12.41
.75	15.22	14.99	14.77	14.56	14.35−	14.14	13.95−	13.76	13.57	13.39	13.21	13.04	12.87	12.71	12.55
−17.00	15.43	15.19	14.97	14.74	14.53	14.32	14.12	13.92	13.73	13.55	13.37	13.19	13.02	12.85+	12.69
.25	15.63	15.39	15.16	14.93	14.71	14.50	14.29	14.09	13.89	13.70	13.52	13.34	13.16	12.99	12.83
.50	15.84	15.59	15.35+	15.12	14.89	14.68	14.46	14.26	14.06	13.86	13.67	13.49	13.31	13.13	12.96
.75	16.04	15.79	15.54	15.30	15.07	14.85+	14.63	14.42	14.22	14.02	13.82	13.64	13.45+	13.27	13.10
−18.00	16.24	15.98	15.73	15.49	15.25+	15.02	14.80	14.59	14.38	14.17	13.97	13.78	13.59	13.41	13.23
.25	16.45+	16.18	15.93	15.68	15.43	15.20	14.97	14.75+	14.54	14.33	14.13	13.93	13.74	13.55+	13.37
.50	16.65+	16.38	16.12	15.86	15.61	15.37	15.14	14.91	14.70	14.48	14.28	14.07	13.88	13.69	13.50
.75	16.85+	16.58	16.31	16.04	15.79	15.54	15.31	15.08	14.85+	14.63	14.42	14.22	14.02	13.83	13.64
−19.00	17.06	16.77	16.49	16.23	15.97	15.72	15.47	15.24	15.01	14.79	14.57	14.36	14.16	13.96	13.77
.25	17.26	16.96	16.68	16.41	16.14	15.89	15.64	15.40	15.16	14.94	14.72	14.50	14.30	14.09	13.90
.50	17.46	17.16	16.87	16.59	16.32	16.06	15.80	15.56	15.32	15.09	14.86	14.65−	14.43	14.23	14.03
.75	17.66	17.35+	17.06	16.77	16.49	16.23	15.97	15.72	15.47	15.24	15.01	14.79	14.57	14.36	14.16
−20.00	17.86	17.54	17.24	16.95−	16.67	16.39	16.13	15.87	15.62	15.38	15.15+	14.93	14.71	14.49	14.29
.25	18.06	17.74	17.43	17.13	16.84	16.56	16.29	16.03	15.78	15.53	15.29	15.06	14.84	14.62	14.41
.50	18.25	17.93	17.61	17.31	17.01	16.73	16.45	16.19	15.93	15.68	15.44	15.20	14.97	14.75+	14.54
.75	18.45+	18.12	17.80	17.49	17.19	16.89	16.61	16.34	16.08	15.83	15.58	15.34	15.11	14.88	14.66

(Contd...)

(Contd...)

	6	7	8	9	10	11	12	13	14	15	16	17	18	19	20
−21.00	18.65–	18.31	17.98	17.66	17.36	17.06	16.77	16.50	16.23	15.97	15.72	15.48	15.24	15.01	14.79
.25	18.85–	18.50	18.16	17.84	17.53	17.22	16.93	16.65–	16.38	16.11	15.86	15.61	15.37	15.14	14.91
.50	19.04	18.69	18.35–	18.01	17.70	17.39	17.09	16.80	16.53	16.26	16.00	15.75–	15.50	15.26	15.04
.75	19.24	18.88	18.53	18.19	17.86	17.55+	17.25–	16.95+	16.67	16.40	16.13	15.88	15.63	15.39	15.16
−22.00	19.43	19.05+	18.71	18.36	18.03	17.71	17.40	17.11	16.82.	16.54	16.27	16.01	15.76	15.51	15.28
.25	19.63	19.25+	18.89	18.54	18.20	17.88	17.56	17.26	16.97	16.68	16.41	16.14	15.89	15.64	15.40
.50	19.82	19.44	19.07	18.71	18.37	18.04	17.72	17.41	17.11	16.82	16.54	16.30	16.01	15.76	15.52
.75	20.02	19.62	19.25–	10.00	18.53	18.20	17.87	17.56	17.25	16.96	16.68	16.40	16.14	15.88	15.63
−23.00	20.21	19.81	19.43	19.05+	18.70	18.36	18.02	17.71	17.40	17.10	16.81	16.53	16.27	16.01	15.75
.25	20.40	20.00	19.60	19.23	18.86	18.52	18.18	17.85+	17.54	17.24	16.95	16.66	16.39	16.13	15.87
.50	20.60	20.18	19.78	19.40	19.03	18.67	18.33	18.00	17.68	17.38	17.08	16.79	16.52	16.25–	15.99
.75	20.79	20.36	19.96	19.57	19.19	18.83	18.48	18.15–	17.82	17.51	17.21	16.92	16.64	16.37	16.10
−24.00	20.98	20.55–	20.13	19.74	19.35+	18.99	18.63	18.29	17.96	17.65–	17.34	17.04	16.76	16.48	16.22
.25	21.17	20.73	20.31	19.90	19.52	19.14	18.78	18.44	18.10	17.78	17.47	17.17	16.88	16.60	16.33
.50	21.36	20.91	20.48	20.07	19.68	19.30	18.93	18.58	18.24	17.91	17.60	17.30	17.00	16.72	16.44
.75	21.55–	21.10	20.66	20.24	19.84	19.45+	19.08	18.73	18.38	18.05	17.73	17.42	17.12	16.83	16.56
−25.00	21.74	21.28	20.83	20.41	20.00	19.61	19.23	18.87	18.52	18.18	17.86	17.54	17.24	16.95–	16.67
.25	21.93	21.46	21.01	20.58	20.16	19.76	19.38	19.01	18.66	18.32	17.99	17.67	17.36	17.06	16.78
.50	22.12	21.64	21.18	20.74	20.32	19.91	19.52	19.15–	18.79	18.44	18.11	17.79	17.48	17.18	16.89
.75	22.31	21.82	21.35+	20.91	20.48	20.07	19.67	19.29	18.93	18.58	18.24	17.91	17.60	17.29	17.00
−26.00	22.49	22.00	21.52	21.07	20.64	20.22	19.82	19.43	19.06	18.71	18.36	18.03	17.71	17.40	17.11

(Contd...)

(Contd...)

	6	7	8	9	10	11	12	13	14	15	16	17	18	19	20
.25	22.68	22.17	21.69	21.23	20.79	20.37	19.96	19.57	19.19	18.83	18.48	18.15	17.83	17.51	17.21
.50	22.86	22.35+	21.86	21.39	20.95–	20.52	20.10	19.71	19.33	18.96	18.61	18.27	17.94	17.62	17.32
.75	23.05+	22.53	22.04	21.56	21.11	20.67	20.25	19.85–	19.46	19.09	18.73	18.39	18.06	17.74	17.43
–27.00	23.23	22.71	22.20	21.72	21.26	20.82	20.39	19.98	19.59	19.22	18.85+	18.50	18.17	17.84	17.53
.25	23.42	22.88	22.37	21.88	21.41	20.96	20.53	20.12	19.72	19.34	18.98	18.62	18.28	17.95+	17.64
.50	23.61	23.06	22.54	22.05–	21.57	21.11	20.68	20.26	19.86	19.47	19.10	18.74	18.40	18.06	17.74
.75	23.79	23.23	22.71	22.20	21.72	21.26	20.82	20.39	19.98	19.59	19.22	18.85+	18.50	18.17	17.84
–28.00	23.97	23.41	22.88	22.36	21.87	21.41	20.96	20.53	20.11	19.72	19.34	18.97	18.62	18.28	17.95–
.25	24.15+	23.58	23.04	22.52	22.03	21.55+	21.10	20.66	20.24	19.84	19.46	19.08	18.73	18.38	18.05+
.50	24.34	23.76	23.21	22.68	22.18	21.70	21.24	20.79	20.37	19.96	19.57	19.20	28.84	18.49	18.15+
.75	24.52	23.93	23.38	22.84	22.33	21.84	21.38	20.93	20.50	20.09	19.69	19.31	18.95–	18.59	18.25+
–29.00	24.70	24.11	23.54	23.00	22.48	21.99	21.51	21.06	20.63	20.21	19.81	19.43	19.05+	18.70	18.36
.25	24.88	24.28	23.70	23.15	22.63	22.13	21.65	21.19	20.75	20.33	19.92	19.54	19.16	18.80	18.45+
.50	25.06	24.45–	23.87	23.31	22.78	22.27	21.79	21.32	20.88	20.45–	20.04	19.65–	19.27	18.90	18.55+
.75	25.25–	24.62	24.03	23.47	22.93	22.42	21.93	21.45+	21.00	20.57	20.16	19.76	19.38	19.01	18.65+
–30.00	25.42	24.79	24.19	23.62	23.08	22.56	22.06	21.58	21.13	20.69	20.27	19.87	19.48	19.11	18.75

Surface Power in Dioptres for Various Radii and Refractive Index Differences				
Radii, r in mm	1.568–1	1.376–1	1.3375–1	1.490–1.336
5.00	113.600	75.200	67.500	30.800
5.10	111.373	73.725	66.176	30.196
5.20	109.231	72.306	64.904	29.615
5.30	107.170	70.943	63.679	29.057
5.40	105.185	69.630	62.500	28.519
5.50	103.273	68.364	61.364	28.000
5.60	101.429	67.143	60.268	27.500
5.70	99.649	65.965	59.211	21.018
5.80	97.931	64.828	58.190	26.552
5.90	96.271	69.729	57.203	26.102
6.00	94.667	62.667	56.250	25.667
6.10	93.115	61.639	55.328	25.246
6.20	91.613	60.645	54.435	24.839
6.30	90.159	59.683	53.571	24.444
6.40	88.750	58.750	52.734	24.063
6.50	87.385	57.846	51.923	23.692
6.60	86.061	56.970	51.136	23.333
6.70	84.776	56.119	50.373	22.985
6.80	83.529	55.294	49.632	22.647
6.90	82.319	54.493	48.913	22.319
7.00	81.143	53.714	48.214	22.000
7.05	80.567	53.333	47.872	21.844
7.10	80.000	52.958	47.535	21.690
7.15	79.441	52.587	47.203	21.538
7.20	78.889	52.222	46.875	21.389
7.25	78.345	51.862	46.552	21.241
7.30	77.808	51.507	46.233	21.096
7.35	77.279	51.156	45.918	20.952
7.40	76.757	50.811	45.608	20.811
7.45	76.242	50.470	45.302	20.671
7.50	75.733	51.133	45.000	20.533
7.55	75.232	49.801	44.702	20.397
7.60	74.737	49.474	44.408	20.263
7.65	74.248	49.150	44.118	20131
7.70	73.766	48.831	43.831	20.000
7.75	73.290	48.516	43.548	19.871
7.80	72.821	48.205	43.269	19.744
7.85	72.357	47.898	42.994	19.618

(Contd...)

(Contd...)

Radii, r in mm	1.568–1	1.376–1	1.3375–1	1.490–1.336
7.90	71.899	47.595	42.722	19.494
7.95	71.447	47.296	42.453	19.371
8.00	71.000	47.000	42.188	19.250
8.05	70.559	46.708	41.925	19.130
8.10	70.123	46.420	41.667	19.012
8.15	69.693	46.135	41.411	18.896
8.20	69.268	45.854	41.159	18.780
8.25	68.848	45.576	40.909	18.667
8.30	68.434	45.301	40.663	18.554
8.35	68.024	45.030	40.419	18.443
8.40	67.619	44.762	40.179	18.333
8.45	67.219	44.497	39.941	18.225
8.50	66.824	44.235	39.706	18.118
8.55	66.433	43.977	39.474	18.012
8.60	66.047	43.721	39.244	17.907
8.65	65.665	43.468	39.017	17.803
8.70	65.287	43.218	38.793	17.701
8.75	64.914	42.971	38.571	17.600
8.80	64.545	42.727	38.352	17.500
8.85	64.181	42.486	38:136	17.401
8.90	63.820	42.247	37.921	17.303
8.95	63.464	42.011	37.709	17.207
9.00	63.111	41.778	37.500	17.111
9.10	62.418	41.319	37.088	16.923
9.20	61.739	40.870	36.685	16.739
9.30	61.075	40.430	36.290	16.559
9.40	60.246	40.000	35.904	16.382
9.50	59.789	39.579	35.526	16.211
9.60	59.167	39.167	35.156	16.042
9.70	58.557	38.763	34.794	15.876
9.80	57.959	38.367	34.438	15.714
9.90	57.374	37.980	34.091	15.556
10.00	56.800	37.600	33.750	15.400
10.10	56.238	37.228	33.416	15.248
10.20	55.686	36.863	33.088	15.098
10.30	55.146	36.505	32.767	14.951
10.40	54.615	36.154	32.452	14.808
10.50	54.095	35.810	32.143	14.667

(Contd...)

(Contd...)

Radii, r in mm	1.568–1	1.376–1	1.3375–1	1.490–1.336
10.60	53.585	35.472	31.840	14.528
10.70	53.084	35.140	31.542	14.393
10.80	52.593	34.815	31.250	14.259
10.90	52.110	34.495	30.963	14.128
11.00	51.636	34.182	30.682	14.000
11.10	51.171	33.874	30.405	13.874
11.20	50.714	33.571	30.134	13.750
11.30	50.265	33.274	29.867	13.628
11.40	49.825	32.982	29.605	13.509
11.50	59.391	32.696	29.348	13.391
11.60	48.966	32.414	29.095	13. 276
11.70	48.547	32.137	28.846	13.162
11.80	48.136	31.864	28.602	13.051
11.90	47.731	31.597	28.361	12.941
12.00	47.333	31.333	28.125	12.833

The Refractive Indices given pertain to the following materials:

1.568	Hyfrax
1.490	Polymethyl methacrylate
1.376	Cornea
1.3375	Most keratometers
1.336	Tears

Surface Powers in Air for n = 1.49 (PMMA), r = radius of curvature, F = surface power

r in mm	F in Dioptres	r in mm	F in Dioptres	r in mm	F in Dioptres	r in mm	F in Dioptres	r in mm	F in Dioptres	r in mm	F in Dioptres	r in mm	F in Dioptres
4.90	100.00	5.30	92.45	5.70	85.96	6.10	80.33	6.50	75.38	6.90	71.01	7.30	67.12
.91	99.80	.31	92.28	.71	85.81	.11	80.20	.51	75.27	.91	70.91	.31	67.03
.92	99.59	.32	92.11	.72	85.66	.12	80.07	.52	75.15	.92	70.81	.32	66.94
.93	99.39	.33	91.93	.73	85.51	.13	79.93	.53	75.04	.93	70.71	.33	66.85
.94	99.19	.34	91.76	.74	85.37	.14	79.80	.54	74.92	.94	70.60	.34	66.76
.95	98.99	.35	91.59	.75	85.22	.15	79.67	.55	74.81	.95	70.50	.35	66.67
.96	98.79	.36	91.42	.76	85.07	.16	79.55	.56	74.70	.96	70.40	.36	66.58
.97	98.58	.37	91.25	.77	84.92	.17	79.42	.57	74.58	.97	70.30	.37	66.49
.98	98.39	.38	91.08	.78	84.78	.18	79.29	.58	74.47	.98	70.20	.38	66.40
.99	98.20	.39	90.91	.79	84.63	.19	79.16	.59	74.36	.99	70.10	.39	66.31
5.00	98.00	5.40	90.74	5.80	84.48	6.20	79.03	6.60	74.24	7.00	70.00	7.40	66.22
.01	97.80	.41	90.57	.81	84.34	.21	78.90	.61	74.13	.01	69.90	.41	66.13
.02	97.61	.42	90.41	.82	84.19	.22	78.78	.62	74.02	.02	69.80	.42	66.04
.03	97.42	.43	90.24	.83	84.05	.23	78.65	.63	73.91	.03	69.70	.43	65.95
.04	97.22	.44	90.07	.84	83.90	.24	78.53	.64	73.80	.04	69.60	.44	65.86
.05	97.03	.45	89.91	.85	83.76	.25	78.40	.65	73.68	.05	69.50	.45	65.77
.06	96.84	.46	89.74	.86	83.62	.26	78.27	.66	73.57	.06	69.41	.46	65.68
.07	96.65	.47	89.58	.87	83.48	.27	78.15	.67	73.46	.07	69.31	.47	65.60
.08	96.46	.48	89.42	.88	83.33	.28	78.03	.68	73.35	.08	69.21	.48	65.51
.09	96.27	.49	89.25	.89	83.19	.29	77.90	.69	73.24	.09	69.11	.49	65.42

(Contd...)

(Contd...)

r in mm	F in Dioptres	r in mm	F in Dioptres	r in mm	F in Dioptres	r in mm	F in Dioptres	r in mm	F in Dioptres	r in mm	F in Dioptres	r in mm	F in Dioptres
5.10	96.09	5.50	89.09	5.90	83.05	6.30	77.78	6.70	73.13	7.10	69.01	7.50	65.33
.11	95.89	.51	88.93	.91	82.91	.31	77.65	.71	73.03	.11	68.92	.51	65.25
.12	95.70	.52	88.77	.92	82.77	.32	77.53	.72	72.92	.12	68.82	.52	65.16
.13	95.52	.53	88.61	.93	82.63	.33	77.41	.73	72.81	.13	68.72	.53	65.07
.14	95.33	.54	88.45	.94	82.49	.34	77.29	.74	72.70	.14	68.63	.54	64.99
.15	95.15	.55	88.29	.95	82.35	.35	77.17	.75	72.59	.15	68.53	.55	64.90
.16	94.96	.56	88.13	.96	82.21	.36	77.04	.76	72.49	.16	68.44	.56	64.81
.17	94.78	.57	87.97	.97	82.08	.37	76.92	.77	72.38	.17	68.34	.57	64.73
.18	94.59	.58	87.81	.98	81.94	.38	76.80	.78	72.27	.18	68.25	.58	64.64
.19	94.41	.59	87.66	.99	81.80	.39	76.68	.79	72.16	.19	68.15	.59	64.56
5.20	94.23	5.60	87.50	6.00	81.67	6.40	76.56	6.80	72.06	7.20	68.06	7.60	64.47
.21	94.05	.61	87.34	.01	81.53	.41	76.44	.81	71.95	.21	67.96	.61	64.39
.22	93.87	.62	87.19	.02	81.40	.42	76.32	.82	71.85	.22	67.87	.62	64.30
.23	93.69	.63	87.03	.03	81.26	.43	76.21	.83	71.74	.23	67.77	.63	64.22
.24	93.51	.64	86.88	.04	81.13	.44	76.09	.84	71.64	.24	67.68	.64	64.14
.25	93.33	.65	86.73	.05	80.99	.45	75.97	.85	71.53	.25	67.59	.65	64.05
.26	93.16	.66	86.57	.06	80.86	.46	75.85	.86	71.43	.26	67.49	.66	63.97
.27	92.98	.67	86.42	.07	80.72	.47	75.73	.87	71.32	.27	67.40	.67	63.89
.28	92.80	.68	86.27	.08	80.59	.48	75.62	.88	71.22	.28	67.31	.68	63.80
.29	92.63	.69	86.12	.09	80.46	.49	75.50	.89	71.12	.29	67.22	.69	63.72

(Contd...)

(Contd...)

r in mm	F in Dioptres	r in mm	F in Dioptres	r in mm	F in Dioptres	r in mm	F in Dioptres	r in mm	F in Dioptres	r in mm	F in Dioptres	r in mm	F in Dioptres
7.70	63.64	8.10	60.49	8.50	57.65	8.90	55.06	9.30	52.69	9.70	50.52	10.10	48.51
.71	63.55	.11	60.42	.51	57.58	.91	54.99	.31	52.63	.71	50.46	.11	48.47
.72	63.47	.12	60.34	.52	57.51	.92	54.93	.32	52.58	.72	50.41	.12	48.42
.73	63.39	.13	60.27	.53	57.44	.93	54.87	.33	52.52	.73	50.36	.13	48.37
.74	63.31	.14	60.20	.54	57.38	.94	54.81	.34	52.46	.74	50.31	.14	48.32
.75	63.23	.15	60.12	.55	57.31	.95	54.75	.35	52.41	.75	50.26	.15	48.28
.76	63.14	.16	60.05	.56	57.24	.96	54.69	.36	52.35	.76	50.20	.16	48.23
.77	63.06	.17	59.98	.57	57.18	.97	54.63	.37	52.29	.77	50.15	.17	48.18
.78	62.98	.18	59.90	.58	57.11	.98	54.57	.38	52.24	.78	50.10	.18	48.13
.79	62.90	.19	59.83	.59	57.04	.99	54.51	.39	52.18	.79	50.05	.19	48.09
7.80	62.82	8.20	59.76	8.60	56.98	9.00	54.44	9.40	52.13	9.80	50.00	10.20	48.04
.81	62.74	.21	59.68	.61	56.91	.01	54.38	.41	52.07	.81	49.95	.21	47.99
.82	62.66	.22	59.61	.62	56.84	.02	54.32	.42	52.02	.82	49.90	.22	47.95
.83	62.58	.23	59.54	.63	56.78	.03	54.26	.43	51.96	.83	49.85	.23	47.90
.84	62.50	.24	59.47	.64	56.71	.04	54.20	.44	51.91	.84	49.80	.24	47.85
.85	62.42	.25	59.39	.65	56.65	.05	54.14	.45	51.85	.85	49.75	.25	47.81
.86	62.34	.26	59.32	.66	56.58	.06	54.08	.46	51.80	.86	49.70	.26	47.76
.87	62.26	.27	59.25	.67	56.52	.07	54.02	.47	51.74	.87	49.65	.27	47.71
.88	62.18	.28	59.18	.68	56.45	.08	53.96	.48	51.69	.88	49.60	.28	47.67
.89	62.10	.29	59.11	.69	56.39	.09	53.91	.49	51.63	.89	49.54	.29	47.62

(Contd...)

(Contd...)

r in mm	F in Dioptres	r in mm	F in Dioptres	r in mm	F in Dioptres	r in mm	F in Dioptres	r in mm	F in Dioptres	r in mm	F in Dioptres	r in mm	F in Dioptres
7.90	62.03	8.30	59.04	8.70	56.32	9.10	53.85	9.50	51.58	9.90	49.49	10.30	47.57
.91	61.95	.31	58.97	.71	56.26	.11	53.79	.51	51.52	.91	49.45	.31	47.53
.92	61.87	.32	58.89	.72	56.19	.12	53.73	.52	51.47	.92	49.40	.32	47.48
.93	61.79	.33	58.82	.73	56.13	.13	53.67	.53	51.42	.93	49.35	.33	47.44
.94	61.71	.34	58.75	.74	56.06	.14	53.61	.54	51.36	.94	49.30	.34	47.39
.95	61.64	.35	58.68	.75	56.00	.15	53.55	.55	51.31	.95	49.25	.35	47.34
.96	61.56	.36	58.61	.76	55.94	.16	53.49	.56	51.25	.96	49.20	.36	47.30
.97	61.48	.37	58.54	.77	55.87	.17	53.43	.57	51.20	.97	49.15	.37	47.25
.98	61.40	.38	58.47	.78	55.81	.18	53.38	.58	51.15	.98	49.10	.38	47.21
.99	61.33	.39	58.40	.79	55.75	.19	53.32	.59	51.09	.99	49.05	.39	47.16
8.00	61.25	8.40	58.33	8.80	55.68	9.20	53.26	9.60	51.04	10.00	49.00	10.40	47.12
.01	61.17	.41	58.26	.81	55.62	.21	53.20	.61	50.99	.01	48.95	.41	47.07
.02	61.10	.42	58.19	.82	55.56	.22	53.15	.62	50.94	.02	48.90	.42	47.03
.03	61.02	.43	58.13	.83	55.49	.23	53.09	.63	50.88	.03	48.85	.43	46.98
.04	60.95	.44	58.06	.84	55.43	.24	53.03	.64	50.83	.04	48.80	.44	46.94
.05	60.87	.45	57.99	.85	55.37	.25	52.97	.65	50.78	.05	48.76	.45	46.89
.06	60.79	.46	57.92	.86	55.30	.26	52.92	.66	50.72	.06	48.71	.46	46.85
.07	60.72	.47	57.85	.87	55.24	.27	52.86	.67	50.67	.07	48.66	.47	46.80
.08	60.64	.48	57.78	.88	55.18	.28	52.80	.68	50.62	.08	48.61	.48	46.76
.09	60.57	.49	57.72	.89	55.12	.29	52.75	.69	50.57	.09	48.56	.49	46.71

(Contd...)

(Contd...)

r in mm	F in Dioptres	r in mm	F in Dioptres	r in mm	F in Dioptres	r in mm	F in Dioptres	r in mm	F in Dioptres	r in mm	F in Dioptres
10.50	46.67	10.90	44.95	11.30	43.36	11.70	41.88	12.10	40.50	12.50	39.20
.51	46.62	.91	44.91	.31	43.32	.71	41.84	.11	40.46	.51	39.17
.52	46.58	.92	44.87	.32	43.29	.72	41.81	.12	40.43	.52	39.14
.53	46.53	.93	44.83	.33	43.25	.73	41.77	.13	40.40	.53	39.11
.54	46.49	.94	44.79	.34	43.21	.74	41.74	.14	40.36	.54	39.08
.55	46.45	.95	44.75	.35	43.17	.75	41.70	.15	40.33	.55	39.04
.56	46.40	.96	44.71	.36	43.13	.76	41.67	.16	40.30	.56	39.01
.57	46.36	.97	44.67	.37	43.10	.77	41.63	.17	40.26	.57	38.98
.58	46.31	.98	44.63	.38	43.06	.78	41.60	.18	40.23	.58	38.95
.59	46.27	.99	44.59	.39	43.02	.79	41.56	.19	40.20	.59	38.92
10.60	46.23	11.00	44.55	11.40	42.98	11.80	41.53	12.20	40.16	12.60	38.89
.61	46.18	.01	44.51	.41	42.95	.81	41.49	.21	40.13		
.62	46.14	.02	44.47	.42	42.91	.82	41.46	.22	40.10		
.63	46.10	.03	44.43	.43	42.87	.83	41.42	.23	40.07		
.64	46.06	.04	44.38	.44	42.83	.84	41.39	.24	40.03		
.65	46.01	.05	44.34	.45	42.80	.85	41.35	.25	40.00		
.66	45.97	.06	44.30	.46	42.76	.86	41.32	.26	39.97		
.67	45.92	.07	44.26	.47	42.72	.87	41.28	.27	39.94		
.68	45.88	0.8	44.22	.48	42.68	.88	41.25	.28	39.90		
.69	45.84	0.9	44.18	.49	42.65	.89	41.21	.29	39.87		
10.70	45.79	11.10	44.14	11.50	42.61	11.90	41.18	12.30	39.84		

(Contd...)

(Contd...)

r in mm	F in Dioptres	r in mm	F in Dioptres	r in mm	F in Dioptres	r in mm	F in Dioptres	r in mm	F in Dioptres
.71	45.75	.11	44.10	.51	42.57	.91	41.14	.31	39.81
.72	45.71	.12	44.07	.52	42.54	.92	41.11	.32	39.77
.73	45.67	.13	44.03	.53	42.50	.93	41.07	.33	39.74
.74	45.62	.14	43.99	.54	42.46	.94	41.04	.34	39.71
.75	45.58	.15	43.95	.55	42.43	.95	41.00	.35	39.68
.76	45.54	.16	43.91	.56	42.39	.96	40.97	.36	39.64
.77	45.50	.17	43.87	.57	42.35	.97	40.94	.37	39.61
.78	45.46	.18	43.83	.58	42.31	.98	40.90	.38	39.58
.79	45.41	.19	43.79	.59	42.28	.99	40.87	.39	39.55
10.80	45.37	11.20	43.75	11.60	42.24	12.00	40.83	12.40	39.52
.81	45.33	.21	43.71	.61	42.21	.01	40.80	.41	39.48
.82	45.29	.22	43.67	.62.	42.17	.02	40.77	.42	39.45
.83	45.25	.23	43.63	.63	42.13	.03	40.73	.43	39.42
.84	45.20	.24	43.60	.64	42.10	.04	40.70	.44	39.39
.85	45.16	.25	43.56	.65	42.06	.05	40.66	.45	39.36
.86	45.12	.26	43.52	.66	42.02	.06	40.63	.46	39.33
.87	45.08	.27	43.48	.67	41.99	.07	40.60	.47	39.29
.88	45.04	.28	43.44	.68	41.95	.08	40.56	.48	39.26
.89	45.00	.29	43.40	.69	41.92	.09	40.53	.49	39.23

SAGITTA in mm

optic diameter (chords in mm)

Redii in mm	3.0	3.2	3.4.	3.6	3.8	4.0	4.2	4.4	4.5	4.6	5.0	5.2	5.4	5.6	5.8	6.0	6.2	6.4	6.6	6.8	7.0
5.00	0.230	0.263	0.298	0.335	0.337	0.417	0.462	0.510	0.560	0.614	0.670	0.729	0.792	0.858	0.927	1.000	1.077	1.158	1.244	1.334	1.429
5.25	0.219	0.250	0.283	0.318	0.356	0.396	0.438	0.483	0.531	0.581	0.633	0.689	0.748	0.809	0.874	0.942	1.013	1.088	1.167	1.250	1.337
5.50	0.209	0.236	0.269	0.303	0.339	0.377	0.417	0.459	0.504	0.551	0.601	0.653	0.706	0.766	0.827	0.890	0.957	1.027	1.100	1.177	1.257
5.75	0.199	0.227	0.267	0.299	0.323	0.359	0.397	0.438	0.480	0.525	0.572	0.621	0.673	0.728	0.765	0.845	0.907	0.973	1.041	1.113	1.186
6.00	0.191	0.217	0.246	0.276	0.309	0.343	0.380	0.418	0.458	0.501	0.546	0.593	0.642	0.693	0.747	0.804	0.863	0.925	0.989	1.066	1.127
6.25	0.183	0.209	0.236	0.265	0.296	0.329	0.364	0.400	0.439	0.479	0.522	0.566	0.613	0.662	0.714	0.767	0.823	0.881	0.942	1.006	1.072
6.50	0.175	0.200	0.226	0.254	0.284	0.315	0.349	0.384	0.421	0.459	0.500	0.543	0.587	0.634	0.683	0.734	0.787	0.842	0.900	0.960	1.023
6.75	0.169	0.193	0.218	0.245	0.273	0.303	0.335	0.369	0.404	0.441	0.480	0.521	0.564	0.604	0.655	0.703	0.754	0.807	0.862	0.919	0.978
7.00	0.163	0.185	0.210	0.235	0.263	0.292	0.322	0.365	0.369	0.424	0.462	0.501	0.542	0.584	0.629	0.675	0.724	0.774	0.827	0.881	0.938
7.10	0.160	0.183	0.207	0.232	0.259	0.289	0.318	0.349	0.363	0.418	0.456	0.493	0.533	0.575	0.619	0.665	0.713	0.762	0.814	0.867	0.923
7.20	0.158	0.180	0.204	0.229	0.255	0.283	0.313	0.344	0.377	0.412	0.448	0.486	0.525	0.567	0.610	0.655	0.702	0.750	0.801	0.853	0.906
7.30	0.156	0.176	0.201	0.225	0.252	0.279	0.309	0.339	0.372	0.406	0.441	0.479	0.518	0.555	0.601	0.645	0.691	0.739	0.768	0.840	0.894
7.40	0.154	0.175	0.196	0.222	0.248	0.275	0.304	0.335	0.367	0.400	0.435	0.472	0.510	0.550	0.592	0.636	0.681	0.728	0.777	0.827	0.890
7.50	0.152	0.173	0.195	0.219	0.245	0.272	0.300	0.330	0.361	0.394	0.429	0.465	0.503	0.542	0.583	0.626	0.671	0.717	0.765	0.815	0.867
7.60	0.150	0.170	0.193	0.216	0.241	0.268	0.296	0.325	0.356	0.399	0.423	0.469	0.496	0.536	0.575	0.617	0.651	0.707	0.754	0.803	0.854
7.70	0.148	0.168	0.190	0.213	0.238	0.264	0.292	0.321	0.352	0.384	0.417	0.452	0.469	0.527	0.567	0.608	0.662	0.696	0.743	0.791	0.841
7.80	0.146	0.166	0.186	0.211	0.235	0.261	0.266	0.317	0.347	0.378	0.411	0.446	0.482	0.520	0.559	0.600	0.642	0.687	0.732	0.780	0.829
7.90	0.144	0.164	0.185	0.208	0.232	0.257	0.284	0.313	0.342	0.373	0.406	0.440	0.476	0.513	0.552	0.592	0.634	0.677	0.722	0.769	0.818

Redii in mm	optic diameter (chords in mm)																				
	7.2	7.4	7.6	7.8	8.0	8.2	8.4	8.6	8.8	9.0	9.2	9.4	9.6	9.8	10.0	10.2	10.4	10.6	10.8	11.0	11.2
5.00	1.530	1.637	1.750	1.873	2.000	2.135	2.287	2.449	2.625	2.821	3.040	3.294	3.600	4.005	5.000						
5.25	1.429	1.525	1.626	1.735	1.850	1.971	2.100	2.236	2.386	2.546	2.720	2.911	3.123	3.365	3.649	4.004	4.527				
5.50	1.342	1.431	1.524	1.622	1.725	1.834	1.949	2.071	2.200	2.338	2.485	2.643	2.815	3.002	3.209	3.441	3.708	4.030	4.458	5.500	
5.75	1.266	1.349	1.435	1.525	1.619	1.719	1.823	1.933	2.048	2.171	2.300	2.436	2.584	2.741	2.911	3.094	3.296	3.520	3.775	4.073	4.445
6.00	1.200	1.277	1.357	1.440	1.528	1.619	1.715	1.816	1.921	2.031	2.148	2.270	2.400	2.537	2.683	2.839	3.007	3.188	3.385	3.602	3.846
6.25	1.141	1.213	1.268	1.365	1.448	1.533	1.622	1.714	1.811	1.913	2.019	2.130	2.247	2.370	2.500	2.637	2.783	2.938	3.103	3.281	3.475
6.50	1.088	1.156	1.226	1.300	1.377	1.456	1.539	1.626	1.716	1.810	1.908	2.010	2.117	2.229	2.347	2.470	2.600	2.737	2.882	3.036	3.200
6.75	1.040	1.104	1.171	1.241	1.313	1.385	1.456	1.547	1.631	1.719	1.810	1.905	2.004	2.108	2.215	2.328	2.446	2.570	2.700	2.837	2.981
7.00	0.997	1.058	1.121	1.187	1.255	1.326	1.400	1.476	1.556	1.638	1.724	1.813	1.905	2.001	2.101	2.205	2.314	2.427	2.546	2.670	2.800
7.10	0.980	1.040	1.103	1.167	1.234	1.303	1.375	1.450	1.528	1.608	1.692	1.778	1.868	1.962	2.059	2.160	2.266	2.376	2.490	2.610	2.735
7.20	0.966	1.023	1.064	1.148	1.213	1.281	1.352	1.425	1.501	1.580	1.661	1.746	1.833	1.925	2.019	2.118	2.220	2.327	2.438	2.553	2.675
7.30	0.949	1.007	1.067	1.129	1.193	1.260	1.329	1.401	1.475	1.562	1.632	1.714	1.800	1.889	1.981	2.077	2.177	2.280	2.368	2.500	2.617
7.40	0.935	0.991	1.050	1.111	1.174	1.240	1.307	1.378	1.450	1.525	1.603	1.664	1.768	1.855	1.945	2.038	2.135	2.236	2.340	2.449	2.563
7.50	0.920	0.976	1.034	1.094	1.156	1.220	1.266	1.365	1.426	1.500	1.576	1.655	1.737	1.822	1.910	2.001	2.095	2.193	2.295	2.401	2.511
7.60	0.907	0.961	1.018	1.077	1.138	1.201	1.266	1.333	1.403	1.475	1.550	1.628	1.708	1.791	1.876	1.965	2.057	2.153	2.252	2.355	2.462
7.70	0.893	0.947	1.003	1.061	1.120	1.182	1.246	1.313	1.381	1.452	1.525	1.601	1.679	1.760	1.844	1.931	2.021	2.114	2.211	2.311	2.415
7.80	0.880	0.933	0.968	1.045	1.104	1.164	1.227	1.292	1.360	1.429	1.501	1.575	1.662	1.731	1.813	1.898	1.986	2.077	2.172	2.269	2.370
7.90	0.868	0.920	0.974	1.030	1.088	1.147	1.209	1.273	1.339	1.407	1.477	1.550	1.625	1.703	1.784	1.867	1.953	2.042	2.134	2.229	2.328

Radii in mm	Optic diameters (chords) in mm																			
	11.4	11.6	11.8	12.00	12.25	12.50	12.75	13.00	13.25	13.50	13.75	14.00	14.25	14.50	14.75	15.00	15.25	15.50	15.75	16.00
5.00																				
5.25																				
5.50																				
5.75	4.993																			
6.00	4.127	4.464	4.909	6.000																
6.25	3.686	3.921	4.188	4.500	5.006	6.250														
6.50	3.376	3.566	3.772	4.000	4.324	4.715	5.231	6.500												
6.75	3.134	3.297	3.471	3.658	3.913	4.200	4.531	4.930	5.457	6.750										
7.00	2.937	3.081	3.233	3.394	3.612	3.848	4.109	4.402	4.740	5.146	5.683	7.000								
7.10	2.867	3.005	3.150	3.304	3.509	3.731	3.974	4.243	4.547	4.898	5.327	5.913								
7.20	2.801	2.934	3.073	3.220	3.415	3.625	3.853	4.103	4.381	4.695	5.061	5.515	6.163							
7.30	2.739	2.867	3.001	3.142	3.328	3.528	3.743	3.977	4.234	4.520	4.846	5.229	5.711	6.447						
7.40	2.681	2.804	2.933	3.069	3.247	3.438	3.642	3.863	4.103	4.367	4.662	5.000	5.401	5.918	6.792					
7.50	2.626	2.745	2.870	3.000	3.172	3.354	3.549	3.759	3.984	4.231	4.503	4.807	5.158	5.580	6.136	7.500				
7.60	2.573	2.689	2.809	2.935	3.101	3.276	3.462	3.662	3.876	4.108	4.360	4.640	4.955	5.320	5.764	6.371				
7.70	2.523	2.635	2.752	2.874	3.034	3.203	3.382	3.572	3.776	3.995	4.232	4.492	4.780	5.106	5.487	5.956	6.628			
7.80	2.476	2.585	2.698	2.818	2.970	3.133	3.306	3.488	3.683	3.891	4.116	4.359	4.626	4.923	5.260	5.658	6.157	6.918		
7.90	2.430	2.536	2.646	2.761	2.911	3.068	3.234	3.410	3.598	3.795	4.008	4.238	4.498	4.762	5.068	5.418	5.834	6.397	7.272	

SAGITTA in mm

Optic diameters (chords) in mm

Radii in mm	3.0	3.2	3.4	3.6	3.8	4.0	4.2	4.4	4.6	4.8	5.0	5.2	5.4	5.6	5.8	6.0	6.2	6.4	6.6	6.8	7.0	7.2
8.00	0.142	0.162	0.183	0.205	0.229	0.254	0.281	0.308	0.338	0.369	0.401	0.434	0.469	0.506	0.544	0.584	0.625	0.668	0.712	0.758	0.806	0.856
8.10	0.140	0.160	0.180	.0203	0.226	0.251	0.277	0.305	0.333	0.364	0.395	0.429	0.463	0.499	0.537	0.576	0.617	0.659	0.703	0.748	0.795	0.844
8.20	0.138	0.158	0.178	0.200	0.223	0.248	0.274	0.301	0.329	0.359	0.390	0.423	0.457	0.493	0.530	0.568	0.609	0.650	0.693	0.738	0.784	0.832
8.30	0.137	0.156	0.176	0.198	0.220	0.245	0.270	0.297	0.325	0.355	0.385	0.418	0.451	0.487	0.523	0.561	0.601	0.642	0.684	0.728	0.774	0.821
8.40	0.135	0.154	0.174	0.195	0.218	0.242	0.267	0.292	0.321	0.350	0.381	0.413	0.446	0.480	0.516	0.554	0.593	0.633	0.675	0.719	0.764	0.811
8.50	0.133	0.152	0.172	0.193	0.215	0.239	0.264	0.290	0.317	0.346	0.376	0.407	0.440	0.474	0.510	0.547	0.585	0.625	0.667	0.710	0.754	0.800
8.60	0.132	0.150	0.170	0.191	0.213	0.236	0.260	0.286	0.313	0.342	0.371	0.402	0.435	0.469	0.504	0.540	0.578	0.618	0.658	0.701	0.744	0.790
8.70	0.130	0.148	0.168	0.188	0.210	0.233	0.257	0.283	0.310	0.338	0.367	0.398	0.430	0.463	0.498	0.534	0.571	0.610	0.650	0.692	0.735	0.780
8.80	0.129	0.147	0.166	0.186	0.208	0.230	0.254	0.279	0.306	0.334	0.363	0.393	0.424	0.457	0.492	0.527	0.564	0.602	0.642	0.683	0.726	0.770
8.90	0.127	0.145	0.164	0.184	0.205	0.228	0.251	0.276	0.302	0.330	0.358	0.388	0.419	0.452	0.486	0.521	0.557	0.595	0.634	0.675	0.717	0.761
9.00	0.126	0.143	0.162	0.182	0.203	0.225	0.248	0.273	0.299	0.326	0.354	0.384	0.415	0.447	0.480	0.515	0.551	0.588	0.627	0.667	0.708	0.751
9.10	0.125	0.142	0.160	0.180	0.201	0.223	0.246	0.270	0.296	0.322	0.350	0.379	0.410	0.441	0.474	0.509	0.544	0.581	0.619	0.659	0.700	0.742
9.20	0.123	0.140	0.158	0.178	0.198	0.220	0.243	0.267	0.292	0.319	0.346	0.375	0.405	0.436	0.469	0.503	0.538	0.574	0.612	0.651	0.692	0.734
9.30	0.122	0.139	0.157	0.176	0.196	0.218	0.240	0.264	0.289	0.315	0.342	0.371	0.401	0.432	0.464	0.497	0.532	0.568	0.605	0.644	0.684	0.725
9.40	0.121	0.137	0.155	0.174	0.194	0.215	0.238	0.261	0.286	0.312	0.339	0.367	0.396	0.427	0.459	0.492	0.526	0.561	0.598	0.636	0.676	0.717
9.50	0.119	0.136	0.153	0.172	0.192	0.213	0.235	0.258	0.283	0.308	0.335	0.363	0.392	0.422	0.453	0.486	0.520	0.555	0.592	0.629	0.668	0.709
9.60	0.118	0.134	0.152	0.170	0.190	0.211	0.233	0.256	0.280	0.305	0.331	0.359	0.388	0.417	0.448	0.481	0.514	0.549	0.585	0.622	0.661	0.701
9.70	0.117	0.133	0.150	0.169	0.188	0.208	0.230	0.253	0.277	0.302	0.328	0.355	0.383	0.413	0.444	0.476	0.509	0.543	0.579	0.615	0.653	0.693
9.80	0.116	0.132	0.149	0.167	0.186	0.206	0.228	0.250	0.274	0.298	0.324	0.351	0.379	0.409	0.439	0.470	0.503	0.537	0.572	0.609	0.646	0.685
9.90	0.114	0.130	0.147	0.165	0.184	0.204	0.225	0.248	0.271	0.295	0.321	0.348	0.375	0.404	0.434	0.465	0.498	0.531	0.566	0.602	0.639	0.678

Optic diameters (Chords) in mm

Radii in mm	7.4	7.6	7.8	8.0	8.2	8.4	8.6	8.8	9.0	9.2	9.4	9.6	9.8	10.0	10.2	10.4	10.6	10.8	11.0	11.2	11.4	11.6
8.00	0.907	0.960	1.015	1.072	1.131	1.191	1.254	1.319	1.386	1.455	1.526	1.600	1.676	1.755	1.836	1.921	2.008	2.097	2.191	2.287	2.387	2.490
8.10	0.894	0.947	1.001	1.057	1.114	1.174	1.236	1.299	1.365	1.433	1.503	1.575	1.650	1.727	1.807	1.890	1.975	2.063	2.154	2.248	2.345	2.446
8.20	0.882	0.934	0.987	1.042	1.099	1.157	1.218	1.280	1.345	1.412	1.481	1.552	1.625	1.701	1.779	1.860	1.943	2.029	2.118	2.210	2.305	2.403
8.30	0.870	0.921	0.973	1.027	1.083	1.141	1.201	1.262	1.326	1.391	1.459	1.529	1.601	1.675	1.752	1.831	1.913	1.997	2.084	2.174	2.267	2.363
8.40	0.859	0.909	0.960	1.014	1.069	1.125	1.184	1.245	1.307	1.371	1.438	1.507	1.577	1.650	1.725	1.803	1.883	1.966	2.051	2.139	2.230	2.324
8.50	0.848	0.897	0.948	1.000	1.054	1.110	1.168	1.227	1.289	1.352	1.418	1.485	1.554	1.626	1.700	1.776	1.855	1.936	2.019	2.105	2.194	2.286
8.60	0.837	0.885	0.935	0.987	1.040	1.095	1.152	1.211	1.271	1.334	1.398	1.464	1.532	1.603	1.675	1.750	1.827	1.907	1.989	2.073	2.160	2.250
8.70	0.826	0.874	0.923	0.974	1.027	1.081	1.137	1.195	1.254	1.316	1.379	1.444	1.511	1.580	1.652	1.725	1.801	1.879	1.959	2.042	2.127	2.215
8.80	0.816	0.863	0.911	0.962	1.013	1.067	1.122	1.179	1.238	1.298	1.360	1.424	1.490	1.558	1.629	1.701	1.775	1.852	1.931	2.012	2.096	2.182
8.90	0.806	0.852	0.900	0.950	1.001	1.053	1.108	1.164	1.221	1.281	1.342	1.405	1.470	1.537	1.606	1.677	1.750	1.825	1.903	1.983	2.065	2.149
9.00	0.796	0.842	0.889	0.938	0.988	1.040	1.094	1.149	1.206	1.264	1.325	1.387	1.451	1.517	1.584	1.654	1.726	1.800	1.876	1.954	2.035	2.118
9.10	0.786	0.831	0.878	0.926	0.976	1.027	1.080	1.134	1.191	1.248	1.308	1.369	1.432	1.497	1.563	1.632	1.703	1.775	1.850	1.927	2.006	2.088
9.20	0.777	0.821	0.868	0.915	0.964	1.015	1.067	1.120	1.176	1.233	1.291	1.351	1.413	1.477	1.543	1.611	1.680	1.752	1.825	1.901	1.979	2.059
9.30	0.768	0.812	0.857	0.904	0.953	1.002	1.054	1.107	1.161	1.217	1.275	1.334	1.396	1.458	1.523	1.590	1.658	1.720	1.801	1.875	1.952	2.030
9.40	0.759	0.802	0.847	0.894	0.941	0.990	1.041	1.093	1.147	1.202	1.259	1.318	1.378	1.440	1.504	1.569	1.637	1.706	1.777	1.850	1.925	2.003
9.50	0.750	0.793	0.837	0.833	0.930	0.979	1.029	1.080	1.133	1.188	1.244	1.302	1.361	1.422	1.485	1.550	1.616	1.684	1.754	1.826	1.900	1.976
9.60	0.742	0.784	0.828	0.873	0.920	0.968	1.017	1.066	1.120	1.174	1.229	1.286	1.345	1.405	1.467	1.530	1.596	1.663	1.732	1.803	1.875	1.950
9.70	0.733	0.775	0.819	0.863	0.909	0.956	1.005	1.055	1.107	1.160	1.215	1.271	1.329	1.388	1.449	1.512	1.576	1.642	1.710	1.780	1.851	1.925
9.80	0.725	0.767	0.809	0.853	0.899	0.946	0.994	1.043	1.094	1.147	1.201	1.256	1.313	1.371	1.432	1.493	1.557	1.622	1.689	1.758	1.828	1.901
9.90	0.717	0.758	0.801	0.844	0.889	0.935	0.983	1.032	1.082	1.134	1.187	1.241	1.298	1.355	1.415	1.476	1.538	1.602	1.668	1.736	1.806	1.877

Redii in mm	Optic diameters (Chords) in mm																					
	11.8	12.00	12.25	12.50	12.75	13.00	13.25	13.50	13.75	14.00	14.25	14.50	14.75	15.00	15.25	15.50	15.75	16.00	17.00	18.00	19.00	20.00
8.00	2.597	2.708	2.854	3.006	3.167	3.336	3.516	3.706	3.909	4.127	4.362	4.618	4.900	5.216	5.579	6.016	6.591	8.000				
8.10	2.550	2.658	2.800	2.948	3.103	3.267	3.440	3.623	3.817	4.024	4.247	4.488	4.750	5.041	5.367	5.745	6.204	6.831				
8.20	2.505	2.611	2.748	2.892	3.043	3.201	3.368	3.544	3.731	3.929	4.141	4.369	4.615	4.885	5.183	5.521	5.914	6.400				
8.30	2.462	2.565	2.699	2.839	2.985	3.139	3.300	3.470	3.650	3.840	4.043	4.259	4.492	4.745	5.021	5.329	5.678	6.089				
8.40	2.421	2.521	2.652	2.788	2.930	3.079	3.236	3.400	3.574	3.757	3.951	4.158	4.379	4.617	4.876	5.160	5.477	5.839				
8.50	2.361	2.479	2.606	2.739	2.878	3.023	3.175	3.334	3.502	3.678	3.865	4.063	4.274	4.500	4.744	5.018	5.301	5.628	8.500			
8.60	2.343	2.439	2.563	2.693	2.828	2.969	3.116	3.271	3.433	3.604	3.784	3.974	4.176	4.392	4.623	4.872	5.144	5.444	7.292			
8.70	2306	2.400	2.522	2.648	2.780	2.917	3.061	3.211	3.369	3.534	3.708	3.891	4.085	4.291	4.511	4.747	5.002	5.281	6.845			
8.80	2.271	2.363	2.481	2.605	2.734	2.868	3.006	3.154	3.307	3.467	3.635	3.812	3.999	4.197	4.407	4.631	4.873	5.134	6.522			
8.90	2.237	2.327	2.443	2.564	2.690	2.821	2.957	3.099	3.248	3.404	3.567	3.738	3.918	4.108	4.310	4.524	4.753	5.000	6.262			
9.00	2.204	2.292	2.406	2.524	2.647	2.775	2.908	3.047	3.192	3.343	3.501	3.667	3.842	4.025	4.210	4.424	4.643	4.877	6.042	9.000		
9.10	2.172	2.258	2.370	2.486	2.605	2.731	2.861	2.997	3.139	3.285	3.439	3.600	3.769	3.946	4.133	4.331	4.540	4.763	5.850	7.755		
9.20	2.141	2.226	2.335	2.449	2.567	2.689	2.817	2.949	3.087	3.230	3.380	3.536	3.700	3.872	4.052	4.242	4.443	4.657	5.680	7.292		
9.30	2.111	2.194	2.302	2.413	2.529	2.649	2.773	2.903	3.037	3.177	3.323	3.475	3.634	3.801	3.976	4.159	4.353	4.558	5.526	6.957		
9.40	2.082	2.164	2.270	2.379	2.492	2.616	2.732	2.858	2.990	3.126	3.269	3.417	3.572	3.733	3.903	4.080	4.267	4.464	5.386	6.687		
9.50	2.054	2.135	2.238	2.345	2.457	2.572	2.691	2.815	2.944	3.077	3.216	3.361	3.512	3.669	3.833	4.006	4.186	4.377	5.257	6.459	9.500	
9.60	2.027	2.106	2.208	2.313	2.422	2.535	2.662	2.774	2.900	3.030	3.166	3.307	3.454	3.608	3.767	3.935	4.110	4.293	5.138	6.259	8.218	
9.70	2.001	2.078	2.178	2.282	2.389	2.500	2.615	2.734	2.857	2.985	3.118	3.256	3.399	3.549	3.704	3.867	4.037	4.215	5.027	6.082	7.740	
9.80	1.975	2.051	2.150	2.252	2.357	2.466	2.579	2.695	2.816	2.941	3.071	3.206	3.346	3.492	3.644	3.802	3.967	4.140	4.923	5.922	7.394	
9.90	1.950	2.025	2.122	2.222	2.326	2.433	2.543	2.658	2.776	2.899	3.027	3.159	3.296	3.438	3.586	3.740	3.900	4.068	4.825	5.776	7.114	

Radii in mm	Optic diameters (chords) in mm																
	5.0	5.2	5.4	5.6	5.8	6.0	6.2	6.4	6.6	6.8	7.0	7.2	7.4	7.6	7.8	8.0	8.2
10.00	0.318	0.344	0.371	0.400	0.430	0.461	0.493	0.526	0.560	0.596	0.633	0.670	0.710	0.750	0.792	0.835	0.879
10.25	0.310	0.335	0.362	0.390	0.419	0.449	0.480	0.512	0.546	0.580	0.616	0.653	0.691	0.730	0.771	0.813	0.856
10.50	0.302	0.327	0.353	0.380	0.408	0.438	0.468	0.500	0.532	0.566	0.601	0.636	0.674	0.712	0.751	0.792	0.834
10.75	0.295	0.319	0.345	0.371	0.399	0.427	0.457	0.487	0.519	0.552	0.586	0.621	0.667	0.694	0.732	0.772	0.813
11.00	0.288	0.312	0.337	0.362	0.389	0.417	0.446	0.476	0.507	0.539	0.572	0.606	0.641	0.677	0.715	0.753	0.793
11.25	0.282	0.305	0.329	0.354	0.380	0.406	0.436	0.465	0.495	0.527	0.559	0.592	0.626	0.661	0.698	0.736	0.774
11.50	0.275	0.298	0.321	0.346	0.372	0.398	0.426	0.454	0.484	0.514	0.546	0.578	0.611	0.646	0.681	0.718	0.756
11.75	0.269	0.292	0.315	0.339	0.364	0.390	0.416	0.444	0.473	0.503	0.534	0.566	0.598	0.632	0.666	0.702	0.739
12.00	0.263	0.285	0.308	0.331	0.356	0.381	0.407	0.435	0.463	0.492	0.522	0.553	0.585	0.618	0.651	0.686	0.722
12.25	0.258	0.279	0.302	0.325	0.349	0.373	0.399	0.426	0.453	0.481	0.511	0.541	0.573	0.605	0.638	0.672	0.707
12.50	0.253	0.273	0.295	0.318	0.041	0.365	0.390	0.417	0.443	0.471	0.500	0.530	0.560	0.592	0.624	0.657	0.692
12.75	0.248	0.268	0.289	0.312	0.335	0.358	0.383	0.408	0.435	0.462	0.490	0.519	0.549	0.580	0.612	0.644	0.677
13.00	0.243	0.263	0.283	0.305	0.328	0.351	0.375	0.400	0.426	0.452	0.480	0.508	0.538	0.568	0.599	0.631	0.663
13.25	0.238	0.258	0.278	0.299	0.322	0.344	0.368	0.393	0.418	0.444	0.471	0.498	0.527	0.557	0.587	0.619	0.651
13.50	0.234	0.253	0.273	0.294	0.315	0.338	0.361	0.385	0.410	0.435	0.462	0.489	0.517	0.546	0.576	0.606	0.638
13.75	0.229	0.248	0.268	0.288	0.309	0.332	0.354	0.378	0.402	0.427	0.453	0.480	0.507	0.536	0.565	0.595	0.626
14.00	0.225	0.244	0.263	0.283	0.304	0.325	0.348	0.371	0.394	0.419	0.445	0.471	0.496	0.526	0.554	0.584	0.614
14.25	0.221	0.239	0.258	0.278	0.298	0.320	0.342	0.364	0.388	0.412	0.437	0.463	0.489	0.516	0.544	0.573	0.603
14.50	0.217	0.235	0.254	0.273	0.293	0.314	0.335	0.358	0.381	0.404	0.429	0.454	0.480	0.507	0.534	0.563	0.592
14.75	0.214	0.231	0.249	0.268	0.288	0.308	0.330	0.352	0.374	0.398	0.422	0.447	0.472	0.498	0.525	0.553	0.581
15.00	0.210	0.227	0.245	0.264	0.283	0.303	0.324	0.345	0.368	0.390	0.414	0.438	0.463	0.489	0.516	0.543	0.571
15.25	0.207	0.224	0.241	0.259	0.278	0.298	0.318	0.340	0.362	0.384	0.407	0.431	0.456	0.481	0.507	0.534	0.562
15.50	0.203	0.220	0.237	0.255	0.274	0.293	0.313	0.334	0.355	0.378	0.400	0.424	0.448	0.473	0.499	0.525	0.552
15.75	0.200	0.216	0.233	0.251	0.269	0.283	0.308	0.329	0.350	0.372	0.394	0.417	0.441	0.466	0.491	0.517	0.543
16.00	0.197	0.213	0.229	0.247	0.265	0.284	0.303	0.323	0.344	0.365	0.388	0.410	0.434	0.458	0.483	0.508	0.534
17.00	0.185	0.200	0.216	0.232	0.249	0.267	0.285	0.304	0.323	0.343	0.364	0.386	0.408	1.430	0.453	0.477	0.502

Radii in mm	Optic diameters (chords) in mm																
	8.4	8.6	8.8	9.0	9.2	9.4	9.6	9.8	10.0	10.2	10.4	10.6	10.8	11.0	11.2	11.4	11.6
10.00	0.925	0.972	1.020	1.070	1.121	1.173	1.227	1.283	1.340	1.398	1.458	1.520	1.583	1.648	1.715	1.784	1.854
10.25	0.900	0.946	0.992	1.041	1.090	1.141	1.193	1.247	1.302	1.359	1.417	1.477	1.536	1.601	1.665	1.731	1.799
10.50	0.877	0.921	0.966	1.013	1.061	1.111	1.161	1.213	1.267	1.322	1.378	1.435	1.495	1.556	1.618	1.682	1.747
10.75	0.854	0.897	0.942	0.987	1.034	1.062	1.131	1.182	1.234	1.287	1.341	1.397	1.455	1.514	1.574	1.636	1.699
11.00	0.833	0.875	0.918	0.963	1.008	1.055	1.103	1.152	1.202	1.254	1.307	1.361	1.417	1.474	1.532	1.592	1.653
11.25	0.814	0.854	0.896	0.940	0.984	1.029	1.076	1.124	1.172	1.223	1.274	1.327	1.361	1.436	1.493	1.551	1.511
11.50	0.794	0.834	0.875	0.917	0.960	1.004	1.050	1.096	1.144	1.193	1.243	1.294	1.347	1.400	1.456	1.513	1.570
11.75	0.777	0.815	0.855	0.896	0.938	0.981	1.025	1.071	1.117	1.165	1.214	1.263	1.315	1.367	1.420	1.475	1.532
12.00	0.759	0.797	0.836	0.876	0.917	0.959	1.002	1.046	1.091	1.138	1.185	1.234	1.284	1.336	1.387	1.440	1.495
12.25	0.743	0.780	0.818	0.857	0.897	0.938	0.980	1.023	1.067	1.112	1.159	1.206	1.255	1.304	1.355	1.407	1.460
12.50	0.727	0.763	0.800	0.838	0.877	0.917	0.958	1.000	1.044	1.088	1.133	1.179	1.227	1.275	1.325	1.375	1.427
12.75	0.712	0.747	0.784	0.821	0.859	0.897	0.938	0.979	1.022	1.065	1.109	1.154	1.200	1.248	1.296	1.345	1.396
13.00	0.697	0.732	0.767	0.804	0.841	0.879	0.919	0.959	1.000	1.042	1.085	1.129	1.175	1.221	1.268	1.316	1.366
13.25	0.684	0.717	0.752	0.766	0.824	0.862	0.900	0.940	0.960	1.021	1.063	1.107	1.151	1.195	1.242	1.289	1.337
13.50	0.670	0.703	0.737	0.772	0.808	0.845	0.882	0.921	0.960	1.000	1.042	1.084	1.127	1.171	1.216	1.262	1.309
13.75	0.668	0.690	0.723	0.757	0.792	0.828	0.866	0.903	0.942	0.961	1.021	1.063	1.106	1.148	1.192	1.237	1.263
14.00	0.645	0.677	0.709	0.743	0.777	0.813	0.849	0.986	0.923	0.962	1.002	1.042	1.083	1.126	1.169	1.213	1.259
14.25	0.633	0.665	0.697	0.729	0.763	0.797	0.833	0.869	0.906	0.944	0.963	1.022	1.063	1.104	1.147	1.190	1.234
14.50	0.622	0.652	0.684	0.716	0.749	0.783	0.818	0.853	0.889	0.926	0.964	1.003	1.043	1.084	1.125	1.167	1.211
14.75	0.611	0.641	0.672	0.704	0.736	0.769	0.803	0.838	0.873	0.910	0.947	0.956	1.024	1.064	1.104	1.146	1.189
15.00	0.600	0.630	0.660	0.691	0.723	0.755	0.789	0.823	0.858	0.894	0.930	0.968	1.006	1.045	1.065	1.125	1.167
15.25	0.590	0.619	0.649	0.679	0.711	0.743	0.775	0.809	0.843	0.878	0.914	0.951	0.969	1.027	1.066	1.105	1.146
15.50	0.580	0.608	0.638	0.668	0.698	0.730	0.762	0.795	0.829	0.863	0.896	0.934	0.971	1.009	1.047	1.088	1.126
15.75	0.570	0.598	0.627	0.657	0.687	0.715	0.750	0.782	0.815	0.849	0.863	0.919	0.956	0.992	1.030	1.066	1.107
16.00	0.561	0.569	0.617	0.646	0.676	0.706	0.737	0.769	0.801	0.835	0.869	0.903	0.936	1.975	1.012	1.050	1.066
17.00	0.527	0.553	0.579	0.606	0.634	0.663	0.692	0.721	0.752	0.783	0.815	0.847	0.830	0.914	0.949	0.984	1.020

Radii in mm	Optic diameters (chords) in mm																
	11.5	12.00	12.25	12.50	12.75	13.00	13.25	13.50	13.75	14.00	14.25	14.50	14.75	15.00	15.25	15.50	15.75
10.00	1.926	2.000	2.025	2.194	2.295	2.401	2.509	2.622	2.738	2.859	2.983	3.113	3.247	3.386	3.530	3.680	3.837
10.25	1.868	1.940	2.031	2.126	2.224	2.325	2.429	2.536	2.640	2.763	2.881	3.004	3.132	3.263	3.400	3.542	3.689
10.50	1.814	1.863	1.972	2.063	2.157	2.254	2.354	2.457	2.564	2.674	2.787	2.905	3.026	3.152	3.281	3.416	3.555
10.75	1.764	1.830	1.916	2.004	2.094	2.188	2.284	2.383	2.486	2.591	2.700	2.813	2.929	3.049	3.172	3.300	3.432
11.00	1.716	1.780	1.863	1.948	2.036	2.126	2.219	2.315	2.413	2.515	2.619	2.727	2.839	2.953	3.072	3.194	3.320
11.25	1.672	1.734	1.814	1.896	1.961	2.068	2.158	2.250	2.345	2.443	2.544	2.648	2.755	2.865	2.978	3.095	3.216
11.50	1.629	1.689	1.767	1.847	1.929	2.013	2.100	2.189	2.281	2.376	2.473	2.573	2.676	2.782	2.891	3.004	3.119
11.75	1.589	1.648	1.723	1.800	1.890	1.962	2.046	2.132	2.221	2.313	2.407	2.503	2.603	2.705	2.810	2.918	3.030
12.00	1.551	1.608	1.681	1.756	1.833	1.913	1.995	2.078	2.165	2.253	2.344	2.438	2.534	2.633	2.734	2.838	2.945
12.25	1.515	1.570	1.641	1.715	1.790	1.867	1.946	2.028	2.111	2.197	2.285	2.376	2.469	2.564	2.662	2.763	2.867
12.50	1.480	1.534	1.603	1.675	1.748	1.823	1.900	1.979	2.060	2.144	2.229	2.317	2.407	2.500	2.595	2.693	2.793
12.75	1.448	1.500	1.568	1.637	1.708	1.781	1.856	1.933	2.012	2.093	2.177	2.262	2.349	2.439	2.531	2.626	2.723
13.00	1.416	1.467	1.533	1.601	1.670	1.742	1.815	1.890	1.967	2.046	2.126	2.209	2.294	2.382	2.471	2.563	2.657
13.25	1.386	1.436	1.501	1.567	1.634	1.704	1.775	1.848	1.923	2.000	2.079	2.159	2.242	2.327	2.414	2.503	2.599
13.50	1.358	1.407	1.469	1.534	1.600	1.668	1.737	1.809	1.882	1.957	2.033	2.112	2.193	2.275	2.360	2.446	2.535
13.75	1.331	1.379	1.440	1.503	1.567	1.633	1.701	1.771	1.842	1.915	1.990	2.067	2.145	2.226	2.308	2.392	2.478
14.00	1.304	1.351	1.411	1.473	1.536	1.600	1.667	1.735	1.804	1.876	1.949	2.023	2.100	2.178	2.259	2.341	2.425
14.25	1.279	1.325	1.363	1.444	1.506	1.569	1.634	1.700	1.768	1.838	1.909	1.982	2.057	2.133	2.212	2.292	2.374
14.50	1.255	1.300	1.357	1.416	1.478	1.539	1.602	1.667	1.733	1.802	1.871	1.943	2.016	2.090	2.167	2.245	2.325
14.75	1.232	1.276	1.332	1.390	1.449	1.509	1.572	1.635	1.700	1.767	1.835	1.905	1.976	2.049	2.124	2.200	2.278
15.00	1.209	1.252	1.308	1.364	1.422	1.482	1.542	1.605	1.668	1.734	1.800	1.868	1.938	2.010	2.083	2.157	2.233
15.25	1.188	1.230	1.284	1.340	1.396	1.455	1.514	1.575	1.638	1.701	1.767	1.834	1.902	1.972	2.043	2.116	2.191
15.50	1.167	1.208	1.262	1.316	1.372	1.429	1.487	1.547	1.608	1.671	1.735	1.800	1.867	1.935	2.005	2.077	2.150
15.75	1.147	1.188	1.240	1.294	1.348	1.404	1.461	1.520	1.580	1.641	1.704	1.768	1.833	1.900	1.969	2.039	2.110
16.00	1.128	1.168	1.219	1.271	1.325	1.380	1.436	1.494	1.552	1.613	1.674	1.737	1.801	1.867	1.934	2.002	2.072
17.00	1.057	1.094	1.142	1.191	1.241	1.292	1.344	1.398	1.452	1.508	1.565	1.623	1.683	1.744	1.806	1.869	1.934

Radii in mm	Optic diameters (chords) in mm														
	16.0	17.0	18.0	19.0	20.0	21.0	22.0	23.0	24.0	25.0	26.0	27.0	28.0	29.0	30.0
10.00	4.000	4.638	5.641	6.878	10.000										
10.25	3.842	4.522	5.345	6.401	8.000										
10.50	3.699	4.336	5.092	6.028	7.298	10.500									
10.75	3.569	4.169	4.871	5.719	6.805	8.445									
11.00	3.450	4.018	4.675	5.455	6.417	7.721	11.000								
11.25	3.340	3.880	4.500	5.224	6.096	7.211	8.892								
11.50	3.239	3.754	4.341	5.019	5.821	6.810	8.221	11.500							
11.75	3.144	3.638	4.196	4.835	5.581	6.476	7.619	9.339							
12.00	3.056	3.529	4.063	4.669	5.367	6.191	7.204	8.572	12.000						
12.25	2.973	3.429	3.940	4.516	5.175	5.940	6.859	8.030	9.788						
12.50	2.895	3.359	3.825	4.376	5.000	5.718	6.563	7.601	9.000	12.500					
12.75	2.822	3.247	3.719	4.246	4.840	5.517	6.303	7.244	8.442	10.238					
13.00	2.753	3.164	3.619	4.126	4.693	5.336	6.072	6.938	8.000	9.429	13.000				
13.25	2.688	3.086	3.526	4.014	4.557	5.168	5.863	6.669	7.632	8.855	10.688				
13.50	2.626	3.012	3.438	3.908	4.431	5.015	5.674	6.429	7.315	8.401	9.860	13.500			
13.75	2.567	2.942	3.355	3.810	4.313	4.872	5.500	6.213	6.937	8.022	9.271	11.140			
14.00	2.511	2.876	3.276	3.717	4.202	4.740	5.340	6.016	6.789	7.695	8.804	10.292	14.000		
14.25	2.458	2.813	3.202	3.629	4.095	4.616	5.191	5.836	6.565	7.408	8.414	9.688	11.592		
14.50	2.407	2.753	3.131	3.546	4.000	4.500	5.061	5.668	6.361	7.152	8.077	9.208	10.725	14.500	
14.75	2.358	2.695	3.064	3.467	3.907	4.361	4.923	5.514	6.173	6.920	7.784	8.808	10.106	12.046	
15.00	2.311	2.641	3.000	3.392	3.820	4.286	4.802	5.369	6.000	6.708	7.517	8.462	9.615	11.159	15.000
15.25	2.267	2.589	2.939	3.321	3.736	4.191	4.688	5.234	5.839	6.514	7.277	8.157	9.203	10.526	12.500
15.50	2.224	2.539	2.881	3.253	3.657	4.098	4.580	5.108	5.689	6.335	7.059	7.884	8.848	10.023	11.595
15.75	2.183	2.491	2.825	3.189	3.582	4.011	4.478	4.988	5.549	6.168	6.858	7.638	8.536	9.601	10.948
16.00	2.144	2.445	2.771	3.126	3.510	3.927	4.381	4.875	5.417	6.013	6.673	7.412	8.254	9.236	10.432
17.00	2.000	2.278	2.578	2.920	3.252	3.630	4.039	4.480	4.958	5.478	6.046	6.668	7.356	8.126	9.000

Index

Page numbers followed by *f* refer to figure, and *t* refer to table